Dopamine Receptor Agonists

NEW HORIZONS IN THERAPEUTICS
Smith Kline & French Laboratories Research
Symposia Series

Series Editors: George Poste and Stanley T. Crooke
Smith Kline & French Laboratories, Philadelphia, Pennsylvania

---

DOPAMINE RECEPTOR AGONISTS
Edited by George Poste and Stanley T. Crooke

Dopamine Receptor Agonists

Edited by

GEORGE POSTE and
STANLEY T. CROOKE

Smith Kline & French Laboratories
Philadelphia, Pennsylvania

PLENUM PRESS · NEW YORK AND LONDON

Library of Congress Cataloging in Publication Data
Main entry under title:

Dopamine receptor agonists.

(New horizons in therapeutics)
Proceedings of the Annual Smith, Kline, and French Research Symposium on New
Horizons in Therapeutics, held in Philadelphia, Feb. 23-24, 1983.
Includes bibliographical references and index.
1. Dopamine — Receptors — Congresses. 2. Dopamine — Agonists — Congresses. I.
Poste, George. II. Crooke, Stanley T. III. Smith, Kline, and French Research Symposium on New Horizons in Therapeutics (1983: Philadelphia, Pa.) IV. Series. [DNLM:
1. Receptors, Dopamine — congresses. WL 102.8 D6917 1983]
QP563.D66D65   1984   615'.78   84-8290
ISBN 978-1-4757-0312-2   ISBN 978-1-4757-0310-8 (eBook)
DOI 10.1007/978-1-4757-0310-8

©1984 Plenum Press, New York
Softcover reprint of the hardcover 1st edition 1984

A Division of Plenum Publishing Corporation
233 Spring Street, New York, N.Y. 10013

Contributors

Sonia Arbilla, Department of Biology, Laboratoires d'Etudes et de Recherches Synthélabo, 75013 Paris, France

Richard J. Barrett, Department of Pharmacology and Institute for Cardiovascular Studies, College of Pharmacy, University of Houston Central Campus, Houston, Texas 77004. *Present address:* Department of Biomedical Research, ICI Americas, Inc., Wilmington, Delaware 19897

Barry A. Berkowitz, Smith Kline & French Laboratories, Philadelphia, Pennsylvania 19101

M. G. Bogaert, Heymans Institute of Pharmacology, University of Gent Medical School, B-9000 Gent, Belgium

W. A. Buylaert, Heymans Institute of Pharmacology, University of Gent Medical School, B-9000 Gent, Belgium

Robert M. Carey, Division of Endocrinology and Metabolism, Department of Internal Medicine, University of Virginia Medical Center, Charlottesville, Virginia 22908

I. Creese, Department of Neurosciences, University of California, San Diego, School of Medicine, La Jolla, California 92093

Robert Erickson, Smith Kline & French Laboratories, Philadelphia, Pennsylvania 19101

Christopher G. Goetz, Department of Neurological Sciences, Rush-Presbyterian St. Lukes Medical Center, Chicago, Illinois 60612

Leon I. Goldberg, Committee on Clinical Pharmacology, Departments of Pharmacological and Physiological Sciences and Medicine, The University of Chicago, Chicago, Illinois 60637

Carl A. Gruetter, Departments of Pharmacology and Surgery, Tulane University School of Medicine, New Orleans, Louisiana 70112. *Present address:* Department of Pharmacology, Marshall University School of Medicine, Huntington, West Virginia 25701

Arthur C. Guyton, Department of Physiology and Biophysics, University of Mississippi Medical Center, Jackson, Mississippi 39216

M. Hadjiconstantinou, Laboratory of Preclinical Pharmacology, National Institute of Mental Health, Saint Elizabeths Hospital, Washington, D.C. 20032

John E. Hall, Department of Physiology and Biophysics, University of Mississippi Medical Center, Jackson, Mississippi 39216

M. W. Hamblin, Department of Neurosciences, University of California, San Diego, School of Medicine, La Jolla, California 92093

Rita M. Huff, Department of Pharmacology, University of Pennsylvania School of Medicine, Philadelphia, Pennsylvania 19104. *Present address:* Division of Cardiology, Brigham and Women's Hospital, Boston, Massachusetts 02115

Albert L. Hyman, Departments of Pharmacology and Surgery, Tulane University School of Medicine, New Orleans, Louisiana 70012

Louis J. Ignarro, Departments of Pharmacology and Surgery, Tulane University School of Medicine, New Orleans, Louisiana 70012

Philip J. Kadowitz, Departments of Pharmacology and Surgery, Tulane University School of Medicine, New Orleans, Louisiana 70012

Carl Kaiser, Smith Kline & French Laboratories, Research and Development Division, Philadelphia, Pennsylvania 19101

John W. Kebabian, Experimental Therapeutics Branch, National Institute of Neurological and Communicative Disorders and Stroke, National Institutes of Health, Bethesda, Maryland 20205

Harold L. Klawans, Department of Neurological Sciences, Rush-Presbyterian St. Lukes Medical Center, Chicago, Illinois 60612

Z. Lackovic, Department of Pharmacology, Medical Faculty University of Zagreb, Zagreb, Yugoslavia

Salomon Z. Langer, Department of Biology, Laboratoires d'Etudes et de Recherches Synthélabo, 75013 Paris, France

R. A. Lefebvre, Heymans Institute of Pharmacology, University of Gent Medical School, B-9000 Gent, Belgium

S. E. Leff, Department of Neurosciences, University of California, San Diego, School of Medicine, La Jolla, California 92093

Thomas E. Lohmeier, Department of Physiology and Biophysics, University of Mississipi Medical Center, Jackson, Mississippi 39216

Mustafa F. Lokhandwala, Department of Pharmacology and Institute for Cardiovascular Studies, College of Pharmacy, University of Houston Central Campus, Houston, Texas 77004

R. Davis Manning, Department of Physiology and Biophysics, University of Mississippi Medical Center, Jackson, Mississippi 39216

Perry B. Molinoff, Department of Pharmacology, University of Pennsylvania School of Medicine, Philadelphia, Pennsylvania 19104

Philip Needleman, Department of Pharmacology, Washington University School of Medicine, St. Louis, Missouri 63110

N. H. Neff, Laboratory of Preclinical Pharmacology, National Institute of Mental Health, Saint Elizabeths Hospital, Washington, D.C. 20032

Eliot H. Ohlstein, Smith Kline & French Laboratories, Philadelphia, Pennsylvania 19101

Herbert S. Ormsbee III, Department of Pharmacology, Smith Kline & French Laboratories, Philadelphia, Pennsylvania 19101

D. R. Sibley, Department of Neurosciences, University of California, San Diego, School of Medicine, La Jolla, California 92093

Jay H. Stein, Department of Medicine, The University of Texas Health Science Center at San Antonio, San Antonio, Texas 78284

Caroline M. Tanner, Department of Neurological Sciences, Rush-Presbyterian St. Lukes Medical Center, Chicago, Illinois 60612

J. L. Willems, Heymans Institute of Pharmacology, University of Gent Medical School, B-9000 Gent, Belgium

Bodgan Zabko-Potavpovich, Smith Kline & French Laboratories,Philadelphia, Pennsylvania 19101

Preface to the Series

The unprecedented scope and pace of discovery in modern biology and clinical medicine present remarkable opportunities for the development of new therapeutic modalities, many of which would have been unimaginable even a few years ago. This situation reflects the unprecedented progress being made not only in disciplines such as pharmacology, physiology, organic chemistry, and biochemistry that have traditionally made important contributions to drug discovery, but also in new disciplines such as molecular genetics, cell biology and immunology that are now of sufficient maturity to contribute significantly to our understanding of the pathogenesis of disease and to the development of novel therapies. Contemporary biomedical research, embracing the entire spectrum of biological organization from the molecular level to whole body function, is on the threshold of an era in which biological processes, including disease, can be analyzed in increasingly precise and mechanistic terms. The transformation of biology from a largely descriptive, phenomenological discipline to one in which the regulatory principles underlying biological organization can be understood and manipulated with ever-increasing predictability brings an entirely new dimension to the study of disease and the search for effective therapeutic modalities. In undergoing this transformation into an increasingly mechanistic discipline, biology and medicine are following the course already charted by the sister disciplines of chemistry and physics, albeit still far behind.

The consequences of these changes for biomedical research are profound: new concepts; new and increasingly powerful analytical techniques; new advances generated at a seemingly ever-rapid pace; an almost unmanageable glut of information dispersed in an increasing number of books and journals; and the task of integrating this information into a realistic experimental framework. Nowhere is the challenge more pronounced than in the pharmaceutical industry. Drug discovery and development have always required the successful coordination of multiple scientific disciplines. The need to assimilate more and more disciplines within the drug discovery process, the extraordinary pace of discovery in all disciplines, and the growing scientific and organizational complexity of coordinating increasingly ultraspecialized and resource-intensive scientific skills in an ever-enlarging framework of collaborative research activities represent formidable challenges for the pharmaceutical industry. These demands are balanced, however, by the excitement and the scale of the potential opportunities for achieving dramatic improvements in health care and the quality of human life over the next twenty years via the development of novel therapeutic modalities for effective treatment of major human and animal diseases.

It is against this background of change and opportunity that the present symposium series, *New Horizons in Therapeutics,* was conceived as a forum for providing critical and up-to-date surveys of important topics in biomedical research in which significant advances were occurring and which offer new approaches to the therapy of disease. Each volume will contain authoritative and topical articles written by investigators who have contributed significantly to their respective research fields. While individual articles will discuss specialized topics, all papers in a single volume will be related to a common theme. The level will be advanced, directed primarily to the needs of the active research investigator and graduate students.

Editorial policy will be to impose as few restrictions as possible on contributors. This is appropriate since each volume is limited to the papers presented at the symposium and no attempt will be made to create a definitive monograph dealing with all aspects of the selected subject. Although each symposium volume will provide a survey of recent research accomplishments, emphasis will also be given to the examination of controversial and conflicting issues, to the presentation of new ideas and hypotheses, to the identification of important unsolved questions and to future directions and possible approaches by which such questions might be answered.

The range of topics for future volumes in the symposium series will be broad and will embrace the full repertoire of scientific disciplines that contribute to modern drug discovery and development. We thus look forward to the publication of what we hope will be viewed as a worthy series of volumes that reflect the excitement and challenge of contemporary biomedical research in defining new horizons in therapeutics.

George Poste
Stanley T. Crooke

Philadelphia

Preface

Dopamine, in addition to its importance as a precursor of norepinephrine, is now known to be an important neurotransmitter in regulating functional activities in a number of major organ systems, including the central nervous system, the cardiovascular system, the kidney, and the gut. Recent advances in our understanding of the functional role of dopamine, its mechanism of action and the pharmacology of dopaminergic agents have occurred on a broad front. The last few years have witnessed significant progress in the identification and classification of central and peripheral dopamine receptors and the factors that affect their responsiveness to inhibitory and stimulatory ligands. These advances have been paralleled by new insights into the contribution of alterations in dopaminergic regulation in causing disease and the utility of dopamine agonists and antagonists as therapeutic modalities.

This volume, the first in a series of publications arising from the annual Smith Kline and French Research Symposium on *New Horizons in Therapeutics*, provides a comprehensive survey of current research on peripheral dopamine receptors and the physiologic and therapeutic consequences of stimulating pre- and postsynaptic dopamine receptors.

Research in dopamine pharmacology mirrors the remarkable advances that are occurring in the field of pharmacology at large as a consequence of the involvement of an ever-larger number of scientific disciplines in the study of drug action. The availability of increasingly sophisticated analytical techniques now enables drug action to be studied across the entire spectrum of biological organization, ranging from new approaches in molecular pharmacology in which drug action can be examined in cell-free systems and in cell, tissue and organ cultures to more traditional experimental and clinical studies in animals and man in both health and disease.

The topics discussed in this volume embrace three interrelated themes: the identification, localization, regulation and classification of dopamine receptor subtypes; the search for new chemical ligands as probes of receptor function with the ultimate aim of elucidating differences in receptor structure; and investigation of the functional consequences of ligand-induced stimulation or inhibition of receptor subtypes in defined target cells.

There is now abundant evidence that dopamine receptors, in common with receptor populations for other neurotransmitters and myriad endogenous biological mediators, can be classified into subtypes on the basis of their differing reactivity to various ligands. Although consensus has still to be achieved regarding the taxonomy of dopamine receptor subtypes, at least two major functional categories of dopamine receptors can be defined: those involved in the inhibition of neurotransmitter release; and those located on the diverse array of cell types that respond to dopamine. An impressive body of experimental evidence has been accumulated documenting the distribution of receptor subtypes in major organ systems. However, successful isolation and reconstitution of dopamine receptors has yet to be achieved and this represents an obvious and important goal for future research.

The ability to study ligand–receptor interactions using purified receptors can reasonably be expected to resolve many of the ambiguities surrounding current classification schemes for dopamine receptors. Reliable identification of cell types bearing homogeneous populations of different receptor subtypes would greatly facilitate this strategy in analogous fashion to the progress made in the isolation and biochemical characterization of the β-adrenergic receptor from frog and turkey erythrocytes, and receptors for polypeptide hormones and growth factors isolated from various cell types maintained in culture. In addition, recent advances in molecular genetics in which the genes coding for specific cell surface receptors can be transferred to cells lacking the receptor to induce receptor expression creates a powerful new technology for analyzing cellular receptors and their properties.

More information is needed about mechanisms of receptor coupling, signal transduction, and receptor regulation in dopaminergic systems. These issues are relevant not merely from the standpoint of improving the identification and taxonomy of dopamine receptor subtypes but because they offer potentially novel targets for therapeutic manipulation. Once again, insight into these questions is not as advanced as knowledge of comparable aspects of adrenergic receptor function, receptor coupling, and signal transduction in a number of hormone receptor systems. We anticipate, however, that this deficiency will be short lived. The substantial momentum of current research on dopamine receptors, and the informative precedents established in other receptor systems, create a climate that is highly conducive to the solution of these questions.

The availability of a suitable panel of chemical ligands for probing the structure and function of different dopamine receptor subtypes is, of course, an essential prerequisite for these studies. Impressive progress has been made in the synthesis of agonists and antagonists for dopamine receptor subtypes in the CNS and in the periphery and in defining the structure–activity relationships that underlie these activities. Nonetheless, in common with investigation of structure–activity relationships in ligands that interact with receptors for other neurotransmitter molecules, current synthetic efforts are still overly dependent on the screening of large numbers of compounds. Neither the chemical skills involved nor the value of the information obtained using such approaches are to be undervalued. However, the ability to study ligand–receptor interactions using purified receptor preparations would generate major new opportunities for improving ligand design. The purification, chemical characterization and determination of the structure of different receptor molecules and the use of computer-generated real time graphics to examine receptor occupation by agonist and antagonist molecules can each be confidently expected to make important contributions to the evolution of improved ligands and the development of new therapeutic agents exhibiting desired selectivities for particular receptor subtypes.

It is no longer an exaggeration to suggest that research efforts in dopamine pharmacology may exceed those devoted to more extensively studied neurotransmitters such as norepinephrine, epinephrine, and acetylcholine. The potential clinical value of dopamine agonists in the treatment of Parkinson's disease, hyperprolactinemia, certain pituitary tumors, and in the therapy of cardiovascular shock continue to attract considerable interest in both academic and industrial research laboratories. However, the findings presented in this volume indicate that the growing recognition of the role of dopamine as a neurotransmitter offers the promise of exciting and novel opportunities for therapeutic manipulation of peripheral dopamine receptors in the gut, the kidney, the heart, and different regions of the vascular bed.

We consider that the topics discussed in this volume fulfill the stated aims of the symposium series in providing a critical survey of a subject in which considerable progress is being made and which heralds new opportunities for improvements in therapy. We anticipate further important advances in this subject in the next few years. We hope this volume will serve in some small measure to chronicle the progress, the challenge, and the aspirations of this segment of modern pharmacology research.

George Poste
Stanley T. Crooke

Philadelphia

Contents

I. DOPAMINE RECEPTORS

Chapter 1

Pharmacological and Biochemical Characterization of Two Categories of Dopamine Receptor

John W. Kebabian

Chapter 2

Radioligand Binding Studies of Agonist Interactions with Dopamine Receptors

I. Creese, S. E. Leff, D. R. Sibley, and M. W. Hamblin

Chapter 3

Quantitative Assay of Dopamine Receptor Subtypes

Rita M. Huff and Perry B. Molinoff

Chapter 4

Structure–Activity Relationships of Dopamine Receptor Agonists

Carl Kaiser

Chapter 5

Peripheral Dopamine Receptors

M. G. Bogaert, W. A. Buylaert, R. A. Lefebvre, and J. L. Willems

Chapter 6

Pharmacological Significance of Pre- and Postsynaptic Dopamine Receptors

Salomon Z. Langer and Sonia Arbilla

II. DOPAMINE AGONIST FUNCTION AND PHARMACOLOGY

Chapter 7

Dopamine: An Endogenous Peripheral Neurotransmitter

N. H. Neff, M. Hadjiconstantinou, and Z. Lackovic

Chapter 8

Vascular Dopamine and Dopamine Receptor Agonists

Barry A. Berkowitz, Robert Erickson, Bodgan Zabko-Potavpovich, and Eliot H. Ohlstein

Chapter 9

Dopamine Receptor Agonists and Hypertension

Mustafa F. Lokhandwala and Richard J. Barrett

III. CRITICAL CONCEPTS OF PHYSIOLOGICAL AND MOLECULAR MECHANISMS OF CARDIOVASCULAR AND RENAL FUNCTION

Chapter 10

Role of Inflammatory Cells in Metabolic and Cellular Alterations Underlying the Exaggerated Renal Prostaglandin and Thromboxane Synthesis in Ureter Obstruction

Philip Needleman

Chapter 11

The Kidney and Hypertension

Arthur C. Guyton, R. Davis Manning, Thomas E. Lohmeier, and John E. Hall

Chapter 12

Molecular Mechanisms of Vasodilatation

Louis J. Ignarro, Carl A. Gruetter, Albert L. Hyman, and Philip J. Kadowitz

IV. CLINICAL APPLICATIONS

Chapter 13

The Relationship of Receptor Actions of Dopamine Agonists to Their Clinical Effects

Leon I. Goldberg

Chapter 14

Hemodynamic Factors Involved in the Regulation of Sodium Balance

Jay H. Stein

Chapter 15

*Dopaminergic Mechanisms in the Control of Aldosterone Secretion: A
.Critical Appraisal*

Robert M. Carey

Chapter 16

*Dopamine Agonists/Antagonists in the Treatment of Gastrointestinal
Diseases*

Herbert S. Ormsbee III

Chapter 17

The Use of Dopamine Agonists and Antagonists in Neurology

Harold L. Klawans, Christopher G. Goetz, and Caroline M. Tanner

DOPAMINE RECEPTORS

Pharmacological and Biochemical Characterization of Two Categories of Dopamine Receptor

*JOHN W. KEBABIAN**

1. Introduction

At present, dopamine is probably the most studied neurotransmitter within the central nervous system (Horn *et al.*, 1979). Anatomically, dopaminergic neuronal pathways have been defined in many brain regions. Biochemically, minute quantities of dopamine or its precursors and metabolites can be quantified. Changes in the concentration of any of these substances can be detected and correlated with alterations in physiological activity of dopaminergic neurons. Physiologically, various roles have been proposed for dopamine in several brain regions. Pharmacologically, drugs mimicking or antagonizing the effects of dopamine have been identified. Because dopamine regulates the physiological activity of human brain, dopaminergic agonists and antagonists are used as therapeutic agents in clinical medicine. L-DOPA, the precursor of dopamine, as well as bromocriptine, a dopaminergic agonist, are effective in treating Parkinsonism; dopaminergic antagonists are used as antiemetics and antipsychotics. Furthermore, because dopamine regulates physiological activity in peripheral tissue, dopamine is used in the treatment of shock, and dopaminergic agonists are used to treat hyperprolactinemia, acromegaly, and to arrest the growth of prolactin-secreting adenomata.

JOHN W. KEBABIAN • Experimental Therapeutics Branch, National Institute of Neurological and Communicative Disorders and Stroke, National Institutes of Health, Bethesda, Maryland 20205. *Affiliation is shown for identification only. This manuscript was prepared by Dr. Kebabian as a private citizen.

The existence of receptor(s) for dopamine is frequently hypothesized to account for the regulation of physiological activity by dopamine, dopaminergic agonists, and dopaminergic antagonists. This chapter describes some of the advances in our understanding of dopamine receptors that have occurred in the past decade and places these advances within the historical development of the understanding of the role of dopamine as a regulator of physiological activity.

1.1. Classification of Receptors: General Comments

Historically, a receptor was a hypothetical entity accounting for the ability of a tissue to respond to minute quantities of drugs or endogenous compounds. The hypothesized receptor recognizes the compound and transmits an intracellular signal that elicits a physiological response or biochemical change detectable by an investigator (Langley, 1906). Receptors are classified on the basis of the endogenous compound stimulating the receptor (e.g., cholinergic receptors respond to acetylcholine, adrenoceptors respond to epinephrine or norepinephrine). Further subdivision of a population of receptors can then be made on the basis of the relative potency of a series of synthetic agonists and antagonists. At the extremes of the potency series are agonists or antagonists discriminating between the two receptors. Further division of each general category of receptor is possible with the development of still more selective drugs.

The classification of receptors is a continuously evolving science. Receptors for the same substance are differentiated on the basis of their responsiveness to the available drugs. The further subdivision of a "unitary" receptor into subcomponents is made on the basis of limited (and often controversial) data. Once the new subdivision is accepted, new drugs providing a more convincing differentiation are synthesized or discovered. The evolution of the classification of adrenoceptors provides an example of the sequential evolution of receptor classification schemata.

In the early part of this century, Dale used ergot to abolish the ability of some tissues to respond to catecholamines (Dale, 1906). This was taken as evidence for the existence of several receptors for catecholamines. In 1948, Ahlquist noted differences in the rank order of potency of catecholamines on different tissues and proposed the existence of two receptors for catecholamines, which he designated as the α and the β receptors (Ahlquist, 1948, 1981). This radical schema was initially rejected because it went against the then popular sympathin theory of Cannon (Bacq, 1981). Subsequently, the schema of Ahlquist was accepted, and each category of receptor was subdivided into two subcategories designated as the α_1

and α_2 adrenoceptors (Langer, 1981) and the β_1 and β_2 adrenoceptors (Lands *et al.*, 1967).

1.2. Dopamine and Dopamine Receptors: History

In the late 1950s, dopamine was shown to occur at high concentration in the brain and peripheral nervous system (Carlsson *et al.*, 1958; Bertler and Rosengren, 1959). This suggested that dopamine might have functions other than serving as an intermediate in the synthesis of norepinephrine or epinephrine. Subsequently, the existence of receptor(s) specific for dopamine was postulated to account for the biochemical, behavioral, and physiological effects of dopamine and other drugs on the central nervous system (Ernst, 1969; Anden *et al.*, 1966; Ungerstedt, 1971). In view of the high concentration of dopamine in the neostriatum, considerable attention was directed toward this brain region and its involvement in the regulation of movement.

During this period, dopamine receptors were also identified in peripheral, nonneural tissues. A dopamine receptor (distinct from the β and α adrenoceptor) was shown to exist in the renal vasculature of the dog by Goldberg (for a historical overview see Goldberg, 1979). Stimulation of this receptor decreases the resistance of the renal vascular bed. Goldberg and his colleagues characterized the pharmacological properties of this receptor (Goldberg, 1972). A dopamine receptor was also shown to exist on the mammotrophs of the anterior pituitary gland; stimulation of this receptor inhibited the release of prolactin (for a historical summary, see MacLeod, 1976). The pharmacological investigations of MacLeod and his colleagues provided the basis for the classic study of Caron *et al.* in which the properties of this dopamine receptor were characterized by physiological or biochemical techniques (Caron *et al.*, 1978).

In the early 1970s, the biochemical consequences of stimulating a dopamine receptor began to be identified. In either the retina or the bovine superior cervical ganglion, dopamine stimulated the accumulation of cAMP (Brown and Makman, 1972; Kebabian and Greengard, 1971). This effect was the consequence of the stimulation of a dopamine-sensitive adenylate cyclase in these tissues. The demonstration of a dopamine-sensitive adenylate cyclase activity in cell-free homogenates of the neostriatum was an especially important discovery (Kebabian *et al.*, 1972). The pharmacological properties of this dopamine receptor could be rapidly and quantitatively characterized with *in vitro* techniques. The availability of the *in vitro* assay prompted the screening of numerous putative agonists and antagonists of dopamine receptor(s). The result of these experiments have been summarized elsewhere by others (Miller and McDermed, 1979).

In the mid 1970s, dopaminergic drugs radiolabeled to high specific activity began to be used to identify dopamine receptors in binding assays. This methodology has been applied to the brain as well as several peripheral tissues. However, over the years more than 28 different ligands have been used to identify dopamine receptors, and a voluminous and often conflicting literature has developed (Seeman, 1980).

The postulate that more than one category of pharmacologically distinct dopamine receptor might exist has been put forward by many investigators. Usually an additional dopamine receptor is invoked to account for discrepancies or ambiguities in whatever assay systems an investigator is using (Cools and Van Rossum, 1976; Costall and Naylor, 1979; Spano *et al.*, 1979; Goldberg and Kohli, 1979; Seeman, 1980). Because different pairs of assay systems are used in different laboratories, considerable controversy has arisen as to how many dopamine receptors exist and how they should be identified. This situation is further confused because in some cases the same name has been used for different entities, whereas in other cases different names have been used for the same entity.

In 1979, Donald Calne and I put forward the two-dopamine-receptor hypothesis to account for the differences we perceived in the pharmacology of dopamine receptors in several peripheral tissues (Kebabian and Calne, 1979). This hypothesis was a consequence of our observation that lergotrile, a dopaminergic agonist in the anterior pituitary gland, was a dopamine antagonist in the striatal dopamine-sensitive adenylate cyclase assay (Kebabian *et al.*, 1977). According to this hypothesis, there are two categories of dopamine receptor (designated the D-1 and the D-2 receptors). The dopamine receptor associated with the mammotroph of the anterior pituitary gland exemplifies the D-2 receptor, whereas the dopamine receptor associated with the parenchymal cells of the bovine parathyroid gland exemplifies the D-1 receptor.

When the two-dopamine-receptor hypothesis was first advanced, an extremely limited number of drugs provided pharmacological discrimination between the two categories of dopamine receptor. Dopamine itself was more potent as a agonist on the D-2 receptor than on the D-1 receptor. Likewise, apomorphine was a potent full agonist on the D-2 receptor but was only a weak partial agonist on the D-1 receptor. Among the ergots, lergotrile and lisuride were potent full agonists on the D-2 receptor but were antagonists on the D-1 receptor. Sulpiride and metoclopramide were the only antagonists discriminating between the two categories of receptor: both of these drugs were selective antagonists of the D-2 receptor. During the past three years, a number of drugs discriminating between the two categories of dopamine receptor have been discovered. These newer, more selective drugs are discussed in greater detail below.

2. The D-1 Receptor

Although dopamine stimulates adenylate cyclase activity in tissues from species as diverse as cockroaches (Grewe and Kebabian, 1982) and humans (Clement-Cormier *et al.*, 1974), the physiological consequences of a dopamine-stimulated accumulation of adenosine-3'.5'-cyclic mono-phosphate (cAMP) are known in only a few tissues. In the parathyroid gland of the cow, dopamine enhances the formation of cAMP as well as the release of parathyroid hormone. E. M. Brown and his colleagues have provided convincing evidence that the enhanced formation of cAMP is causally related to the enhanced release of hormone (Brown *et al.*, 1980; Brown and Dawson-Hughes, 1983). Because the bovine parathyroid gland is the only tissue in which a physiological role for the dopamine-stimulated accumulation of cAMP has been established, this is also the only tissue in which the pharmacological properties of the D-1 receptor have been characterized on the basis of physiological and biochemical responses. In the external horizontal cells of the carp retina, dopamine stimulates cAMP formation and reduces the electrical coupling between these cells (Teranishi *et al.*, 1983; Watling, 1983). Although it is tempting to speculate that these events are causally related, there is, at present, no experimental evidence to support this possibility. Although the most extensively studied dopamine-sensitive adenylate cyclase is in the neostriatum, there is (at present) no known role for this enzyme.

The pharmacological properties of the D-1 receptor have been extensively characterized on the basis of the ability of drugs to mimic or antagonize the stimulatory effect of dopamine on adenylate cyclase activity. The numerous studies using this enzyme assay system have been summarized by Miller and McDermed (1979).

Several interesting biochemical observations have emerged from the striatal D-1 system. For example, GTP is obligatory for the demonstration of the stimulation by dopamine of striatal adenylate cyclase activity (Clement-Cormier *et al.*, 1975; Kebabian *et al.*, 1979).

3. The Intermediate Lobe of the Rat Pituitary Gland: A Model of the D-2 Receptor

The D-2 receptor can be studied with considerable precision in simple peripheral tissues. Although the D-2 receptor on the mammotroph of the anterior pituitary gland was designated as the prototype of this category of receptor, the melanotrophs of intermediate lobe (IL) also possess this category of receptor (Cote *et al.*, 1982c). Furthermore, the melanotroph offers several practical advantages. First, the IL is composed exclusively of melanotrophs; the cellular homogeneity of the IL contrasts with the cellular heterogeneity of the anterior pituitary gland and facilitates biochemical investigations. Second, the rat IL secretes melanotrophic peptides detectable by bioassay or by radioimmunoassay. Although α-melanocyte stimulating hormone (N-acetyl-ACTH$_{1-13}$amide, αMSH) is widely believed to be the predominant melanotrophic peptide in the rat IL, recent studies have shown that N,0-diacetyl-αMSH is the predominant molecular species contained within and secreted by the rat IL (Goldman *et al.*, 1983). (In rodents, the melanotrophic hormones of the IL are known to control coat color; therefore, the release of such peptides from the IL provides a readily detectable sign of physiological activity in this tissue.) Third, the IL of the rat possesses not only a dopamine receptor but also a β$_2$ adrenoceptor (Bower *et al.*, 1974; Munemura *et al.*, 1980b; Meunier and Labrie, 1982a; Cote *et al.*, 1980). Stimulation of the dopamine receptor inhibits the release of αMSH-like peptides, whereas stimulation of the β$_2$ adrenoceptor enhances the release of these substances.

3.1. The IL β Adrenoceptor

Modern biochemical techniques can identify the β$_2$ adrenoceptor in the IL and establish a role for cAMP in the rat IL. This β$_2$ adrenoceptor can be identified in binding studies using the radiolabeled ligand [^{125}I]-monoiodohydroxybenzylpindolol (Cote *et al.*, 1980). As is the case in many other tissues, stimulation of this receptor enhances adenylate cyclase activity; GTP is obligatory for demonstrating this stimulatory effect of β-adrenergic agonists (Cote *et al.*, 1982a) The requirement of GTP for the demonstration of the stimulation of enzyme activity together with the stimulatory effect of cholera toxin on adenylate cyclase activity (Tsuruta *et al.*, 1981, 1982; Cote *et al.*, 1982a,b) suggests the presence of a stimulatory guanyl nucleotide component (N$_s$ in the schema of Rodbell, 1980). The arrangement of the β adrenoceptor, N$_s$, and adenylate cyclase in the IL is shown in Fig. 1. The participation of GTP in the β-adrenergic enhancement of adenylate cyclase is also shown in Fig. 1.

Stimulation of the β$_2$ adrenoceptor also increases the release of αMSH-like peptides from the IL; the predominant molecular species release is N,0-diacetyl-αMSH. The presence of calcium ions in the bathing medium is obligatory to demonstrate the stimulated release of hormones (Tsuruta *et al.*, 1982). The β-adrenergic agonist (*R*)-isoproterenol is strik-

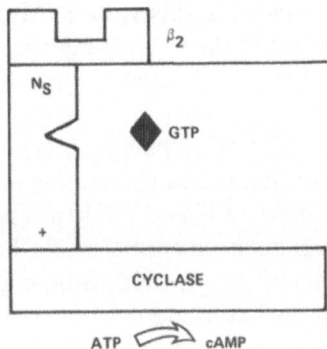

Figure 1. Organization of the β₂-adrenoceptor–adenylate cyclase complex in the intermediate lobe of the rat pituitary gland. Top: The β₂-adrenoceptor (β₂) is coupled to adenylate cyclase (cyclase) by a stimulatory guanyl nucleotide component (N_s). In the absence of a β-adrenergic agonist, GTP (filled diamond) cannot interact with N_s to increase adenylate activity. Bottom: Occupancy of the β₂ adrenoceptor by an agonist (filled square) alters the properties of N_s so that GTP can interact with the guanyl nucleotide recognition site and enhance enzyme activity.

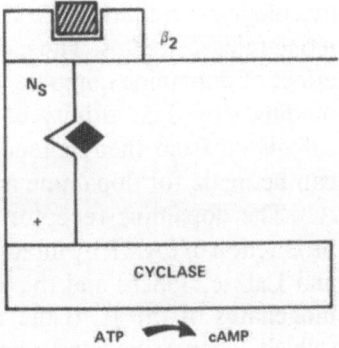

ingly more potent in stimulating the release of hormones from intact cells than it is in any of the biochemical models of the β adrenoceptor (i.e., receptor occupancy, stimulation of cAMP production by intact cells, or stimulation of adenylate cyclase by cell-free homogenates of IL tissue). Future investigations of the factors underlying this discrepancy will probably add to our understanding of the biochemical mechanisms underlying the physiological consequences of receptor activation.

3.2. The IL D-2 Receptor

The presence of a dopamine receptor in the IL can be inferred from the effects of drugs on hormone release. Thus, dopamine and other dopaminergic agonists inhibit the release of IR-αMSH from the IL. The pharmacology of this IL receptor is distinct from that of the D-1 receptor. Most notably, ergot antagonists of the D-1 receptor (e.g., lergotrile; Kebabian *et al.*, 1977) are potent agonists mimicking the inhibitory effect of dopamine in this system (Munemura *et al.*, 1980a). A dopamine receptor occurs in the IL of many species as diverse as amphibians (Peng Loh and Gainer, 1977) and mammals (Stephanini *et al.*, 1980; Sibley and Creese, 1980).

The IL dopamine receptor can be studied with modern biochemical procedures complementing the classical endocrinological studies. The radiolabeled ligand [^{3}H]-spiroperidol has frequently been used to identify dopamine receptors in the brain as well as in the pituitary gland (Stephanini *et al.*, 1980; Sibley and Creese, 1980; Frey *et al.*, 1982). In the IL, as in these other tissues, [^{3}H]-spiroperidol binds with high affinity to a specific binding site. The density of specific spiroperidol binding sites in the IL is as great as the density in the neostriatum (Frey *et al.*, 1982; Lightman *et al.*, 1982). This specific binding site displays many pharmacological similarities to the dopamine receptor identified in the hormone release studies. Thus, dopamine and drugs mimicking the inhibitory effect of dopamine compete with the ligand for occupancy of the specific binding site. The affinity of drugs for the specific binding site can be calculated from their potency in this competition; a similar calculation can be made for dopamine antagonists (Fig. 2, ordinate).

The dopamine receptor in the IL also is capable of regulating the production of cAMP by intact IL cells (Munemura *et al.*, 1980a,b; Meunier and Labrie, 1982b) and the activity of adenylate cyclase in cell-free homogenates of the IL (Cote *et al.*, 1981, 1982b). Unlike the β receptor (which when stimulated increases either parameter), the IL dopamine receptor decreases the capacity of IL cells to synthesize cAMP and decreases the activity of adenylate cyclase. The inhibitory effect of dopamine can also be demonstrated in IL tissue previously treated with cholera toxin (Tsuruta *et al.*, 1981; Cote *et al.*, 1982b). In this latter system, the potency of dopaminergic agonists can be readily determined. Dopaminergic antagonists compete with agonists for the receptor inhibiting adenylate cyclase activity (Frey *et al.*, 1982). Assuming a kinetic competition between agonist and antagonist for the receptor, the affinity of an antagonist can be calculated. There is a reasonable agreement between the potency of agonists and antagonist in the [^{3}H]-spiroperidol binding assay and the adenylate cyclase assay, thereby suggesting that some (or all) of the specific binding sites are the receptors inhibiting adenylate cyclase activity (Fig. 2).

Guanyl nucleotides participate in the functioning of the IL dopamine receptor. GTP diminishes the potency of dopamine and most other dopaminergic agonists for the specific [^{3}H]-spiroperidol binding site (Sibley and Creese, 1980; Frey *et al.*, 1982). [GTP affects the binding properties of the D-2 receptor in the anterior pituitary gland (DeLean *et al.*, 1982;

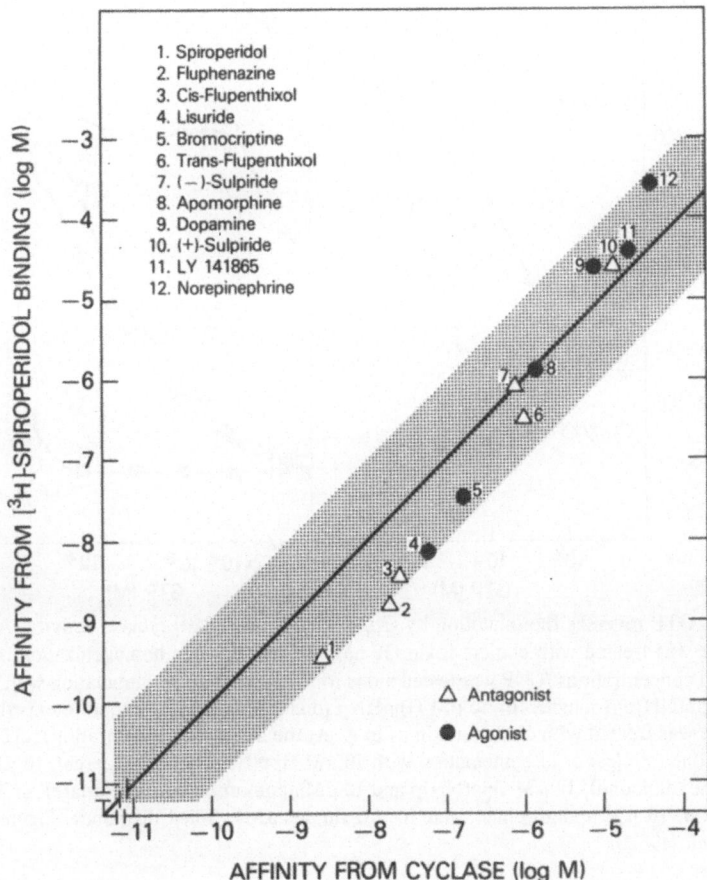

Figure 2. Comparison of the potency of dopaminergic agonists and antagonists toward the IL dopamine receptor. The affinity of the indicated dopaminergic drugs for the dopamine receptor in the IL was determined in either a [³H]-spiroperidol binding assay or an assay of adenylate cyclase activity in IL tissue previously treated with cholera toxin. The shaded area indicates one order of magnitude variation from a perfect correlation (solid line). Data from Frey *et al.* (1982); figure modified from Cote *et al.* (1982c).

Sibley *et al.*, 1982a).] GTP is also obligatory for the demonstration of the dopaminergic inhibition of IL adenylate cyclase activity (Cote *et al.*, 1982b). Nonhydrolyzable analogues of GTP [e.g., 5′-guanylyl imidodiphosphate, Gpp(NH)p] mimic the inhibitory effect on adenylate cyclase of a dopaminergic agonist in the presence of GTP. However, the inhibitory effect of Gpp(NH)p is not reversed by dopaminergic antagonists, suggesting that it is not a consequence of an interaction between the guanyl

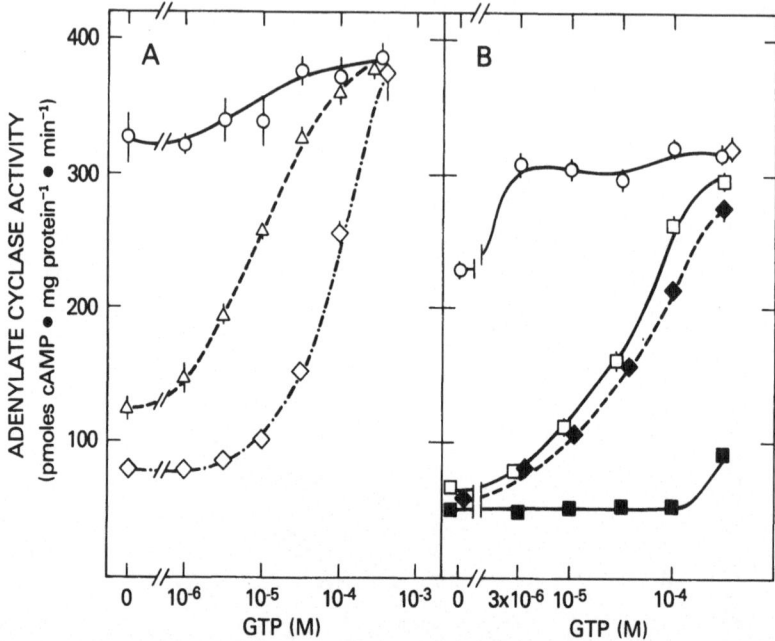

Figure 3. GTP reverses the inhibition by Gpp(NH)p of adenylate cyclase activity. A: The IL tissue was treated with cholera toxin (30 nM) for 2 hr prior to homogenization. At the indicated concentrations. GTP was tested alone (open circles) or in combination with either 2 μM Gpp(NH)p (triangles) or 20 μM GppHNp (diamonds). B: In a separate experiment, IL tissue was treated with cholera toxin as in A. At the indicated concentrations, GTP was tested alone (circles) or in combination with 10 μM Gpp(NH)p (open squares), 10 μM fluphenazine (diamond), 10 μM Gpp(NH)p and 10 μM apomorphine (filled square), or 10 μM Gpp(NH)p, 10 μM apomorphine, and 10 μM fluphenazine (filled diamond). Figure from Cote *et al.* (1982b).

nucleotide and the receptor. The inhibitory effect of Gpp(NH)p is reversed by GTP (Fig. 3A). Apomorphine, a dopaminergic agonist, prevents this reversal by GTP; fluphenazine, a dopaminergic antagonist prevents this effect of apomorphine (Fig. 3B). Together, these two observations suggest that stimulation of the dopamine receptor affects the ability of guanyl nucleotides to regulate adenylate cyclase activity.

The model presented in Fig. 4 accounts for the inhibitory effects of guanyl nucleotides and dopaminergic agonists (Cote *et al.*, 1982b). In accord with Rodbell's model of receptors, guanyl nucleotide components, and adenylate cyclase, the D-2 receptor can be envisioned as being coupled to adenylate cyclase via an inhibitory guanyl nucleotide component (N_i in Rodbell's model). N_i possesses a guanyl nucleotide regulatory site recognizing both GTP and Gpp(NH)p. In the absence of a dopaminergic agonist, Gpp(NH)p can interact with the site and thereby inhibit enzyme activity. Although GTP can interact with the site, it does not inhibit enzyme activity (in the absence of an agonist); this accounts for the ability of GTP to reverse the inhibitory effect of Gpp(NH)p. Stimulation of the D-2 receptor in some way alters N_i so that occupancy by GTP causes an inhibition of enzyme activity. This would account for the ability of a dopaminergic agonist to prevent the reversal by GTP of the Gpp(NH)p-induced inhibition of enzyme activity. Although this model accounts for the experimental observations, there is no direct evidence for the existence of N_i or an alteration in any of its physical properties as a consequence of receptor stimulation. Nonetheless, the model serves as the basis for further experimentation.

The IL provides a model of the D-2 receptor. In addition, the IL provides a model of dopaminergic neurotransmission. Dopaminergic neurons originating in the arcuate nucleus project via the pituitary stalk to the IL, where they arborize into a network of nerve terminals. "Synapselike" connections occur between the dopamine-containing neurons and the parenchymal cells of the IL (Baumgarten *et al.*, 1972). There are two examples of the biochemical and physiological phenomena occurring in the IL being demonstrated in the dopaminergic regions of the CNS. First, the neostriatum possesses a D-1 receptor capable of enhancing adenylate cyclase activity. A D-2 receptor may also occur on these cells; stimulation of the D-2 receptor decreases the responsiveness of the D-1 receptor (Stoof and Kebabian, 1981). This resembles the decreased responsiveness of the β adrenoceptor in the IL that occurs as a consequence of stimulation of the D-2 receptor. Second, a D-2 receptor exists on some of the cholinergic interneurons in the neostriatum (Sethy, 1979; Scatton, 1982). Stimulation of this receptor inhibits the release of acetylcholine from the cholinergic neurons (Stoof and Kebabian, 1982). This latter effect resembles the dopaminergic inhibition of the release of αMSH-like peptides from the IL. These two examples demonstrate the utility of the IL as a model of the dopaminergic phenomena in the CNS.

4. Ramifications of the Two-Dopamine-Receptor Hypothesis

4.1. Drugs Discriminating between the D-1 and the D-2 Receptors

The two-dopamine-receptor hypothesis is strengthened by the identification of drugs discriminating between the two receptors. A number of compounds are potent agonists on the D-2 receptor but are devoid of agonist activity on the D-1 receptor. For example, RU 24213 and RU 24926 are potent D-2 agonists, yet they display no agonist activity on the

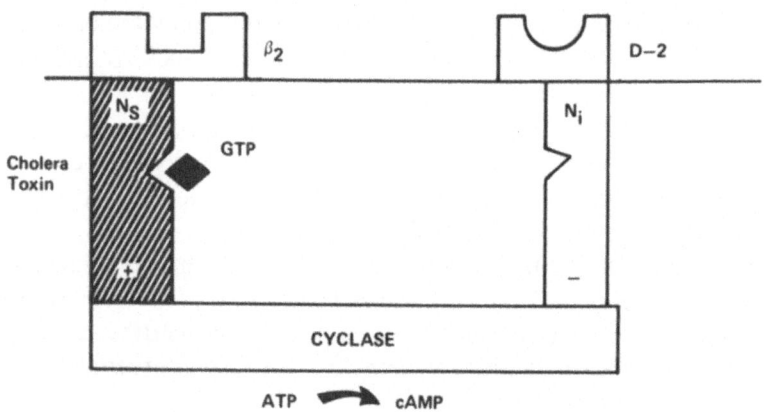

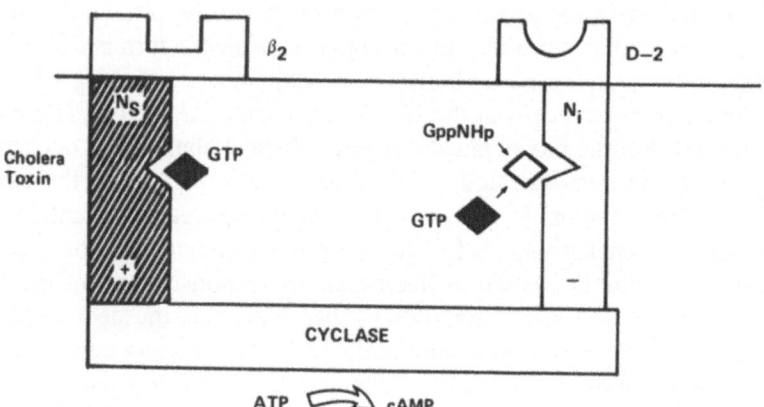

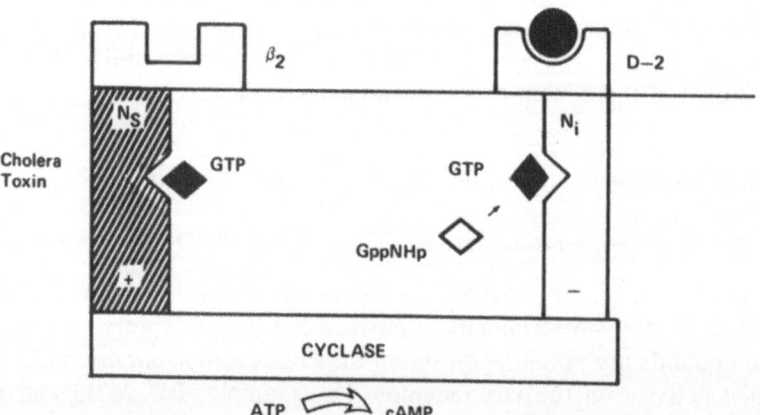

D-1 receptor (Euvrard *et al.*, 1980). Likewise, LY-141865 is a D-2 agonist devoid of activity on the D-1 receptor (Tsuruta *et al.*, 1981; Hahn *et al.*, 1983). Similarily, antagonists discriminate between the two receptors. Domperidone is a potent antagonist of the D-2 receptor in the pituitary gland, but it is virtually devoid of antagonist activity on the D-1 receptor (Denef and Follebouckt, 1978; Watling and Dowling, 1981). Among the substituted benzamides, YM-09151-2 is an extremely potent D-2 antagonist (Grewe *et al.*, 1982; Meltzer *et al.*, 1983); the drug is equipotent with fluphenazine as an antagonist of the D-2 receptor in the rat IL. However, YM-09151-2 is 1000-fold less potent that fluphenazine as a D-1 antagonist.

The D-1 receptor is selectively stimulated by several compounds synthesized by SK&F Laboratories. Either SK&F 38393 or SK&F 82526 stimulates the D-1 receptor (Brown *et al.*, 1980; Brown and Dawson-Hughes, 1983; Setler *et al.*, 1978; Hahn *et al.*, 1982). Because neither of these compounds inhibits the release of prolactin, it has been concluded that they do not interact with the D-2 receptor. However, in biochemical assays of the D-2 receptor (i.e., inhibition of IL cAMP production, inhibition of IL adenylate cyclase activity, or binding of [^{3}H]-spiroperidol to anterior pituitary tissue), either of these compounds displays agonist activity. The reasons for this discrepancy between the physiological and biochemical models of the D-2 receptor are not understood (Munermura *et al.*, 1980a; Sibley *et al.*, 1982b; Itoh, M. E. Goldman, and J. W. Kebabian, unpublished data). Nonetheless, the inactivity of these two compounds in the physiological models of the D-2 receptor coupled with their activity on the D-1 receptor makes them useful research tools.

There are several antagonists favoring the D-1 receptor. $S(+)$Bulbocapnine blocks the DA-1 receptor in the cardiovascular sys-

←

Figure 4. Organization of the β_2 adrenoceptor and the D-2 dopamine receptor in the intermediate lobe of the rat pituitary gland. Top: The organization of the β_2-adrenoceptor–adenylate cyclase complex is as shown in Fig. 1. The inhibitory effect of D-2 agonists is most readily seen in IL tissue treated with cholera toxin, which interacts with N_s and permits GTP (filled diamond) to stimulate adenylate cyclase (cyclase) activity in the absence of a β-adrenergic agonist. The D-2 dopamine receptor (D-2) is coupled to adenylate cyclase by the inhibitory guanyl nucleotide component (N_i). Middle: In the absence of a D-2 agonist, Gpp(NH)p (open diamond) can interact with N_i and diminish the adenylate cyclase activity. GTP can compete with Gpp(NH)p for occupancy of the guanyl nucleotide recognition site on N_i; however, GTP is unable to inhibit enzyme activity. This accounts for the ability of GTP to reverse the inhibitory action of Gpp(NH)p (see Fig. 3A). Bottom: Occupancy of the D-2 receptor by an agonist (filled circle) alters the properties of the guanyl nucleotide recognition site on N_i so that when GTP occupies the site, adenylate cyclase activity is inhibited. Because GTP is able to inhibit enzyme activity, it can no longer reverse the inhibitory effect of Gpp(NH)p.

tem as well as the D-1 receptor in the rat caudate nucleus or carp retina (Goldberg *et al.*, 1979; Shepperson *et al.*, 1982; Miller and McDermed, 1979; Itoh, M. E. Goldman, and J. W. Kebabian, unpublished data). $S(+)$Bulbocapnine is significantly less potent as an antagonist of either the DA-2 receptor in the cardiovascular system or the D-2 receptor in the IL (Shepperson *et al.*, 1982; Itoh, M. E. Goldman, and J. W. Kebabian, unpublished data). Recently, a second D-1 antagonist of higher specificity than $S(+)$bulbocapnine has been identified. SCH 23390 [R-($+$)-8-chloro-2,3,4,5-tetrahydro-3-methyl-5-phenyl-1H-3-benzazepin-7-ol] has a K_i of 0.66 nM at the D-1 receptor but is inactive on the D-2 receptor (Iorio *et al.*, 1981, 1983). The availability of antagonists favoring the D-1 receptor may facilitate investigations of the "physiological role" of the D-1 receptor in the central nervous system as well as the cardiovascular system.

4.2. The "DA Receptors" versus the "D Receptors"

Following his extensive studies of the dopamine receptors in the cardiovascular system, Leon Goldberg proposed the existence of two categories of dopamine receptor, designated as the DA-1 and the DA-2 receptors (Goldberg and Kohli, 1979). He was unable to utilize the nomenclature D-1 and D-2 because of two differences between the pharmacology of the DA-1 receptor and that of the D-1 receptor. First, *in vivo*, ($+$)-sulpiride is a potent antagonist of the DA-1 receptor; however, sulpiride is virtually inactive as an antagonist of the D-1 receptor. Second, the ergots (e.g., lisuride and lergotrile) do not block the DA-1 receptor but do antagonize the D-1 receptor. The first of these discrepancies may not be as great as envisioned by Goldberg. Thus, although ($+$)-sulpiride is a potent DA-1 antagonist *in vivo*, the drug is a weak antagonist of this receptor in *in vitro* studies of dog mesenteric artery (Kohli *et al.*, 1979). This latter observation complements the recent report that ($+$)-sulpiride is an extremely weak antagonist ($K_i = 13$ μm) of the prototype D-1 receptor in the bovine parathyroid gland (Brown and Dawson-Hughes, 1983). The validity of the second of the discrepancies remains unclear; ergots antagonizing the D-1 receptor have not been tested *in vitro* on the DA-1 receptor in the dog mesenteric artery.

There are several other compounds apparently discriminating between the dopamine receptor in the renal vasculature and the D-1 receptor in the neostriatum. Thus, Weinstock and his colleagues at SK&F Laboratories report that the 6-iodo and 6-methyl analogues of SK&F 82526 are antagonists of the D-1 receptor but remain potent renal vasodilators (Weinstock *et al.*, 1983). By analogy with the α and β adrenoceptors, the existence of two subcategories of D-1 (or DA-1) receptor remains a possibility worthy of consideration when attempting to account for such discrepancies. There are no striking pharmacological discrepancies between the pharmacology of the DA-2 receptor and the D-2 receptor (Goldberg and Kohli, 1983).

4.3. Is the Prejunctional Dopamine Receptor a Distinct Entity?

Dopamine receptors have been classified by anatomic criteria. According to this schema, the prejunctional dopamine receptor residing on the nigroneostrital dopaminergic neurons is a distinct entity from the dopamine receptors occurring postjunctional to these neurons. Assuming the validity of this classification schema, TL-99 (6,7-dihydroxy-2-dimethylaminotetralin) has been identified as a dopaminergic agonist selective for the prejunctional dopamine receptor (Goodale *et al.* 1980). However, when tested in biochemical models of postjunctional dopamine receptors, TL-99 displays agonist activity. Thus, in the fish retina, the D-1 receptor occurs on the external horizontal cells; these cells are postjunctional to the dopaminergic amacrine cells, which innervate them. TL-99 is an agonist on this postjunctional D-1 receptor (Watling and Williams, 1982; Kebabian *et al.*, 1982). Similarily, in the rat IL, the D-2 receptor occurs on the melanotrophs; these cells are postjunctional to the dopaminergic neurons originating in the hypothalamus that innervate the IL. TL-99 is also an agonist on this postjunctional D-2 receptor (Kebabian *et al.*, 1982). These observations do not support the conclusion that TL-99 is an agonist selective for the prejunctional receptor. Indeed, in view of the pharmacological similarities between the presynaptic and postsynaptic D-2 receptors, it is difficult to envision the existence of an agonist discriminating between these two entities.

5. Conclusions

The two-dopamine-receptor hypothesis has attracted much attention and has served as the motivating factor for much research. The hypothesis has guided the investigations of my own group into the properties of the dopamine receptor in the intermediate lobe of the rat pituitary gland and the D-2 dopamine receptor in the striatum. The investigations of the dopamine receptors in the cardiovascular system have also been aided by the hypothesis that there are two categories of dopamine receptor. Although there are still apparent discrepancies between the properties of the D-1 and DA-1 receptors and the D-2 and the DA-2 receptors, I anticipate that time will minimize (rather than magnify) these discrepancies.

References

Ahlquist, R. P., 1948, A study of the adrenotopic receptors, *Am. J. Physiol.* **153**:586–600.
Ahlquist, R. P., 1981, Adrenoceptors, in: *Towards Understanding Receptors* (J. W. Lamble, ed.), Elsevier North Holland, Amsterdam, pp. 49–52.
Anden, N. E., Dahlstrom, A., Fuxe, K., and Larsson, K., 1966, Functional role of the nigro-neostriatal dopamine neurons, *Acta Pharmacol. Toxicol.* (*Kbh.*) **24**:263–274.
Bacq, Z. M., 1981, Early work on the adrenergic mediator: How to go wrong, in: *Towards Understanding Receptors* (J. W. Lamble, ed.), Elsevier North Holland, Amsterdam, pp. 44–48.
Baumgarten, G., Bjorklund, A., Holstein, A. F., and Nobin, A., 1972, Organization and ultrastructural identification of the catecholamine nerve terminals in the neural lobe and pars intermedia of the rat pituitary, *Z. Zellforsch.* **126**:483–517.
Bertler, A., and Rosengren, E., 1959, Occurrence and distribution of dopamine in brain and other tissues, *Experientia* **15**:10–11.
Bower, A., Hadley, M. E., and Hruby, V. J., 1974, Biogenic amines and control of melanophore stimulating hormone release, *Science* **184**:70–72.
Brown, E. M., Attie, M. F., Reen, S., Gardner, D. G., Kebabian, J. W., and Aurbach, G. D., 1980, Characterization of dopaminergic receptors in dispersed bovine parathyroid cells, *Mol. Pharmacol.* **18**:335–340.
Brown, E. M., and Dawson-Hughes, B. F., 1983, Dopamine receptor-mediated activation of adenylate cyclase, cAMP accumulation and PTH secretion in dispersed bovine parathyroid cells, in: *Multiple Dopamine Receptors and Modulation of Peripheral Dopamine Receptors* (J. W. Kebabian and C. Kaiser, eds.), American Chemical Society, Washington pp. 1–21.
Brown, J. H., and Makman, M., 1972, Stimulation by dopamine of adenylate cyclase in retinal homogenates and of adenosine-3',5'-cyclic monophosphate formation in intact retina, *Proc. Natl. Acad. Sci. U.S.A.* **69**:539–543.
Carlsson, A., Lindqvist, M., Magnusson, T., and Waldeck, B., 1958, On the presence of 3-hydroxytyramine in brain, *Science* **127**:471.
Caron, M. G., Beaulieu, M., Raymond, V., Gagne, B., Drouin, J., Lefkowitz, R. J., and Labrie, F., 1978, Dopaminergic receptors in the anterior pituitary gland. Correlation of [^{3}H]-dihydroergocryptine binding with the dopaminergic control of prolactin release, *J. Biol. Chem.* **253**:2244–2253.
Clement-Cormier, Y. C., Kebabian, J. W., Petzold, G. L., and Greengard, P., 1974, Dopamine-sensitive adenylate cyclase in mammalian brain: A possible site of action of antipsychotic drugs, *Proc. Natl. Acad. Sci. U.S.A.* **71**:1113–1117.
Clement-Cormier, Y. C., Parrish, R. G., Petzold, G. L., Kebabian, J. W., and Greengard, F., 1975, Characterization of a dopamine-sensitive adenylate cyclase in the rat caudate nucleus, *J. Neurochem.* **25**:143–149.
Cools, A. R., and Van Rossum, J. M., 1976, Excitation-mediating and inhibition-mediating dopamine receptors: A new concept towards a better understanding of electrophysiological, biochemical, pharmacological, functional and clinical data, *Psychopharmacologia* (Berl.) **45**:243–254.
Costall, B., and Naylor, R. J., 1979, Behavioural aspects of dopamine agonists and antagonists, in: *The Neurobiology of Dopamine* (A. S. Horn, J. Korf, and B. H. C. Westerink, eds.), Academic Press, London, pp. 555–576.
Cote, T. E., Munemura, M., Eskay, R. L., and Kebabian, J. W., 1980, Biochemical identification of the β-adrenoceptor and evidence for the involvement of an adenosine 3',5'-monophosphate system in the β-adrenergically induced release of α-melanocyte-stim-

ulating hormone in the intermediate lobe of the rat pituitary gland, *Endocrinology* **107**:108–116.

Cote, T. E., Grewe, C. W., and Kebabian, J. W., 1981, Stimulation of a D-2 dopamine receptor in the intermediate lobe of the rat pituitary gland decreases the responsiveness of the β-adrenoceptor: Biochemical mechanism, *Endocrinology* **108**:420–426.

Cote, T. E., Grewe, C. W., and Kebabian, J. W., 1982a, Guanyl nucleotides participate in the β-adrenergic stimulation of adenylate cyclase activity in the intermediate lobe of the rat pituitary gland, *Endocrinology* **110**:805–811.

Cote, T. E., Grewe, C. W., Tsuruta, K., Stoof, J. C., Eskay, R. L., and Kebabian, J. W., 1982b, D-2 dopamine receptor-mediated inhibition of adenylate cyclase activity in the intermediate lobe of the rat pituitary gland requires GTP, *Endocrinology* **110**:812–819.

Cote, T. E., Eskay, R. L., Frey, E. A., Grewe, C. W., Munemura, M., Stoof, J. C., Tsuruta, K., and Kebabian, J. W., 1982c, Biochemical and physiological studies of the beta-adrenoceptor and the D-2 dopamine receptor in the intermediate lobe of the rat pituitary gland: A review, *Neuroendocrinology* **35**:217–224.

Dale, H. H., 1906, On some physiological actions of ergot, *J. Physiol. (Lond.)* **34**:163–206.

DeLean, A., Kilpatrick, B. F., and Caron, M., 1982, Guanine nucleotides regulate both dopaminergic agonist and antagonist binding in porcine anterior pituitary, *Endocrinology* **110**:1064–1066.

Denef, C., and Follebouckt, J.-J., 1978, Differential effects of dopamine antagonists on prolactin secretion from cultured rat pituitary cells, *Life Sci.* **22**:431–435.

Ernst, A. M., 1969, The role of biogenic amines in the extra-pyramidal system, *Acta Physiol Pharmacol. (Neerl.)* **15**:141–154.

Euvrard, C., Ferland, L., Di Paolo, T., Beaulieu, M., Labrie, F., Oberlander, C., Raynaud, J. F., and Boissier, J. R., 1980, Activity of two new potent dopaminergic agonists at the striatal and anterior pituitary levels, *Neuropharmacology* **19**:379–386.

Frey, E. A., Cote, T. E., Grewe, C. W., and Kebabian, J. W., 1982, [³H]Spiroperidol identifies a D-2 dopamine receptor inhibiting adenylate cyclase activity in the intermediate lobe of the rat pituitary gland, *Endocrinology* **110**:1897–1904.

Goldberg, L. I., 1972, Cardiovascular and renal actions of dopamine: Potential clinical applications, *Pharmacol. Rev.* **24**:1–29.

Goldberg, L. I., 1979, Introductory lecture: The dopamine vascular receptor: Agonists and Antagonists, in: *Peripheral Dopaminergic Receptors. Advances in the Biosciences. Volume 20* (J.-L. Imbs and J. Schwartz, eds.), Pergamon Press, Oxford, pp. 1–12.

Goldberg, L. I., and Kohli, J. D., 1979, Peripheral pre- and postsynaptic dopamine receptors: Are they different from dopamine receptors in the central nervous system?, *Commun. Psychopharmacol.* **3**:447–456.

Goldberg, L. I., Musgrave, G. E., and Kohli, J. D., 1979, Antagonism of dopamine-induced renal vasodilation in the dog by bulbocapnine and sulpiride, in: *Sulpiride and Other Benzamides* (P. F. Spano, M. Trabucchi, G. U. Corsini, and G. L. Gessa, eds.), Italian Brain Research Foundation Press, Milan, pp. 73–81.

Goldberg, L. I., and Kohli, J. D., 1983, Peripheral dopamine receptors: A classification based on potency series and specific antagonism, *Trends Pharmacol. Sci.* **4**:64–66.

Goldman, M. E., Beaulieu, M., Kebabian, J. W., and Eskay, R. L., 1983, α-Melanocyte-stimulating hormone-like peptides in the intermediate lobe of the rat pituitary gland: Characterization of content and release *in vitro*, *Endocrinology* **112**:435–441.

Goodale, D. E., Rusterholz, D. B., Long, J. P., Flynn, J. R., Walsh, B., Cannon, J. G., and Lee, T. L., 1980, Neurochemical and behavioral evidence for a selective presynaptic dopamine receptor agonist, *Science* **210**:1141–1143.

Grewe, C. W., and Kebabian, J. W., 1982, Dopamine stimulates production of cyclic AMP by the salivary gland of the cockroach, *Nauphoeta cinerea*, *Cell. Mol. Neurobiol.* **2**:65–69.

Grewe, C. W., Frey, E. A., Cote, T. E., and Kebabian, J. W., 1982, YM-09151-2: A potent antagonist for a peripheral D_2-dopamine receptor, *Eur. J. Pharmacol.* **81**:149–152.

Hahn, R. A., Wardell, J. R., Sarau, H. M., and Ridley, P. T., 1982, Characterization of the peripheral and central effects of SK&F 82526, a novel dopamine receptor agonist, *J. Pharmacol. Exp. Ther.* **223**:305–313.

Hahn, R. A., MacDonald, B. R., and Martin, M. A., 1983, Antihypertensive activity of LY 141865, a selective presynaptic dopamine receptor agonist, *J. Pharmacol. Exp. Ther.* **224**:206–214.

Horn, A. S., Korf, J., and Westerink, B. H. C. (eds.), 1979, *The Neurobiology of Dopamine*, Academic Press, London.

Iorio, L. C., Houser, V., Korduba, C. A., Leitz, F., and Barnett, A., 1981, SCH 23390, a benzazepine with atypical effects on dopaminergic systems, *Pharmacologist* **23**:137.

Iorio, L. C., Barnett, A., Leitz, F. H., Houser, V. P., and Korduba, C. A., 1983, SCH 23390, a potential benzazepine antipsychotic with unique interactions on dopaminergic systems, *J. Pharmacol. Exp. Ther.* **226**:462–468.

Kebabian, J. W., and Calne, D. B., 1979, Multiple receptors for dopamine, *Nature* **277**:93–96.

Kebabian, J. W., and Greengard, P., 1971, Dopamine-sensitive adenyl cyclase: Possible role in synaptic transmission, *Science* **174**:1346–1349.

Kebabian, J. W., Petzold, G. L., and Greengard, P., 1972, Dopamine-sensitive adenylate cyclase in the caudate nucleus of rat brain, and its similarity to the "dopamine receptor." *Proc. Natl. Acad. Sci. U.S.A.* **69**:2145–2149.

Kebabian, J. W., Calne, D. B., and Kebabian, P. R., 1977, Lergotrile mesylate: An *in vivo* dopamine agonist which blocks dopamine receptors *in vitro*, *Commun. Psychopharmacol.* **1**:311–318.

Kebabian, J. W., Chen, T. C., and Cote, T. E., 1979, Endogenous guanyl nucleotides: Components of the striatum which confer dopamine sensitivity to adenylate cyclase, *Commun. Psychopharmacol.* **3**:421–428.

Kebabian, J. W., Miyazaki, K., and Grewe, C. W., 1982, 6,7-dihydroxy-2-dimethylaminotetralin (TL-99) stimulates postjunctional D-1 and D-2 dopamine receptors, *Neurochem. Int.* **2**:227–229.

Kohli, J. D., Takeda, H., Ozaki, N., and Goldberg, L. I., 1979, *In vitro* study with semirigid rotomeric conformational analogues of dopamine, in: *Peripheral Dopaminergic Receptors, Advances in the Biosciences*, Volume 20 (J.-L. Imbs and J. Schwartz, eds.), Pergamon Press, Oxford, pp. 143–149.

Lands, A. M., Arnold, A., McAuliff, Luduena, F. P., and Brown, T. G., 1967, Differentiation of receptor systems activated by sympathomimetic amines, *Nature* **214**:597–598.

Langer, S. Z., 1981, Presynaptic regulation of the release of catecholamines, *Pharmacol. Rev.* **32**:337–362.

Langley, J. N., 1906, On nerve endings and on special excitable substances in cells, *Proc R. Soc. (Lond.) [Biol.]* **78**:170–194.

Lightman, S. L., Ninkovic, M., and Hunt, S. P., 1982, Localization of [^{3}H]spiperone binding sites in the intermediate lobe of the rat pituitary gland, *Neurosci. Lett.* **32**:99–102.

MacLeod, R. M., 1976, Regulation of prolactin release, in: *Frontiers in Neuroendocrinology*, Volume 4 (L. Martini and W. F. Ganong, eds.), Raven Press, New York, 169–194.

Meltzer, H. Y., Mikuni, M., Simonovic, M., and Gudelsky, G. A., 1983, Effect of a novel benzamide, YM-09151-2, on rat serum prolactin levels, *Life Sci.* **32**:1015–1021.

Meunier, H., and Labrie, F., 1982a, Specificity of the β₂-adrenergic receptor stimulating cyclic AMP accumulation in the intermediate lobe of the rat pituitary gland, *Eur. J. Pharmacol.* **81**:411–420.

Meunier, H., and Labrie, F., 1982b, The dopamine receptor in the intermediate lobe of the rat pituitary gland is negatively coupled to adenylate cyclase, *Life Sci.* **30**:963–968.

Miller, R. J., and McDermed, J. D., 1979, Dopamine-sensitive adenylate cyclase, in: *The Neurobiology of Dopamine* (A. S. Horn, J. Korf, and B. H. C. Westerink, eds.), Academic Press, New York, pp. 159–177.

Munemura, M., Cote, T. E., Tsuruta, K., Eskay, R. L., and Kebabian, J. K., 1980a, The dopamine receptor in the intermediate lobe of the rat pituitary gland: Pharmacological characterization, *Endocrinology* **107**:1676–1683.

Munemura, M., Eskay, R. L., and Kebabian, J. W., 1980b, Release of α-melanocyte-stimulating hormone from dispersed cells of the intermediate lobe of the rat pituitary gland: Involvement of catecholamines and adenosine 3',5'-monophosphate, *Endocrinology* **106**:1795–1803.

Peng Loh, Y., and Gainer, H., 1977, Biosynthesis, processing, and control of release of melanotropic peptides in the neurointermediate lobe of *Xenopus laevis*, *J. Gen. Physiol.* **70**:37–58.

Rodbell, M., 1980, The role of hormone receptors and GTP-regulatory proteins in membrane transduction, *Nature* **284**:17–22.

Scatton, B., 1982, Effect of dopamine agonists and neuroleptic agents on striatal acetylcholine transmission in the rat: Evidence against dopamine receptor multiplicity, *J. Pharmacol. Exp. Ther.* **220**:197–202.

Seeman, P., 1980, Brain dopamine receptors, *Pharmacol. Rev.* **32**:229–313.

Sethy, V. H., 1979, Regulation of striatal acetylcholine concentration by D-2 dopamine receptors, *Eur. J. Pharmacol.* **60**:397–398.

Setler, P. E., Sarau, H. M., Zirkle, C. L., and Saunders, H. L., 1978, The central effects of a novel dopamine agonist, *Eur. J. Pharmacol.* **50**:419–430.

Shepperson, N. B., Duval, N., Massingham, R., and Langer, S. Z., 1982, Differential blocking effects of several dopamine receptor antagonists for peripheral pre- and postsynaptic dopamine receptors in anesthetized dogs, *J. Pharmacol. Exp. Ther.* **221**:753–761.

Sibley, D. R., and Creese, I., 1980, Dopamine receptor binding in bovine intermediate lobe pituitary membranes, *Endocrinology* **107**:1405–1409.

Sibley, D. R., DeLean, A., and Creese, I., 1982a, Anterior pituitary dopamine receptors. Demonstration of interconvertible high and low affinity states of the D-2 dopamine receptor, *J. Biol. Chem.* **257**:6351–6361.

Sibley, D. R., Leff, S. E., and Creese, I., 1982b, Interactions of novel dopaminergic ligands with D-1 and D-2 dopamine receptors, *Life Sci.* **31**:637–645.

Spano, P. F., Frattola, L., Govoni, S., Tonon, G. C., and Trabucchi, M., 1979, Dopaminergic ergot derivatives: Selective agonists of a new class of dopamine receptors, in: *Dopaminergic Ergot Derivatives and Motor Function, Wenner-Gren Center International Symposium Series*, Volume 31 (K. Fuxe and D. B. Calne, eds.), Pergamon Press, Oxford, pp. 159–171.

Stephanini, E., Devoto, F., Marchisio, A. M., Vernaleone, F., and Collu, R., 1980, [³H]-Spiroperidol binding to a putative dopaminergic receptor in rat pituitary gland, *Life Sci.* **26**:583–587.

Stoof, J. C., and Kebabian, J. W., 1981, Opposing roles for D-1 and D-2 dopamine receptors in efflux of cyclic AMP from rat neostriatum, *Nature* **294**:366–368.

Stoof, J. C., and Kebabian, J. W., 1982, Independent *in vitro* regulation by the D-2 dopamine receptor of dopamine-stimulated efflux of cyclic AMP and K⁺-stimulated release of acetylcholine from rat neostriatum, *Brain Res.* **250**:263–270.

Teranishi, T., Negishi, K., and Kato, S., 1983, Dopamine modulates S-potential amplitude and dye-coupling between external horizontal cells in carp retina, *Nature* **301**:243–246.

Tsuruta, K., Frey, E. A., Grewe, C. W., Cote, T. E., Eskay, R. L., and Kebabian, J. W., 1981, Evidence that LY-141865 specifically stimulates the D-2 dopamine receptor, *Nature* **292**:463–465.

Tsuruta, K., Grewe, C. W., and Cote, T. E., Eskay, R. L., and Kebabian, J. W., 1982, Coordinated action of calcium ion and cyclic adenosine 3',5'monophosphate upon the release of α-melanocyte stimulating hormone from the intermediate lobe of the rat pituitary gland, *Endocrinology* **110**:1133–1140.

Ungerstedt, U., 1971, Postsynaptic supersensitivity after 6-hydroxydopamine induced degeneration of the nigro-striatal dopamine system, *Acta Physiol. Scand.* [*Suppl.*] **367**:69–93.

Watling, K. J., and Dowling, J. E., 1981, Dopaminergic mechanisms in teleost retina I. Dopamine-sensitive adenylate cyclase in homogenates of carp retina; effects of agonists, antagonists and ergots, *J. Neurochem.* **36**:559–568.

Watling, K. J., and Williams, M., 1982, Interaction of the putative dopamine autoreceptor agonists, 3-PPP and TL-99, with the dopamine-sensitive adenylate cyclase of carp retina, *Eur. J. Pharmacol.* **77**:321–326.

Watling, K. J., 1983, A function for dopamine-sensitive adenylate cyclase in the retina?, *Trends Pharmacol. Sci.* **4**:328–329.

Weinstock, J., Wilson, J. W., Ladd, D. L., Brenner, M., Ackerman, D. M., Blumberg, A. L., Brennan, F. T., Hahn, R. A., Heible, J. P., Sarau, H. M., and Wiebelhaus, V. D., 1983, Dopaminergic benzazepines with divergent cardiovascular profiles, in: *Multiple Dopamine Receptors and Modulation of Peripheral Dopamine Receptors* (J. W. Kebabian and C. Kaiser, eds.), American Chemical Society, Washington pp. 157–169.

2

Radioligand Binding Studies of Agonist Interactions with Dopamine Receptors

I. CREESE, S. E. LEFF, D. R. SIBLEY, and M. W. HAMBLIN

1. Direct Receptor Characterization: Radioligand Binding Studies

Since 1975, the elegantly simple radioligand binding technique has allowed direct examination of neurotransmitter and drug interactions with dopamine receptors. The simplification obtained through elimination of factors such as alteration of neurotransmitter synthesis or other regulators of dopamine's second messenger systems is the chief advantage of this approach to the study of receptor biochemistry and pharmacology. This simplification, however, also presents a major challenge—to demonstrate that the binding sites identified *in vitro* have functional relevance in the physiological milieu. It is a task of utmost importance, and often of considerable difficulty, to demonstrate that receptor binding sites can be clearly associated with some biological function. Although problems remain, this correspondence between binding sites and their function, on both the behavioral and biochemical level, is steadily being established for the dopamine receptors.

In studies of radioligand binding, it is of utmost importance to demonstrate that the binding under measurement involves a physiological or pharmacological receptor. Since receptors are present in extremely small numbers, and radioligands can adhere to many membrane components,

I. CREESE, S. E. LEFF, D. R. SIBLEY, and M. W. HAMBLIN • Department of Neurosciences, University of California, San Diego, School of Medicine, La Jolla, California 92093.

uptake sites, other "irrelevant" neurotransmitter receptors, and even inorganic materials, considerable caution must be exercised in the interpretation of data. Radioligand binding studies should therefore satisfy the following criteria to reduce the probability of a false positive receptor identification. These criteria have been discussed in detail elsewhere (Burt, 1978).

Briefly, specific binding must be saturable and reversible. In this regard, specific binding must be established with a competitive agent of high affinity and high specificity for the putative receptor of interest. For example, the neuroleptic dopamine antagonists spiroperidol and (+)butaclamol bind with high affinity not only to dopamine receptors but also to serotonin receptors (*vide infra*). Therefore, in tissues where both types of receptors may be present, butaclamol does not provide a satisfactory "blank" for the determination of specific [^{3}H]-spiroperidol binding to dopamine receptors. Under ideal conditions, specific binding should be significantly greater than nonspecific binding. Signal-to-noise ratios greater than or equal to 1 are adequate, and without such, little reliance can be placed on the data. Further criteria are that the regional localization of [^{3}H]-ligand binding sites correspond to known innervation and that these sites are absent from regions lacking innervation or physiological sensitivity to the neurotransmitter. The pharmacological specificity of antagonists should not greatly differ from *in vivo* pharmacological or behavioral responses. Drugs that are inactive in pharmacological measurements of receptors should show little affinity for the [^{3}H]-ligand binding sites. Furthermore, it is important to demonstrate that uptake mechanisms have not confounded the assays and that the radioligand itself, not a metabolite, is bound.

A typical radioligand binding assay consists of incubating membranes with low concentrations of a [^{3}H]-ligand of high specific activity. After binding has reached equilibrium, the [^{3}H]-ligand bound to the membranes is separated from the free ligand in the incubation mix. This is commonly done by centrifugation or by rapid filtration under vacuum over glass fiber filters. The [^{3}H]-ligand remaining on the membranes is the total of both specific binding to the putative receptor and nonspecific binding to the various possible components described above. Nonspecific binding alone is measured in parallel sets of test tubes containing, in addition, excess of a nonradioactive drug known to block the receptors of interest [(+)butaclamol more often than not for dopamine receptors]. Specific binding is then determined by simple subtraction. Receptor number and affinity for the radioligand are determined by conducting saturation experiments utilizing increasing concentrations of radioligand. The affinity of nonradioactive drugs is determined in "competition" experiments in which

Table I. Functional Classification of Dopamine Receptor Subtypes[a]

	D-1	D-2
Prototype receptor location	Parathyroid gland	Anterior and intermediate pituitary glands
Adenylate cyclase linkage	Stimulatory	Inhibitory or unlinked
Agonists		
Dopamine	Full agonist (μmolar potency)	Full agonist (nmolar potency)
Apomorphine	Partial agonist (μmolar potency)	Full agonist (nmolar potency)
Antagonists		
Phenothiazines	nmolar potency	nmolar potency
Thioxanthenes	nmolar potency	nmolar potency
Butyrophenones	μmolar potency	nmolar potency
Substituted benzamides	Inactive	n-μmolar potency
Dopaminergic ergots	Antagonists or partial agonists (μmolar potency)	Full agonists (nmolar potency)

[a] Modified from Kebabian and Calne (1979).

increasing concentrations of the nonradioactive drug are incubated with a fixed concentration of radioligand.

In the standard filtration assay technique, a radiolabeled agent is only useful for identifying receptors for which it has approximately nanomolar affinity (see Bennett, 1978). Thus, it is apparent from the classification described by Kebabian in the previous chapter and summarized in Table I that D-1 receptors should be labeled by radioactive phenothiazines and thioxanthenes. However, these agents would also bind D-2 sites. The butyrophenones [^{3}H]-spiroperidol, [^{3}H]-haloperidol, and [^{3}H]-domperidone should be fairly selective ligands for D-2 receptors since they have lower affinities for D-1 receptors. At first approximation, one might predict that only the D-2 receptor would be labeled by [^{3}H]-agonists such as apomorphine or the ergots. However, other factors must be considered. Agonist affinity for a particular receptor-mediated response may not quantitatively predict agonist affinity for that receptor determined by radioligand binding studies in membrane preparations because of factors such as spare receptors or differing intrinsic activities. Indeed, we shall see that D-2 receptors can exist in two conformational states having low or high affinity for agonists in membrane preparations The existence of a third dopamine receptor subtype termed "D-3," which is characterized as having high affinity for agonists, has been suggested to label autoreceptors (Titeler *et al.*, 1979) and will also be considered.

2. The Pituitary D-2 Receptor

2.1. Binding Studies

The pituitary provides a good and relatively simple starting point for the discussion of CNS dopamine receptors. In contrast to the multiple receptor subtypes in the brain, the pituitary contains only D-2 dopamine receptors. This receptor exhibits two agonist binding states, which are controlled by the presence or absence of guanine nucleotides and various cations. Our understanding of the pituitary dopamine receptor is a recent development and has been instructive in the delineation of other dopamine receptor subtypes.

Accordingly, several groups (Creese *et al.*, 1977a; Caron *et al.*, 1978; Cronin *et al.*, 1978; Calabro and MacLeod, 1978) have used radioactive dopamine agonists and antagonists to identify high-affinity, stereoselective, and saturable D-2 dopamine receptor binding in anterior pituitary membrane preparations. The rank order of agonists and antagonists for competing with radioligand binding to the dopamine receptor agrees closely with their rank order in inhibiting or disinhibiting prolactin release. In addition, one group has provided immunocytochemical evidence that these dopamine receptors are largely confined to the mammotroph cells (Weiner *et al.*, 1979; Goldsmith *et al.*, 1979).

The radiolabeled dopamine antagonist [^{3}H]-spiroperidol has previously been shown to bind exclusively to dopamine receptors in the anterior pituitary of cattle (Creese *et al.*, 1977a), sheep (Cornin and Weiner, 1979), and rats (Stefanini *et al.*, 1980). In bovine anterior pituitary membranes, the specific binding of [^{3}H]-spiroperidol is saturable and of high affinity. Analysis of the saturation data indicates a homogeneous population of binding sites with a dissociation constant (K_D) of approximately 0.3 nM. The maximum number of binding sites (B_{max}) is about 4 pmole/g tissue—only 20% of the number of sites detected in bovine caudate. By use of [^{3}H]-spiroperidol as the radioligand, it can be demonstrated that antagonist competition curves exhibit monophasic, mass-action characteristics with pseudo-Hill coefficients equal to 1. For example, Fig. 1 shows the experimental data and the resulting computer-modeled competition curve for the antagonist (+)butaclamol. The computer analysis employed is a nonlinear least-squares curve-fitting program that can analyze the data in terms of one or more classes of binding sites (De Lean *et al.*, 1980; Munson and Rodbard, 1980). The (+)butaclamol curve models best to a single homogeneous receptor state with a K_D of 1.1 nM.

In contrast, agonist/[^{3}H]-spiroperidol competition curves exhibit heterogeneous characteristics with pseudo-Hill coefficients less than unity.

BUTACLAMOL/[3H]SPIRO

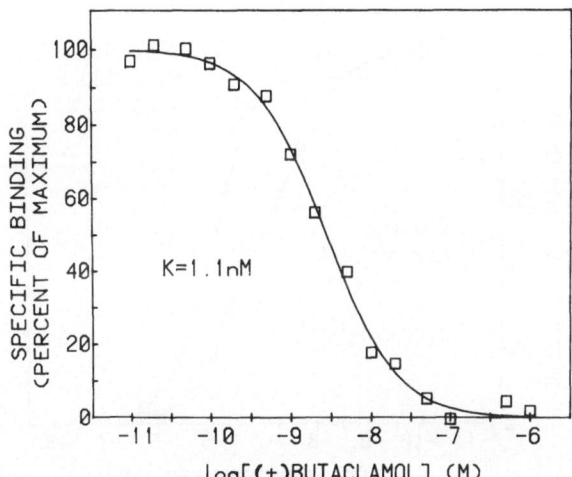

Figure 1. Computer-fitted curve for a (+)butaclamol/[³H]-spiroperidol competition experiment on bovine anterior pituitary membranes. The data points are shown by open squares and are from a single representative experiment. The computer-drawn curve represents the best fit to the data assuming a single homogeneous binding site. The assumption of a two-site model does not improve the fit. The pseudo-Hill coefficient is 0.99.

As shown in Fig. 2, in the absence of guanine nucleotides, the (−)apomorphine/[³H]-spiroperidol curve is shallow (pseudo-Hill coefficient = 0.58), with computer analysis indicating that the data are best explained by a two-site/state binding model. The K_D for the high- and low-affinity binding sites/states (R_H and R_L) have been designated K_H and K_L, respectively. Interestingly, the two sites/states are present in approximately equal proportions in the membranes. In the presence of a saturating concentration of Gpp(NH)p, a nonmetabolizable analogue of GTP, the (−)apomorphine curve is shifted to the right and is steepened (pseudo-Hill coefficient = 0.94). Moreover, computer analysis of the data now indicates a single homogeneous population of binding sites whose affinity for (−)apomorphine is not significantly different from the K_L value of the control curve (Fig. 2). Three additional agonists, (±)ADTN, (−)NPA,* and dopamine, have been investigated and give qualitatively identical results.

Recently, we have characterized the binding of the radiolabeled agonist [³H]-NPA to dopamine receptors in bovine anterior pituitary membranes (Sibley and Creese, 1979, 1982). The identification of high-affinity

---

* ADTN, 2-amino-6,7-dihydroxytetrahydronaphthalene; NPA, N-*n*-propylnorapomorphine.

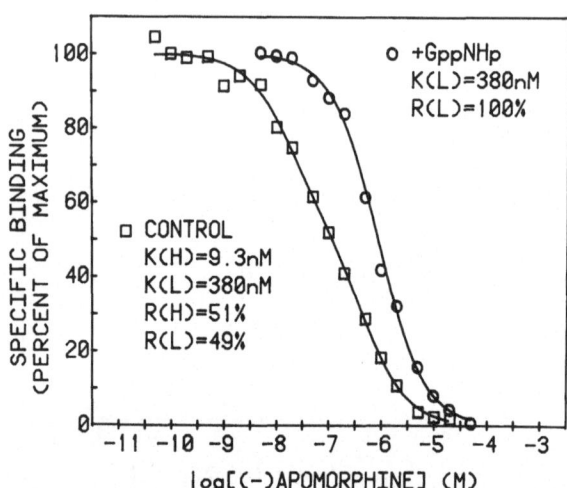

APOMORPHINE/[3H]SPIRO

Figure 2. Computer-fitted curves for a (−)apomorphine/[³H]-spiroperidol competition experiment in bovine anterior pituitary membranes. The (−)apomorphine control curve is best fitted by assuming a two-site model, whereas in the presence of 10^{-4} M guanyl-5'-yl imidodiphosphate (GppNHp), a one-site model is sufficient to explain the data. When the two curves are analyzed simultaneously and constrained to share the same K_L value, there was no worsening of the fit. R_H and R_L represent the high- and low-affinity binding sites, respectively.

[³H]-agonist binding in a tissue with no direct dopaminergic innervation reinforces our hypothesis that under our assay conditions [³H]-agonists can label "postsynaptic" receptors (Creese and Sibley, 1979). One of the more striking findings with this radioligand is that its B_{max} is approximately 50% that of [³H]-spiroperidol, suggesting that it labels the high-affinity agonist site/state (R_H) seen in agonist/[³H]-NPA agonist/[³H]-spiroperidol curves. This is further suggested by the finding that agonist/[³H]-NPA competition curves are homogeneous with single affinities that are not significantly different from the K_H values obtained from the corresponding agonist/[³H]-spiroperidol curve. Furthermore, saturating concentrations of guanine nucleotides completely abolish the specific [³H]-NPA binding to pituitary membranes as they do the high-affinity agonist displacement of [³H]-spiroperidol binding.

Two major explanations for the data are available. One is that the R_H and R_L sites represent two discrete dopamine receptors, i.e., two separate protein molecules. The two receptors would have identical affinity for all antagonists but differential affinity for all agonists. In addi-

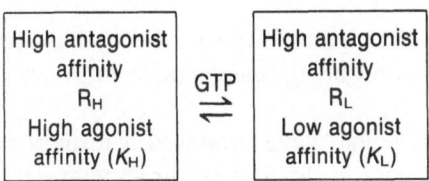

Figure 3. Model of anterior pituitary D-2 receptor.

tion, guanine nucleotides would inhibit agonist binding to the R_H receptor in some "allosteric" fashion. The second possibility is that the R_H and R_L sites actually represent high- and low-affinity agonist binding states of a single receptor molecule (Fig. 3). In this model, guanine nucleotides regulate an interconversion between the high- and low-affinity states. Evidence supporting this latter possibility was seen in experiments in which bovine anterior pituitaries were first dispersed into single whole cells via collagenase treatment and then used directly in the binding experiment (Sibley *et al.*, 1983). Strikingly, the $(-)$apomorphine/$[^3H]$-spiroperidol curve is now steep (pseudo-Hill coefficient = 0.86) and comparable to the $(-)$apomorphine/$[^3H]$-spiroperidol + Gpp(NH) curve in Fig. 2.

Additionally, exogenously added guanine nucleotides no longer affect the $(-)$apomorphine/$[^3H]$-spiroperidol curve. The finding that the $(-)$ apomorphine competition curve does not appear to be maximally shifted and steepened in intact cells may be attributable to a nonsaturating intracellular GTP concentration at the receptor. Thus, in whole cells, endogenous GTP regulates agonist binding in a fashion identical to that of exogenously added GTP in membrane preparations. Importantly, it should also be noted that specific $[^3H]$-NPA binding is not detectable in intact cells, directly confirming the absence of a detectable R_H state in these cells. However, membranes prepared from these cells exhibit identical binding properties to membranes directly prepared from the whole gland, indicating that the lack of high-affinity agonist binding is not the result of receptor degradation occurring during the collagenase-mediated dispersion. Thus, the R_H and R_L sites are presumably not functionally discrete receptor molecules, since if they were, they would both be demonstrable in whole cells as well as in membranes.

Recently, Lefkowitz and co-workers examined in detail the radioligand–receptor binding characteristics of the frog erythrocyte β-adrenergic receptor system (reviewed in Lefkowitz, 1980; Hoffman and Lefkowitz, 1980). Their data with the frog erythrocyte β receptor are qualitatively identical to our anterior pituitary dopamine receptor data. That is, agonist/$[^3H]$-antagonist competition curves model to two affinity states in membranes with the high-affinity state being dispelled with exogenous guanine nucleotides and being undetectable in intact cells (Kent *et al.*, 1980).

De Lean *et al.* (1980) have proposed a ternary complex model to explain the binding data in the frog erythrocyte system.

$$A + R \rightleftharpoons AR$$

$$AR + N \rightleftharpoons ARN$$

This model is similar to the floating-receptor (Jacobs and Cuatrecasas, 1976) or two-step (Boeynaems and Dumont, 1977) models previously described. Briefly, agonists (A) or antagonists can bind to the receptor (R) to form an initial drug–receptor complex (AR). The binding of agonists, however, induces a conformational change in the receptor so that it can now couple to a third membrane component (N). It is this ternary complex (ARN) that is responsible for the high-affinity agonist binding state. Limbird *et al.* (1980) have provided evidence that the third component is the guanine nucleotide-binding protein of the adenylate cyclase complex. Presumably, it is the ternary complex of agonist, receptor, and nucleotide-binding protein that is responsible for activating adenylate cyclase in the presence of GTP. This complex is formed only transiently, however, since the endogenous GTP rapidly induces its dispersal in intact cells.

The application of this model to the anterior pituitary dopamine receptor system is extremely attractive. However, dopamine does not appear to elicit an increase in anterior pituitary adenylate cyclase activity (Schmidt and Hill, 1977; Clement-Cormier *et al.*, 1977; Mowles *et al.*, 1978; MacLeod *et al.*, 1980; however, see Ahn *et al.*, 1979). On the contrary, recent evidence suggests that dopamine may actually decrease cAMP formation in the anterior pituitary (De Camilli *et al.*, 1979; Pawlikowski *et al.*, 1979, 1981; LaBrie *et al.*, 1980; Giannattasio *et al.*, 1981; Ray and Wallis, 1980) and can reverse the activation of adenylate cyclase by vasoactive intestinal peptide (VIP) (Onali *et al.*, 1981). Thus, the consequences of agonist-receptor complexation may be to decrease mammotroph cAMP content and thus to decrease prolactin release. This hypothesis is additionally supported by recent work that suggests that increased mammotroph cAMP leads to an enhancement of prolactin release (Dannies *et al.*, 1976; Naor *et al.*, 1980). Assuming that ternary complex formation is necessary for agonist function, then the data are consistent with the hypothesis that in the presence of GTP the ternary complex is a continually formed but transient intermediate that never accumulates to an extent measurable in our binding assays. This model would be similar to a collision coupling model proposed by Levitski (1978) for adenylate cyclase activation, only in the D-2 receptor system, the functional result is adenylate cyclase inhibition.

One of the major questions concerning our previously proposed ternary complex model for the D-2 receptor is what regulates the proportions of high- and low-affinity agonist binding states. One possible explanation for our finding that dopamine agonists induce the high-affinity state in only 50–55% of the total receptor population is that residual amounts of endogenous guanine nucleotides are present in our membrane tissue preparation. This is unlikely for the following reasons. First, extensive washing of our tissue preparation leads to no further increases in detectable R_H. Second, preincubation with various combinations of agonists, EDTA, divalent cations, and GMP, treatments shown to induce the release of tightly bound GDP in some receptor systems (Lad *et al.*, 1980; Shane *et al.*, 1981), has no effect on the proportion of R_H in our system. Finally, when membrane tissue is preincubated with 1 mM GTP and then washed as in our normal tissue preparation, there is no diminution in subsequent [^{3}H]-NPA binding compared to control, suggesting that GTP can be entirely washed out using this procedure.

Another potential regulatory factor for the formation of the high-affinity receptor state is the concentration of divalent cations in the assay medium. We have found that divalent cations such as Mg^{2+} and Ca^{2+} increase both the proportion of R_H and its affinity for agonists in a graded fashion (Fig. 4) (Sibley and Creese, 1983a). Monovalent cations are without effect, suggesting that this phenomenon is not simply a result of changes in ionic strength. Furthermore, the presence of cations in the assay medium has no effect on radiolabeled antagonist binding, demonstrating the agonist-specific nature of this phenomenon. It is interesting to note that the effects of divalent cations on the D-2 receptor R_H and K_H parameters are reciprocal to those of guanine nucleotides (Sibley *et al.*, 1982). This suggests that divalent cations and guanine nucleotides may exert their opposing effects on a common component or reaction. Consistent with this hypothesis is recent evidence suggesting that a binding site for Mg^{2+} exists on the guanine nucleotide binding protein (Cech *et al.*, 1980). Nevertheless, even with maximally effective divalent cation concentrations, we find that agonists still promote only 50–55% of the high-affinity state, suggesting that additional regulatory factors must be considered.

It was interesting to find that Na^+ had no effect on [^{3}H]-NPA binding in either the absence or presence of a maximally effective Mg^{2+} concentration. It has been hypothesized that a general feature of receptor systems linked to the attentuation of adenylate cyclase activity is their regulation

APOMORPHINE/[3H]SPIRO

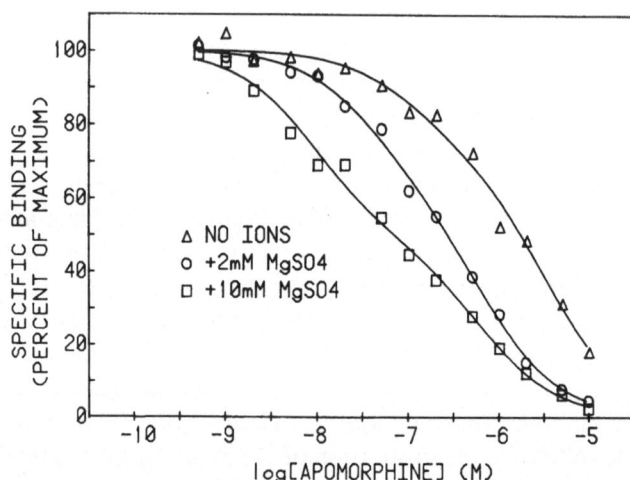

Figure 4. Computer-modeled curves for apomorphine/[³H]-spiroperidol competition experiments with varying MgSO₄ concentrations. All curves were generated with the same membrane preparation using 0.25 nM [³H]-spiroperidol. The data points shown are experimentally
determined, and the drawn lines represent the computer-modeled best fit to the data. In the
presence of 10 mM MgSO₄, the curve is fitted best by assuming a two-site binding model.
The K_D values for the high- (K_H) and the low- (K_L) affinity sites are 4.8 and 320 nM, and
the percent R_H is 53. When the MgSO₄ concentration is reduced to 2 mM, the curve also
assumes a two-site fit with the following parameters: K_H = 22 nM, K_L = 330 nM, and
percent R_H = 39. In the absence of MgSO₄, the curve is still best fitted to two sites with
the following parameters: K_H = 63 nM, K_L = 1600 nM, and percent R_H = 29.

by Na⁺ (Limbird, 1981). Indeed, [³H]-dopamine binding to brain D-2
receptors has been shown to be decreased by Na⁺ (Hamblin and Creese,
1982b). Recently, it has been demonstrated that Na⁺ is not regulatory in
all hormone-inhibitable adenylate cyclase systems (Garcia-Sainz et al.,
1981). Furthermore, the binding of a radiolabeled agonist to β-adrenergic
receptors involved in stimulating adenylate cyclase activity has been
shown to be Na⁺ sensitive (Heidenreich et al., 1980). Thus, the fact that
Na⁺ does not regulate agonist binding to the pituitary D-2 receptor is not
inconsistent with the observation that this receptor can attenuate vasoactive intestinal polypeptide-induced (Onali et al., 1981) as well as basal
(De Camilli et al., 1979; Giannattasio et al., 1981) adenylate cyclase activity in this tissue.

   In order to ascertain what roles the different components of the D-2
receptor system might play in regulating high-affinity agonist binding,
we utilized as chemical probes the sulfhydryl-group-alkylating reagents

Figure 5. Effect of NEM pretreatment on subsequent [³H]-NPA (□) and [³H]-spiroperidol (△) binding. Various concentrations on NEM were added prior to incubating at 37°C for 10 min. After incubation, the samples were diluted fourfold with ice-cold tris buffer and centrifuged at 50,000 × *g* for 10 min. The membranes were then resuspended in assay buffer and used immediately in the binding experiment. This procedure was judged sufficient to terminate the NEM reaction, as when 1 mM DTT was used to quench the reaction prior to

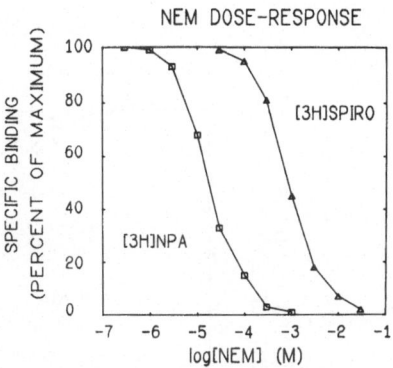

centrifugation, the results did not differ. The data points represent means from two to six experiments, each performed in triplicate. Nonspecific binding of both radioligands was unaffected by NEM.

N-ethylmaleimide (NEM) and parahydroxymercuribenzamide (POMB) (Sibley and Creese, 1983a). The data obtained with these agents indicate the existence of at least two functionally distinct sulfhydryl groups involved in the regulation of receptor binding. One sulfhydryl group appears to regulate the binding of both antagonist and agonist ligands to the receptor moiety. When this sulfhydryl group is inactivated with POMB or with low affinity by NEM, there is an irreversible loss in receptor binding capacity (Fig. 5). The fact that this loss can be protected against by coincubation with either antagonists or agonists suggests that this sulfhydryl is located at or near the ligand-binding site. The second sulfhydryl group appears to play a critical role in regulating the formation of the high-affinity agonist binding state. If this sulfhydryl group is alkylated with high affinity by either NEM or POMB, there is a direct reduction in the extent of ternary complex formation as detected with [³H]-NPA binding (Fig. 6). Neither antagonist nor agonist coincubation can protect against this inactivation. Indeed, the addition of NEM to the assay medium rapidly induces the dissociation of [³H]-NPA from its binding sites.

These findings are in dramatic contrast to the role described for sulfhydryl groups in regulating agonist binding to β-adrenergic receptors (Heindenreich *et al.*, 1982; Vauquelin *et al.*, 1980a,b; Vauquelin and Maguire, 1980). In the β-adrenergic system, free sulfhydryl groups are not required for ligand occupancy of the receptor binding site, nor do sulfhydryl reagents alone inactivate subsequent agonist binding. Instead, agonist occupancy and formation of the high affinity state are required for receptor inactivation by free sulfhydryl alkylation. Once the reactive sulfhydryl group is alkylated, the agonist is "locked" on the receptor, and the ternary complex is resistant to dissociation (Korner *et al.*, 1982). Further

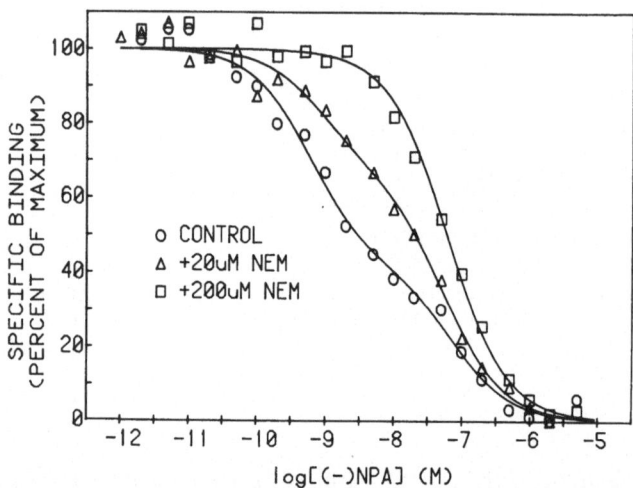

(-)NPA/[3H]SPIROPERIDOL

Figure 6. Computer-modeled competition curves for a (-)NPA/[³H]-spiroperidol experiment after pretreatment with NEM. All curves were generated in the same membrane preparation using 0.34 nM [³H]-spiroperidol. The NEM preincubations were performed as described in Fig. 5. The control curve assumed a two-site fit with the following parameters: $K_H = 0.3$ nM, $K_L = 36$ nM, and percent $R_H = 59$. The +20 μM NEM curve also assumed two sites with the following parameters: $K_H = 0.39$, $K_L = 26$ nM, and percent $R_H = 35$. After treatment with 200 μM NEM, however, the curve assumed a single-site fit exhibiting a dissociation constant (K_L) of 29 nM.

structural differences between D-2 dopaminergic and β-adrenergic receptors are suggested by their different sensitivities to dithiothreitol (DTT) treatment. β-adrenergic receptors have been suggested to possess an essential disulfide bond that, if reduced with DTT, prevents ligand occupancy of the receptor (Vauquelin *et al.*, 1979). In contrast, D-2 dopamine receptor binding is unaffected by DTT pretreatment, suggesting the absence of essential disulfide bonds for this receptor.

Although our present data cannot distinguish if the sulfhydryl group regulating ternary complex formation is located on the D-2 receptor or on the third binding component, the observation that agonist coincubation fails to protect against inactivation suggests that this group is not located at the receptor–third component interface. Recent evidence suggests that the reactive sulfhydryl group regulating β-adrenergic agonist binding is located on the guanine nucleotide binding protein (Korner *et al.*, 1982). However, it should be noted that the guanine nucleotide regulatory protein involved in receptor systems that potentiate adenylate cyclase activity (e.g., β-adrenergic receptors) may differ from that involved in receptor systems that attenuate such activity (e.g., D-2 dopaminergic receptors) (Smith and Limbird, 1982). In this regard, it is interesting to note that opiate receptors linked to inhibition of adenylate cyclase activity demonstrate a similar regulation of ligand binding by sulfhydryl group modification as shown here for D-2 receptors (Larsen *et al.*, 1981).

The observation that functional uncoupling of the receptor–third component interaction by sulfhydryl modification leads to a decrease in the proportion of inducible R_H suggests that this reaction is rate limiting in R_H formation. There are two major explanations as to how this limitation can be achieved. One possibility is that the membrane concentration of the third binding component is stoichiometrically limiting. A second possibility is that the dissociation constant of the second binding step is not favorable enough for this reaction to proceed to completion.

In order to distinguish between these two potential mechanisms, we employed the irreversible antagonist phenoxybenzamine (Hamblin and Creese, 1982a) to decrease the membrane concentration of receptor subunits. Our reasoning was as follows: if N is stoichiometrically limiting, then a proportion of R subunits could be considered "spare" with respect to the ability of agonists to induce ternary complex formation. Indeed, a 50% or greater reduction in R subunits would bring the R/N ratio to unity or less. This should result in agonist/[^{3}H]-spiroperidol competition curves becoming monophasic and of high affinity. If, instead, the second binding reaction is equilibrium limited, then there should be no change in the relative proportions of R_H and R_L even though their absolute membrane concentrations are reduced. Our data clearly support this latter hypothesis (Sibley and Creese, 1983a). Recently, on the basis of computer simulations, De Lean *et al.* (1980) have proposed a similar regulation for the formation of the high-affinity β-adrenergic receptor state. However, in their system, agonists with high intrinsic activity can form high-affinity complexes representing up to 90% of the total receptor population (De Lean *et al.*, 1980).

2.2. Ergot Interactions with Pituitary D-2 Dopamine Receptors

In general dopaminergic ergots are highly potent agonists with full intrinsic activity at D-2 receptors, whereas they are fairly weak antagonists or partial agonists at D-1 receptors (Kebabian and Calne, 1979; Creese *et al.*, 1983). Ergot alkaloids have been well established as potent inhibitiors of prolactin secretion in all vertebrate species tested including man (Shaar and Clemens, 1972; Caron *et al.*, 1978; Muller *et al.*, 1977). Their therapeutic potential has been well demonstrated in the treatment of hyperprolactinemia and pathological lactation in both women and men (Muller *et al.*, 1977). More recently, several ergot derivatives have been shown to additionally possess agonist activity in diminishing anterior pituitary adenylate cyclase activity (De Camilli *et al.*, 1979; Giannattasio *et al.*, 1981; Onali *et al.*, 1981). Ergot alkaloids also exhibit agonist activity at the intermediate pituitary D-2 dopamine receptor, where they decrease α-MSH release and attenuate β-adrenergic receptor-induced cAMP production (Munemura *et al.*, 1980a,b; Tsurata *et al.*, 1981; Meunier and Labrie, 1982; Sibley and Creese, 1983b).

We have recently investigated the ligand-binding properties of D-2 dopamine receptors on anterior pituitary membranes using radioligand binding techniques and computer-assisted data analysis (Sibley *et al.*, 1982). We found that the ergot alkaloid bromocriptine did not differentiate between the high- and low-affinity D-2 receptor binding states (Sibley *et al.*, 1982). Bromocriptine thus exhibits the binding characteristics of an antagonist even though it is a potent, highly efficacious agonist at D-2 receptors. In contrast, the ergot alkaloid pergolide was observed to demonstrate the receptor binding characteristics of an agonist in keeping with its pharmacologically demonstrated agonist properties at the pituitary D-2 receptor (Sibley *et al.*, 1982). These preliminary findings with ergot alkaloid agonists might suggest that a drug's efficacy is not correlated with its ability to differentiate between the two D-2 receptor binding states.

Ergot alkaloids can be divided into two broad categories, the ergopeptines and the ergolines, both of which contain the tetracyclic ergoline nucleus (Rutschmann and Stadler, 1978). Ergopeptines are of high molecular weight and include *d*-lysergic acid, which is linked by an amide bridge to a cyclic peptide component. Ergolines are of lower molecular weight and are derivatives of the tetracyclic skeleton of lysergic acid (Fig. 7). The major structural differences between the ergopeptines relate to their substituents at the R_1 and R_2 positions. Conversely, the ergolines differ mainly in their R_1 substitutions. All of the ergopeptines and ergolines in Fig. 7 have been shown to exhibit agonist activity at either the anterior pituitary D-2 dopamine receptor (De Camilli *et al.*, 1979; Giannattasio *et al.*, 1981 Shaar and Clemens, 1972; Caron *et al.*, 1978; Muller *et al.*, 1977; Delitala *et al.*, 1980) or at D-2 receptor systems in the central nervous system (Tamminga and Schaffer, 1979; Fuxe *et al.*, 1981; Markstein, 1981).

Figure 8 shows representative ergoline competition experiments with the radiolabeled antagonist [^{3}H]-spiroperidol and the agonist [^{3}H]-NPA. The ergoline CF25397/[^{3}H]-spiroperidol curve exhibits heterogeneous characteristics (pseudo-Hill coefficient < 1) with computer analysis, in-

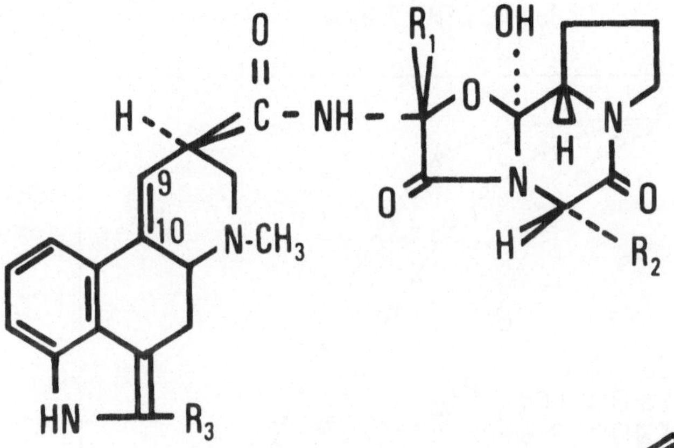

Ergopeptine skeleton

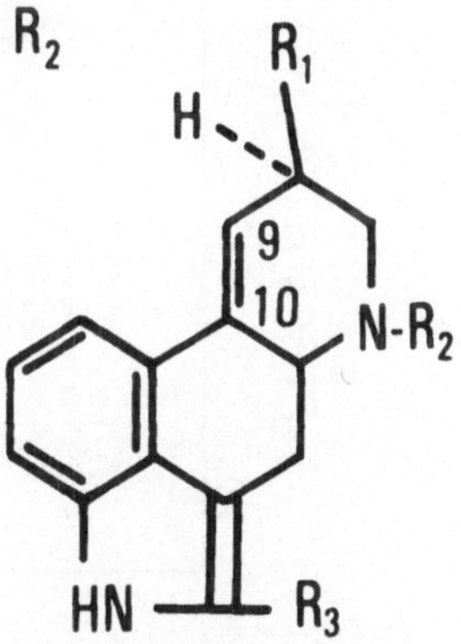

Ergoline skeleton

Ergopeptines	R_1	R_2	R_3
Ergocornine	$CH(CH_3)_2$	$CH(CH_3)_2$	H
Ergocristine	$CH(CH_3)_2$	$CH_2C_6H_5$	H
Ergosine	CH_3	$CH_2CH(CH_3)_2$	H
Ergotamine	CH_3	$CH_2C_6H_5$	H
*Dihydroergotamine	CH_3	$CH_2C_6H_5$	H
*Dihydroergocriptine	$CH(CH_3)_2$	$CH_2CH(CH_3)_2$	H
*Bromocriptine	$CH(CH_3)_2$	$CH_2CH(CH_3)_2$	Br
Ergolines			
Ergometrine	$CONHCH(CH_3)CH_2OH$	CH_3	H
Lisuride	$NHCON(C_2H_5)_2$	CH_3	H
CF 25397	$CH_2SC_5H_4N$	CH_3	H
*CH 29717	$NHSO_2N(CH_3)_2$	CH_3	H
*CQ 32084	$NHSO_2N(C_2H_5)_2$	CH_3	H
*CM 29712	CH_2CN	CH_3	H
*Lergotrile	CH_2CN	CH_3	Cl
*Pergolide	CH_2SCH_3	$CH_2CH_2CH_3$	H

Figure 7. Structural formulas of the ergot alkaloids utilized in this study. The ergot alkaloids are divided into two classes, the ergopeptines and the ergolines, with the backbone skeletons and different substituents of each being designated. Those compounds marked with an asterisk are reduced at the 9–10 double bond.

CF25397/[3H]LIGAND

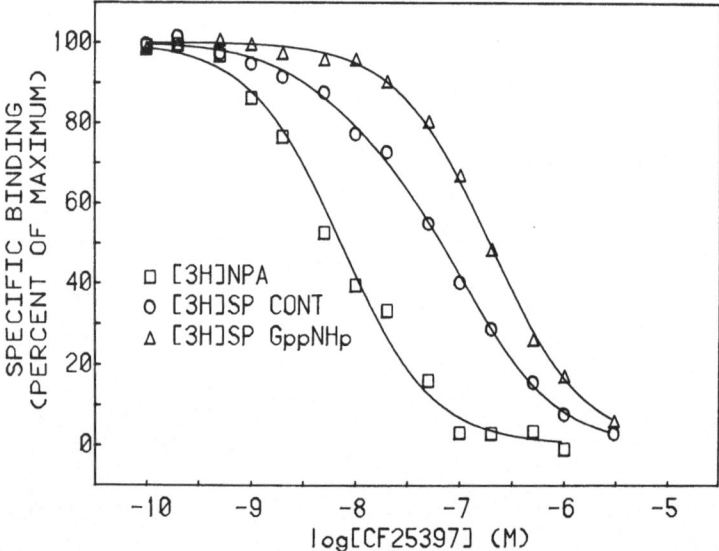

Figure 8. Computer-fitted CF25397/[³H]-ligand competition curves. The data points shown are experimentally determined, and the drawn lines represent the computer-modeled best fit to the data. The CF25397/[³H]-NPA curve (□) exhibits a pseudo-Hill coefficient of 0.94 and fits best to one binding site with an affinity of 5.3 nM. The control CF25397/[³H]-spiroperidol curve (O) has a pseudo-Hill coefficient of 0.66 and is best fitted to two binding sites with the following binding parameters: K_H = 5.9 nM, K_L = 80 nM, and percent R_H = 47. In the presence of 0.1 mM GppNHp (△), the curve's pseudo-Hill coefficient increases to 1.0, and the curve models best to a single binding site with an affinity (K_L) of 75 nM.

dicating that the data are best explained by assuming a two-state binding model. The dissociation constants for the high-affinity (R_H) and the low-affinity (R_L) agonist-binding states have been designated K_H and K_L, respectively. In the presence of the guanine nucleotide, 5'-guanylylimi-dodiphosphate (GppNHp), however, the high-affinity component of the CF25397/[³H]-spiroperidol curve is abolished, resulting in a rightward shift and steepening (pseudo-Hill coefficient = 1) of the curve. Computer modeling now indicates the presence of a single homogeneous binding state whose affinity is similar to that of the low-affinity state observed in the control curve (Fig. 8) (Sibley and Creese, 1983b). As we have previously shown that low concentrations of [³H]-NPA selectively label the high-affinity D-2 receptor binding state (Sibley *et al.*, 1982), it is not surprising that the CF25397/[³H]-NPA competition curve is homogeneous and fits best to a single binding state whose affinity agrees well with the K_H value from the [³H]-spiroperidol curve (Fig. 8).

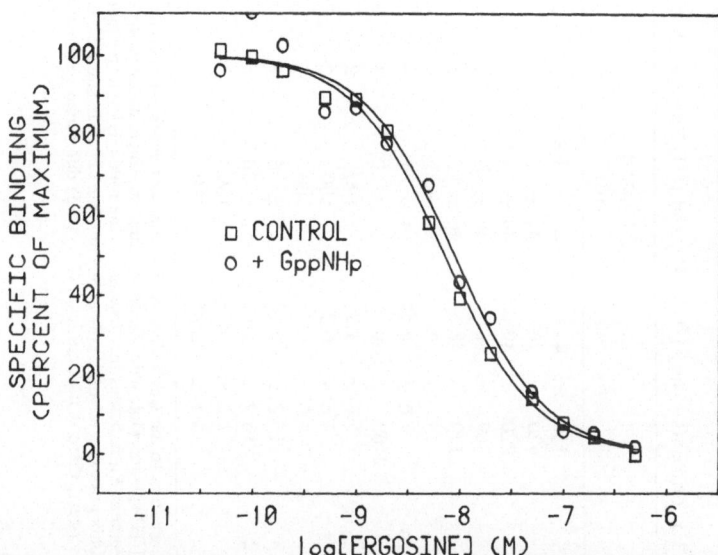

ERGOSINE/[3H]SPIRO

Figure 9. Computer-modeled ergosine/[³H]-spiroperidol competition curves. The control curve (□) represents the fit to a single binding site with a pseudo-Hill coefficient of 0.9 and a dissociation constant (K_D) of 3.8 nM. With the addition of 0.1 mM GppNHp (○), the curve is also sufficiently well fit using a one-site binding model and exhibits a pseudo-Hill coefficient of 0.95 and a K_D of 4.1 nM. When the two curves are analyzed simultaneously, there is no significant ($P > 0.1$) difference between the two K_D values.

Illustrated in Fig. 9 are representative ergopeptine/[³H]-spiroperidol competition experiments using the ergopeptine ergosine. In contrast to the ergolines, the ergosine/[³H]-spiroperidol curve is steep (pseudo-Hill coefficient = 1) and is best described by a single-binding-site model (Fig. 9). Furthermore, the addition of GppNHp has no significant effect on the ability of ergosine to compete with [³H]-spiroperidol binding (Fig. 9).

The computer-derived parameters for all the ergoline and ergopeptine competition experiments have been compiled in Table II (Sibley and Creese, 1983b). All of the ergoline agonists demonstrate the ability to differentiate between the high- and low-affinity receptor binding states. In each case, the affinities derived from [³H]-NPA binding are statistically indistinguishable from the K_H parameters derived from [³H]-spiroperidol binding. Similarly, the [³H]-spiroperidol competition curves are shifted by guanine nucleotides such that their single affinities are indistinguishable from the control K_L values.

Furthermore, with the exception of lergotrile and ergometrine, the high- and low-affinity receptor binding states are induced or detected in

Table II. Computer-Derived Parameters for Ergot Alkaloid Competition Experiments Using [³H]-NPA and [³H]-Spiroperidol[a]

Drug	K_{NPA}	K_H	K_L	K_G	Percent R_H	n	K_L/K_H
Pergolide	3.8 ± 0.59	4.1 ± 1.6	137 ± 14	120 ± 47	45 ± 3.8	3	33
Lergotrile	13.0 ± 1.7	10 ± 1.2	370 ± 67	420 ± 26	31 ± 2	5	37
CM 29712	83 ± 15	90 ± 31	1230 ± 99	1220 ± 39	46 ± 4.5	3	14
CQ 32084	5.0 ± 0.7	6.3 ± 0.9	71 ± 10	69 ± 6	49 ± 5	3	11
CH 29717	8.8 ± 2.6	10 ± 3.2	180 ± 69	170 ± 48	46 ± 5	3	18
CF 25397	5.4 ± 1.4	6.5 ± 2.5	78 ± 11	75 ± 2	51 ± 2.4	4	12
Lisuride	0.5 ± 0.03	0.62 ± 0.1	4.8 ± 0.74	4.0 ± 0.17	51 ± 1	5	8
Ergometrine	87 ± 12	73 ± 21	2200 ± 320	2100 ± 630	32 ± 2	3	31
Ergocornine	4.2 ± 0.62	5.6 ± 1.2	—	5.6 ± 1.2	100	2	—
Ergocristine	4.9 ± 0.62	5.3 ± 1.8	—	4.6 ± 0.7	100	2	—
Ergosine	2.4 ± 0.1	2.6 ± 0.4	—	3.0 ± 0.1	100	3	—
Ergotamine	1.6 ± 0.57	1.1 ± 0.32	12.9 ± 1.8	11.2 ± 0.64	55 ± 6	3	12
Dihydroergotamine	1.4 ± 0.25	1.8 ± 0.5	17.9 ± 1.2	16.9 ± 1.6	51 ± 10	3	10
Dihydroergocriptine	0.91 ± 0.1	1.3 ± 0.14	—	1.2 ± 0.24	100	3	—
Bromocriptine	2.4 ± 0.33	3.2 ± 0.64	—	3.4 ± 0.85	100	3	—

[a] Competition experiments were performed and analyzed as described in Figs. 8 and 9. K_{NPA} refers to the single dissociation constant observed in competing for [³H]-NPA binding. K_H, K_L, and K_G represent dissociation constants for competing with [³H]-spiroperidol, with K_G designating the single dissociation constant observed in th presence of 0.1 mM GppNHp. All dissociation constants are nanomolar. Percent R_H indicates that fraction of the total [³H]-spiroperidol binding sites observed in the high-affinity state. The data are presented as mean ± S.E., with the number of experimental replications indicated by n. In some experiments, incubation times were increased to 30 min with no difference in the results. By Student's t-test, there is no significant ($P > 0.05$) difference between any pair of K_{NPA} and K_H or K_L and K_G values.

about equal proportions. These ergoline binding characteristics are qualitatively similar to those for classical dopamine agonists previously demonstrated (Sibley *et al.*, 1982). An important exception, however, is the ratio of affinities for the two receptor binding states. Catecholamine dopamine agonists exhibit K_L/K_H ratios approaching 100 (Sibley *et al.*, 1982). However, the ergolines demonstrate much less selectivity, with K_L/K_H ratios ranging between 8 and 37 (Table II). In contrast to the ergolines, ergopeptine agonists, in general, do not discriminate between the two receptor binding states (Table II). For these agonists, the homogeneous affinities in competing for [^{3}H]-NPA binding and for [^{3}H]-spiroperidol binding in the absence and presence of GppNHp are all identical. There are, however, two ergopeptines that are exceptional, ergotamine and dihydroergotamine, which, interestingly, exhibit binding characteristics similar to the ergolines (Table II).

The availability of both ergopeptine and ergoline compounds radiolabeled to a high specific activity has enabled us to examine their receptor binding properties directly. The radiolabeled ergopeptine [^{3}H]-dihydroergocriptine ([^{3}H]-DHE) has been previously characterized as labeling dopaminergic receptors in anterior pituitary membrane preparations (Caron *et al.*, 1978; Cronin *et al.*, 1978). The binding of [^{3}H]-DHE to anterior pituitary membranes is homogeneous and saturable, exhibiting a maximum binding capacity (B_{max}) identical to that for [^{3}H]-spiroperidol. Furthermore, the binding of [^{3}H]-DHE is unaffected by guanine nucleotides. The binding characteristics of [^{3}H]-DHE are thus "antagonistlike" and similar to those exhibited in the unlabeled DHE competition experiments (Table II).

The radiolabeled ergoline [^{3}H]-lisuride has been shown previously to label dopaminergic receptors as well as serotonergic and α_2-adrenergic receptors in the central nervous system (Fujita *et al.*, 1979; Reynolds and Riederer, 1981; Battaglia and Titeler, 1981). There are no known α_2-adrenergic or serotonergic receptors in the anterior pituitary, however, and our experiments have indicated that [^{3}H]-lisuride binding to bovine anterior pituitary membranes is exclusively dopaminergic. Saturation isotherms for this radiolabeled ergoline are shown in Fig. 10. In the absence of nucleotides, the [^{3}H]-lisuride isotherm is curvilinear when plotted in Scatchard coordinates. Computer analysis of this data indicates the presence of two binding components present in approximately equal proportions in the membranes (Fig. 10). With the addition of GppNHp, the [^{3}H]-lisuride isotherm becomes homogeneous, indicating a uniform population of binding sites whose affinity is similar to the low-affinity sites defined in the control isotherm (Fig. 10). It is important to note that the total receptor binding capacity of [^{3}H]-lisuride is similar to that for [^{3}H]-spi-

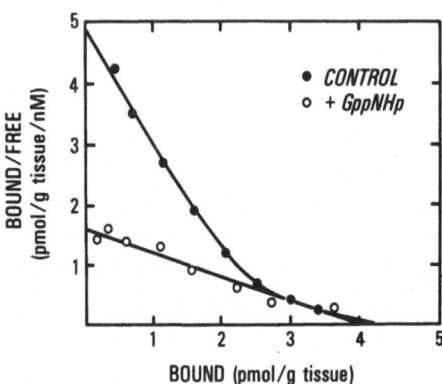

Figure 10. [³H]-Lisuride saturation isotherms in bovine anterior pituitary membranes. Both isotherms were conducted in the same membrane preparation using [³H]-isuride concentrations from 0.1 to 14.2 nM. The control isotherm (●) was found to optimally fit to two binding sites with the following parameters: K_H = 0.40 nM, K_L = 2.6 nM, R_H = 1.9 pmole/g tissue (47% of total), and R_L = 2.2 pmole/g tissue (53% of total). In the presence of 0.1 mM GppNHp (○), the [³H]-lisuride saturation isotherm fits best to a single binding site with a K_D = 2.4 nM and a B_{max} of 4.0 pmole/g tissue.

roperidol and [³H]-DHE. Furthermore, the dissociation constants for the high- and low-affinity components of [³H]-lisuride binding agree reasonably well with the K_H and K_L values for lisuride shown in Table II. It is thus reasonable to assume that the two binding components of the ergoline [³H]-lisuride represent the high- and low-affinity receptor binding states of the D-2 receptor.

One possible explanation for the fact that ergopeptine agonists exhibit the binding characteristics of antagonist ligands is that they interact with the receptor in an irreversible fashion. Indeed, Bannon *et al.* (1980) have suggested this possibility based on the long duration of bromocriptine's agonist action *in vivo* and on subsequent radioligand binding experiments. To evaluate the reversibility of ergopeptine ligands in a more direct fashion, [³H]-DHE kinetic experiments were performed. [³H]-Dihydroergocriptine binding achieves equilibrium by 30 min, and the pseudo-first-order association rate constant, k_{obs}, equals 0.16 min⁻¹. The dissociation of [³H]-DHE was evaluated by adding excess bromocriptine after equilibrium was achieved. The [³H]-DHE binding is completely reversible, with the dissociation occurring as a first-order process. The dissociation rate constant was determined to equal 0.0071 min⁻¹. Other unlabeled compounds, such as spiroperidol and apomorphine, that were used to measure dissociation gave similar results. The second-order association rate constant, k_1, can be calculated from the equation $k_1 = (k_{obs} - k_2/[³H]\text{-DHE})$ and equals 0.40 nM⁻¹ min⁻¹. The ratio of the rats constants (k_2/k_1) provides a kinetic estimate of the equilibrium dissociation constant (K_D) for [³H]-DHE binding of 18 pM. This is approximately 50-fold lower than values determined either directly from saturation data or indirectly from displacement of [³H]-spiroperidol binding. Thus, although DHE is a competitive and reversible ligand, its interactions with the receptor exhibit anomalous kinetics. This is additionally suggested by a comparison of the [^{3}H]-DHE and [^{3}H]-spiroperidol dissociation experiments. [^{3}H]-Spiroperidol dissociates from the receptor almost 20-fold faster than [^{3}H]-DHE and exhibits kinetics in accordance with its equilibrium-determined K_D (Sibley and Creese, 1983b).

Several explanations for the anomalous binding characteristics of ergopeptines can be considered. One possibility may be that the radioligand binding sites under investigation in the anterior pituitary bear no relationship to the pharmacologically identified D-2 receptors. In this case, the "nondiscriminating" ergopeptines would actually be antagonists at the D-2 receptor labeled with radioligands. This explanation is unlikely, since there is excellent agreement between the affinities determined for ligands in radioligand binding studies and those obtained in pharmacological investigations (Caron *et al.*, 1978; Sibley *et al.*, 1982; Bethea *et al.*, 1982). Thus, the receptors identified in these two experimental paradigms appear to be identical.

Another explanation, mentioned earlier, may be that the ergopeptines bind to the receptor in an irreversible fashion. This hypothesis seems to be discounted by the finding that the ergopeptine DHE interacts in a competitive fashion with [^{3}H]-spiroperidol and that [^{3}H]-DHE binding is completely reversible. These data appear to conflict with the observations of Bannon *et al.* (1980), who observed that 2 hr after a peripheral injection of bromocriptine, there was a decrease in the binding capacity of [^{3}H]-spiroperidol to rat striatal membranes. However, since bromocriptine was administered *in vivo*, it is possible that the observed loss in binding reflected an agonist-induced receptor down-regulation (Creese and Sibley, 1981). Other conceivable mechanisms for ergopeptine binding include the possibility that they do not bind at the same "active" site on the receptor as other ligands or that they bind to more than one receptor site. The former possibility appears to be excluded by the observation that [^{3}H]-DHE and [^{3}H]-spiroperidol bind to sites that qualitatively and quantitatively exhibit the same pharmacological specificity. The latter possibility is ruled out by the fact that [^{3}H]-DHE and [^{3}H]-spiroperidol possess the same binding capacity.

Finally, one may speculate that although ergopeptines bind at the same site on the receptor as other ligands, their cyclic peptide side chain undergoes an additional binding reaction with adjacent receptor sites (Sibley and Creese, 1983b). This latter reaction is proposed to provide a major portion of the ergopeptine–receptor binding energy. In our model, ergopeptines would exert their agonist activity by inducing ternary complex formation; however, in contrast to low-molecular-weight agonists, little additional binding energy is derived from this reaction. Thus, since er-gopeptines exhibit the same affinity for the receptor whether or not it is coupled to N, guanine nucleotides would not be predicted to affect their binding affinity. This model is also consistent with the extremely slow dissociation of [^{3}H]-DHE from its binding sites, which, presumably, is limited by the dissociation of the peptide side chain. These observations could account for several reports in the literature documenting extremely long-lasting pharmacological effects of ergopeptine agonists on dopamine receptors (Bannon et al., 1980; Fuxe et al., 1974; Yeo et al., 1979; Delitala et al., 1980).

This proposed model for ergopeptine binding is additionally consis-tent with several experimental observations. First, the ability of ergot agonists to discriminate between the high- and low-affinity receptor states is generally correlated with the absence or presence of a high-molecular-weight peptide side chain. For instance, the ergopeptines ergocornine, ergocristine, and ergosine are structurally homologous with the ergolines ergometrine, lisuride, and CF25397 (Fig. 7). All of these compounds pos-sess the same tetracyclic ergoline nucleus containing the proposed do-paminergic pharmacophore (Weber, 1980; Bach et al., 1980; Camerman and Camerman, 1981; Cannon et al., 1981), which presumably interacts with the "active site" on the receptor. However, in contrast to the er-golines, the ergopeptines do not differentiate between the two receptor binding states. Secondly, even though the ergoline compounds were able to differentiate between R_H and R_L, they did not exhibit as great a se-lectivity as the smaller catecholamine agonists (Table II) (Sibley et al., 1982). Thus, the ergolines can be placed in the middle of a general struc-tural continuum in which the K_L/K_H ratio is dependent on the size of an agonist and thus on the number of potential attachment points on the receptor. Finally, since dopaminergic ergot alkaloids are generally sug-gested to possess full intrinsic agonist activity at D-2 receptors, those ergots that discriminate between R_H and R_L would be expected to exhibit about 50% R_H, as do other full agonists (Sibley et al., 1982). This pre-diction is generally fulfilled for both ergoline and ergopeptine agonists (Table II).

Although this model can successfully explain the binding character-istics of most of the ergot alkaloids, there do, however, appear to be some exceptions. For instance, it was interesting to observe that ergotamine and dihydroergotamine exhibited the binding characteristics of ergolines despite the fact that they possess cyclic peptide side chains (Table II). A simple explanation for this phenomenon is not immediately apparent. However, these two ergopeptines are the only ergots that have their par-ticular substituents at both the R_1 and R_2 positions (Fig. 7). This substituted R_1 and R_2 combination may serve to place the peptide side chain in such a three-dimensional conformation as to preclude an extremely avid binding reaction so that the binding characteristics of an ergoline is observed. Another exceptional finding was that lergotrile and ergometrine both exhibited about 30% R_H in their [^{3}H]-spiroperidol competition curves (Table II). We have previously suggested that the percentage of R_H may be correlated with the intrinsic activity of a dopaminergic agonist (Sibley *et al.*, 1982). These findings would thus appear in conflict with the proposal that dopaminergic ergot agonists exhibit full intrinsic activity at D-2 receptors. However, the efficacy of lergotrile and ergometrine has not yet been investigated in the bovine anterior pituitary D-2 receptor system. It will be especially important to examine the efficacy of these compounds in *in vitro* systems such as the dopaminergic-mediated inhibition of VIP-induced adenylate cyclase activity in anterior pituitary membranes (Onali *et al.*, 1981).

Our present findings suggest that the K_L/K_H ratio or the "fold shift" of agonist competition curves induced by guanine nucleotides is not correlated with or predictive of the intrinsic activity of a dopaminergic agonist. Previous reports have indicated a dissociation of β-adrenergic agonist activity and the ability of GTP to affect agonist competitive curves in the rat reticulocyte and turkey erythrocyte systems; however, these findings have been shown to result from incomplete washout of GDP (Lad *et al.*, 1980; Shane *et al.*, 1981). However, Lefkowitz and co-workers have demonstrated that an agonist's K_L/K_H ratio is highly correlated with its efficacy in the frog erythrocyte β-adrenergic and the human platelet α_2-adrenergic receptor systems (De Lean *et al.*, 1980; Kent *et al.*, 1980; Hoffman *et al.*, 1982). In addition, the percentage of R_H was also correlated with the agonist's intrinsic activity at β-adrenergic receptors (De Lean *et al.*, 1980; Kent *et al.*, 1980) but not at α_2-adrenergic receptors (Hoffman *et al.*, 1982). These differences in the binding characteristics of β-adrenergic, α_2-adrenergic, and D-2 dopaminergic catecholamine receptor systems may be reflective of structural differences in the receptors themselves or in other membrane components with which they interact.

3. Dopamine Receptors in the CNS

The very first dopamine receptor binding studies utilized [^{3}H]-dopamine and [^{3}H]-haloperidol as ligands (Creese *et al.*, 1975; Burt *et al.*, 1975; Seeman *et al.*, 1975) in the examination of receptors in mammalian striatum. [^{3}H]-Haloperidol bound to a site with high affinity very much like the D-2 receptor since described in anterior pituitary (Seeman *et al.*,

1975; Creese *et al.*, 1975). Bovine striatum also possessed high-affinity sites for [^{3}H]-dopamine and other agonist ligands that, unlike the R_H state of the pituitary D-2 receptor, had very low (approximately micromolar) affinity for butyrophenones (Creese *et al.*, 1975; Burt *et al.*, 1976; Seeman *et al.*, 1976a). This led to the suggestion that mammalian striatum contained two district dopaminergic binding sites (Furchgott, 1978). Much of the controversy of the last few years within this area of research has centered around the neuronal localization of these two sites and their relationship to the dopamine-stimulated adenylate cyclase and autoreceptors.

3.1. [^{3}H]-Butyrophenone Binding: Labeling D-2 Receptors

Several lines of evidence suggest that at least the majority of high-affinity binding sites for [^{3}H]-butyrophenones in the striatum are identical to the D-2 pituitary receptor. The K_D for [^{3}H]-spiroperidol binding to dopamine receptors in striatum determined under a variety of conditions in rat, bovine, and human striatal membranes has been reported as 0.1–0.3 nM (Fields *et al.*, 1977; Creese *et al.*, 1977a; Howlett and Nahorski, 1978; Leysen *et al.*, 1978; Quik and Iversen, 1979), in excellent agreement with the value obtained in bovine anterior pituitary.

Early equilibrium studies produced linear Scatchard plots for [^{3}H]-haloperidol (Burt *et al.*, 1976) and [^{3}H]-spiroperidol (Creese *et al.*, 1977a), and kinetic analysis yielded association and dissociation rates consistent with the existence of homogeneous binding sites. This evidence indicated that, as in the pituitary, there existed one D-2 receptor. As in pituitary, [^{3}H]-agonist ligands can, under appropriate conditions, label these same sites with high affinity (*vide infra*), and the affinity of agonists is reduced by guanine nucleotides with a specificity similar to that of pituitary (Zahniser and Molinoff, 1978; Creese *et al.*, 1979c). These D-2 sites are present in considerably higher numbers in striatum than pituitary, as mentioned above, with B_{max} values for [^{3}H]-butyrophenones typically reported from 25 to 50 pmole/g tissue (Creese *et al.*, 1977a; Leysen *et al.*, 1978) or 250 to 600 fmole/mg protein (Fields *et al.*, 1977; Howlett and Nahorski, 1978; Quik and Iversen, 1979). All D-2 receptors appear to be postsynaptic to the nigrostriatal terminals since they are not decreased by 6-hydroxy-dopamine lesions that remove this pathway (Creese *et al.*, 1977b). A striatal kainic acid lesion that destroys the intrinsic striatal neurons removes about 50% of the D-2 receptors (Schwarcz *et al.*, 1978). The remaining D-2 receptors are located on the presynaptic terminals of the cortical input to the striatum and may regulate glutamate release from these neurons. The sensitivity of these D-2 receptors to GTP may be different from that of the D-2 receptors in the pituitary or on the intrinsic striatal neurons (Creese *et al.*, 1979b).

Biochemically, the function of the striatal D-2 receptor is not known, although it now seems certain that it is not positively linked to the dopamine-stimulated adenylate cyclase. This D-2 site displays a much different pharmacological specificity (Creese *et al.*, 1975; Hyttel, 1978b), ontogenetic time course (Pardo *et al.*, 1977), and regional (Quik and Iversen, 1979) and cellular (*vide infra*) distribution than the dopamine-stimulated adenylate cyclase. This contention has further been supported by irreversible inhibition studies with phenoxybenzamine (Hamblin and Creese, 1982a). That the striatal D-2 receptor mediates the inhibition of a hormone-stimulated adenylate cyclase (as suggested for the pituitary D-2 receptors) is purely conjectural at this time. It should be borne in mind, however, that guanine nucleotide sensitivity is at least consistent with such a hypothesis.

On the behavioral level, by contrast, the functional relevance of the striatal D-2 receptors is extremely well documented. The affinities of a number of structurally diverse dopamine antagonists for butyrophenone binding sites correlate highly with their molar potencies in antagonism of apomorphine ($r = 0.94$, $p < 0.001$) and amphetamine-induced ($r = 0.92$, $p < 0.001$) stereotyped behavior in rat (Creese *et al.*, 1978a). Blockade of apomorphine-induced emesis in dog also correlates closely with D-2 binding site affinities. This latter test may avoid the complicating factor of differential drug distribution, since it is presumed to involve dopamine receptors in the area postrema of the brainstem, an area where the blood–brain barrier is less effective. Of greatest clinical importance is the highly significant correlation ($r = 0.8–0.9$) between the potency of these drugs as antipsychotic agents in man and their potency in competition for [³H]-butyrophenone binding (Creese *et al.*, 1976; Seeman *et al.*, 1976b). The affinity of an antagoinst for [³H]-butyrophenone binding is thus a powerful predictor of *in vivo* dopamine receptor antagonism and antipsychotic activity. The nanomolar affinity of the antipsychotic drugs for dopamine receptor binding sites is also commensurate with the plasma concentrations of these drugs at therapeutic dose levels as measured by the neuroleptic radioreceptor assay and by other methods (Creese and Snyder, 1977). A similar analysis has indicated that the antiparkinsonian effects of dopamine agonists are also mediated through the butyrophenone-labeled D-2 receptors (Titeler and Seeman, 1978; Schachter *et al.*, 1980).

3.2. Solubilization and Isolation of D-2 Receptors

Complete characterization of the various dopamine receptors will ultimately require the isolation and purification of the receptor constituents involved, followed by successful reconstitution. The initial steps in this direction have already been taken. The solubilization of [³H]-butyrophenone binding sites as reported by Gorissen and Laduron (1979) employed digitonin treatment of dog striatal membranes. Subsequent ultracentrifugation results in a supernatant containing binding sites for [³H]-spiroperidol, assayable using gel filtration to separate bound from free [³H]-ligand. These solubilized sites possess affinities for a large number of dopaminergic and nondopaminergic compounds close to those observed for membrane-bound [³H]-spiroperidol sites, with the displacement by the isomers of butaclamol being stereospecific.

Affinities of the dopaminergic antagonists also correlate well with the potencies of these compounds in antagonizing apomorphine-induced emesis in dogs. The solubilized binding sites show a regional distribution consistent with a dopaminergic nature. Similar results have now been reported using rat (Gorrisen *et al.*, 1980) and human (Madras *et al.*, 1980) striatum. In a similar solubilized receptor preparation, we have found that unlike striatal membrane homogenates, agonist displacement of [³H]-spiroperidol binding is steep (pseudo-Hill slope 1) and of low affinity. Sensitivity to guanine nucleotides is correspondingly lost, suggesting that guanine nucleotide binding protein is unavailable for functional coupling following this solubilization procedure (Leff and Creese, 1982). However, if D-2 receptors are solubilized in the presence of dopamine, subsequent guanine nucleotide sensitivity is maintained. This suggests that under these conditions the presence of dopamine induces the formation of the ternary complex that can then be solubilized intact. Subsequent addition of GTP leads to the disruption of the complex with a loss of affinity for dopamine and its rapid dissociation (Leff and Creese, 1982).

3.3. [³H]-Thioxanthene Binding: Labeling D-1 Receptors

A high-affinity striatal binding site for [³H]-flupenthixol (Hyttel, 1978a,b; Cross and Owen, 1980; Hyttel, 1980) and [³H]-piflutixol (Hyttel, 1981) has been identified that appears from competition studies to be the D-1 (adenylate cyclase stimulatory linked) receptor. The potencies of a number of dopaminergic antagonists from a variety of structural classes in inhibiting dopamine-stimulated adenylate cyclase activity correlate well with their potencies in displacing [³H]-thioxanthenes. For example, thioxanthenes, which possess very high affinity for [³H]-flupenthixol binding sites, also have nanomolar potency in the inhibition of the dopamine-stimulated adenylate cyclase. Butyrophenone affinities for both the dopamine-stimulated adenylate cyclase and [³H]-flupenthixol binding sites are one to two orders of magnitude lower. Agonists are active both in displacing [³H]-flupenthixol and in stimulating cyclase in the micromolar range. It is interesting to note that the density of stereospecific binding sites is approximately three to four times the number seen for [³H]-butyrophenone binding sites. Detailed displacement studies have revealed that a minor portion, about 20%, of the specific binding of these thioxanthene ligands is to D-2 receptors (Cross and Owen, 1980; Hyttel, 1981). [³H]-Thioxanthene binding can be directed to exclusively label the putative D-1 receptor by the inclusion of an appropriate "masking" drug, i.e., a low concentration of unlabeled butyrophenones in the assay to saturate the D-2 receptors, allowing competition studies of the D-1 sites selectively. Agonist interactions with [³H]-flupenthixol binding sites are discussed below.

3.4. [³H]-Agonist Binding Sites

Putative dopamine receptors in striatum have also been identified by the binding of the tritiated dopamine agonists including [³H]-dopamine itself. Unlike the binding of the [³H]-butyrophenone ligands, that of the [³H]-agonist ligands is markedly dependent on assay conditions. Under some conditions, [³H]-agonist ligands bind to striatal D-2 receptors with high affinity, as they do in anterior pituitary. A subset of the [³H]-agonist binding sites, however, differ from both the butyrophenone-labeled D-2 binding sites and the dopamine-stimulated adenylate cyclase in that butyrophenones have micromolar affinities, whereas agonists have nanomolar affinities for these sites. Thus, it has been proposed that these agonist binding sites, termed "D-3," represent yet another distinct dopamine receptor, the autoreceptor (Titeler *et al.*, 1979).

The "D-3" binding sites are operationally defined as possessing high affinity for [³H]-dopamine, [³H]-apomorphine, [³H]-NPA, or [³H]-ADTN and low affinity for butyrophenones. Although "D-3" binding sites are not observed in pituitary, they are present in mammalian striatum at 10–40 pmole/g wet weight tissue (Burt *et al.*, 1976; Thal *et al.*, 1978; Komiskey *et al.*, 1978; Creese and Snyder, 1978; Creese *et al.*, 1979a) or about 50–700 fmole/mg membrane protein (Seeman *et al.*, 1975; Cronin *et al.*, 1978; Titeler and Seeman, 1979; List *et al.*, 1980) depending on the conditions employed. At 37°C in bovine striatal membranes in the presence of "physiological" (extracellular) concentrations of ions, [³H]-dopamine labels "D-3" sites with a K_D of about 10–20 nM (Creese *et al.*, 1975; Burt *et al.*, 1976). Such sites have also been labeled in both calf and rat striatum under various conditions with [³H]-apomorphine (Thal *et al.*, 1978; Seeman *et al.*, 1979), [³H]-NPA (Creese *et al.*, 1979a; Titeler and Seeman, 1979), and [³H]-ADTN (Creese and Snyder, 1978; Seeman *et al.*, 1979) with affinities in the nanomolar range. Oddly, under these same roughly physiological conditions, high-affinity [^{3}H]-dopamine binding to rat striatal membranes is not reproducibly found (Creese et al., 1979d), although Seeman and co-workers have been able to obtain such binding under other conditions (Titeler et al., 1979; List et al., 1980). We have recently explained these divergent results by characterizing the effects of varying temperature and ionic conditions on [^{3}H]-dopamine binding in rat caudate membranes (Hamblin and Creese, 1982b).

Preincubation of tissue in buffer at 37°C and in the absence of metal cations and chelating agents produces specific [^{3}H]-dopamine binding at 22°C that is entirely to the "D-3" sites. Addition of millimolar Ca^{2+}, Mg^{2+}, Mn^{2+}, or Co^{2+} allows [^{3}H]-dopamine labeling of both the D-2 and "D-3" sites with approximately equal affinity (Hamblin and Creese, 1982b). This in part reflects prevention by these cations of an irreversible degradation of D-2 sites as previously described using [^{3}H]-spiroperidol binding (Usdin et al., 1980). EDTA and EGTA (0.1 μM to 10 mM) paradoxically have a similar but incomplete effect. Chelators and divalent cations have a further effect in greatly decreasing nonspecific binding of [^{3}H]-dopamine. Sodium (10–150 mM), on the other hand, decreases [^{3}H]-dopamine binding to D-2 and "D-3" sites by decreasing [^{3}H]-dopamine but not [^{3}H]-spiroperidol affinity. Such a Na^+-mediated decrease in agonist affinity is also observed for the opiate receptor (Pert et al., 1973), the α_1 (Glossman and Hornung, 1980) and the α_2 (Tsai and Lefkowitz, 1978) adrenergic receptors, and the histamine-1 receptor (Chang and Snyder, 1980).

[^{3}H]-Dopamine binding to both D-2 and "D-3" sites is also reduced by increasing incubation temperature, although [^{3}H]-butyrophenone binding to D-2 sites is not. The combined effects of sodium and temperature are sufficient to place the affinity of [^{3}H]-dopamine for "D-3" sites in rat membranes outside the range detectable in filtration assays, with a K_D for unlabeled dopamine of about 200–300 nM at 37°C (Creese et al., 1979d). At 22–25°C in the absence of sodium, however, [^{3}H]-dopamine displays a K_D of about 2 nM for "D-3" sites. On the other hand, [^{3}H]-NPA (Titeler and Seeman, 1979) and [^{3}H]-apomorphine (Thal et al., 1978; Titeler et al., 1978) also label D-2 receptors, as they do in anterior pituitary, as well as "D-3" sites under these conditions. Thus, dopaminergic [^{3}H]-agonists can label either D-2 or "D-3" binding sites, simultaneously or selectively, depending on the tissue preparation and incubation conditions.

The function of the "D-3" sites is unclear. Drug affinities at these sites do not correlate with antipsychotic (Creese et al., 1976) or antiparkinsonian (Titeler and Seeman, 1978) activities. Lesion studies have suggested that the "D-3" site may represent autoreceptors on nigrostriatal terminals. In the rat striatum, "D-3" sites were decreased 50% by 6-hydroxydopamine (6-OHDA) lesions of the nigrostriatal dopamine pathway (Nagy *et al.*, 1978; Sokoloff *et al.*, 1980a,b), suggesting that such "D-3" binding labels presynaptic dopamine autoreceptors on the degenerated nigrostriatal terminals (Seeman, 1980; Nagy *et al.*, 1978; Sokoloff *et al.*, 1980a,b). However, nigrostriatal denervation produces a concomitant depletion of striatal dopamine. We have demonstrated that a reserpine-induced depletion of dopamine produces a comparable decrease in "D-3" binding independent of presynaptic terminal degeneration (Leff *et al.*, 1982; Leff and Creese, 1983) This loss in binding, or that caused by 6-OHDA lesions, is recovered by preincubating the striatal membranes with dopamine or with the supernatant from control striatal membrane preparations. Therefore, we suggest that the loss of "D-3" binding following 6-OHDA lesions results from the depletion of endogenous DA rather than from the degeneration of terminals and their putatively associated autoreceptors.

As shown above, [^{3}H]-agonists can label both the classical postsynaptic D-2 receptors and "D-3" binding sites (Hamblin and Creese, 1982b). Figure 11 shows that [^{3}H]-dopamine/butyrophenone competition curves are biphasic. Computer analysis of these competition curves to quantify binding parameters demonstrates that about 40–50% of [^{3}H]-dopamine binding is to D-2 receptors and 50–60% is to putative "D-3" binding sites as defined by high or low butyrophenone affinity. Six to eight weeks following a 6-OHDA lesion of the nigrostriatal tract (Fig. 11, dashed lines), the proportion of D-2 [^{3}H]-dopamine binding is unchanged or slightly increased with a concomitant decrease of 64 ± 4% of "D-3" [^{3}H]-dopamine binding. The total amount of [^{3}H]-dopamine binding decreases under this protocol by 27 ± 4%. The decrease in "D-3" binding was related to a decrease in B_{max} for these sites.

Figure 12 demonstrates that similar changes in displacement curves are obtained following a 20-hr reserpine-induced catecholamine depletion of normal rats. This treatment produces a 42 ± 6% decrease in "D-3" binding. This phenomenon is not the result of a direct reserpine interaction with "D-3" receptors, since *in vitro* reserpine is a poor inhibitor of "D-3" binding (IC_{50} ~ 10 μM). Furthermore, preincubating membranes from reserpine-treated animals with either dopamine (100 nM) or the supernatant from a membrane preparation of a normal striatum reverses the loss in "D-3" [^{3}H]-dopamine binding. Similarly, preincubating striatal membranes from 6-OHDA-denervated striata with dopamine also reverses the "lesion-induced" loss in "D-3" [^{3}H]-dopamine binding. Thus, the loss in striatal "D-3" binding produced by both reserpine treatment

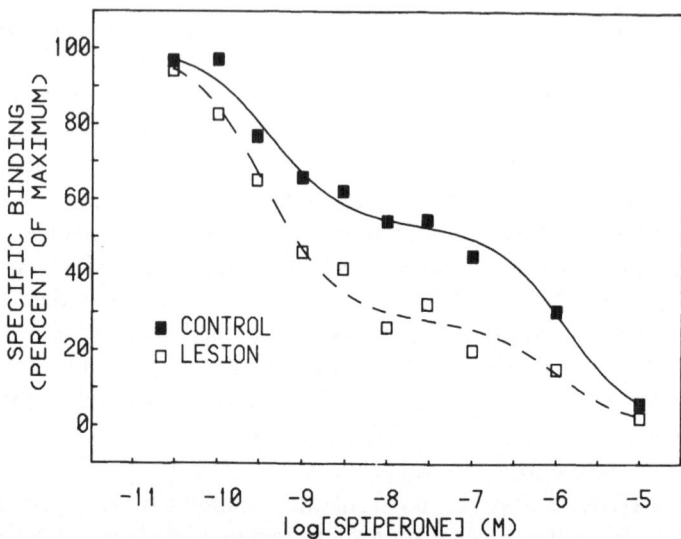

Figure 11. Unilateral 6-OHDA lesions: representative fitted curves for [³H]-DA/spiroperidol competition in contralateral (■) and ipsilateral (□) striata. Representative spiroperidol competition for [³H]-DA binding experiments in control striatum were analyzed showing a best-fit curve modeling to two sites. The K_is for spiroperidol for the two sites were estimated to be 213 pmole and 0.65 μM for the high-affinity (D-2) and low-affinity (D-3) sites, respectively. D-3 sites comprised 53% of the total at this [³H]-DA concentration (1.3 nM) in the nonlesioned striatum. On the lesioned side, D-3 sites comprised only 28% of the total [³H]-DA binding or 47% of the concentration of D-3 sites observed in the contralateral side. Final parameter estimates for the curves shown were: contralateral, K_{D-2} = 213 pM, R_{D-2} = 9.1 fmole/mg tissue, K_{D-3} = 0.65 μM, R_{D-3} = 10.2 fmole/mg tissue; lesion, K_{D-2} = 176 pM, R_{D-2} = 12.6 fmole/mg tissue; K_{D-3} = 0.50 μM, R_{D-3} = 4.8 fmole/mg tissue. Mean values ± S.E.M. (n = 6): contralateral, K_{D-2} = 140 ± 23 pM, R_{D-2} = 8.84 ± 0.36 fmole/mg tissue; K_{D-3} = 1.45 ± 0.39 μM, R_{D-3} = 10.36 ± 0.59 fmole/mg; lesion, K_{D-2} = 104 ± 42 nM, R_{D-2} = 10.28 ± 0.79 fmole/mg tissue; K_{D-3} = 0.75 ± 0.24 μM, R_{D-3} = 3.71 ± 0.35* fmole/mg tissue, [*P < 0.005 (paired t-test) compared to contralateral R_{D-3}]. The [³H]-DA saturation experiments indicated that the decrease in D-3 binding reflected a decrease in B_{max}. Values for control and contralateral striatum did not differ significantly. Qualitatively identical results were found for the agonist [³H]-apomorphine. (From Leff and Creese, 1983.)

and 6-OHDA denervation results from a depletion of dopamine in the treated tissues (Leff *et al.*, 1982; Leff and Creese, 1983).

Other recent studies have suggested that the addition of dopamine to preincubations of washed or dopamine-depleted striatal membrane homogenates produces increased ''D-3'' binding (Hamblin and Creese, 1982b; Bacopolous, 1981). In these studies, the preincubation of the membrane homogenates was a crucial variable in the improved expression of all [³H]-dopamine specific binding. As has been suggested by Hamblin and Creese (1982b), this preincubation in the presence of (endogenous)

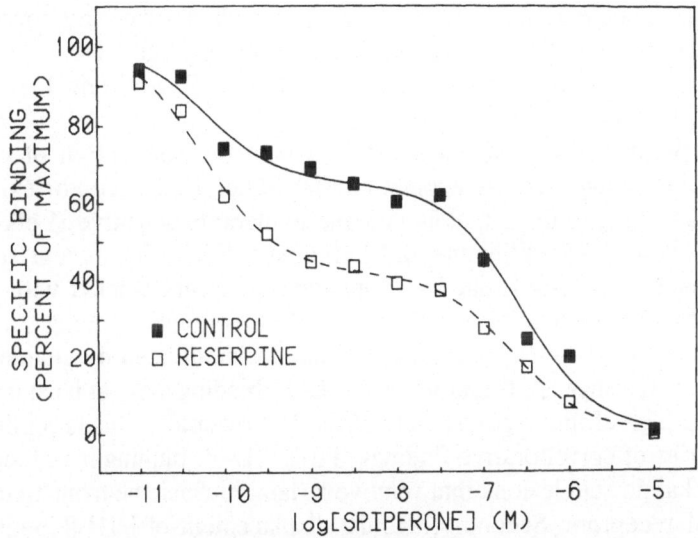

Figure 12. Fitted curves for [³H]-DA/spiroperidol competition in the striatum of saline- (■) and reserpine- (□) injected rats. Similar changes in the D-3 component of [³H]-DA binding were seen in reserpine-injected rats as for 6-OHDA denervated striatum. Mean values ± S.E.M. ($n = 6$) were: control, $K_{D-2} = 86 ± 34.9$ pM, $R_{D-2} = 2.81 ± 0.24$ fmole/mg tissue, $K_{D-3} = 130.2 ± 14.5$ nM, $R_{D-3} = 4.88 ± 0.23$ fmole/mg tissue; reserpine, $K_{D-2} = 62.3 ± 23.8$ pM, $R_{D-2} = 3.14 ± 0.45$ fmole/mg tissue; $K_{D-3} = 133.8 ± 23.4$ nM, $R_{D-3} = 2.83 ± 0.26^*$ fmole/mg tissue [$^*P < 0.001$ (paired *t*-test) compared to control R_{D-3}]. Experiments for Figs. 11 and 12 were conducted at different times, which contributed to the differences seen in the absolute binding parameters of the control striata. (From Leff and Creese, 1983.)

dopamine and divalent cations may act to promote the dissociation and washout of endogenous guanine nucleotides from guanine nucleotide binding sites that regulate dopamine agonist binding to D-2 and "D-3" binding sites by decreasing agonist affinity. This resembles the mechanism by which agonist preincubations appear to enhance agonist binding to some β-adrenergic receptors (Lad *et al.*, 1980).

Irrespective of mechanism, these data indicate that 6-OHDA denervation and reserpine treatments appear to reduce specific "D-3" binding by eliminating the usual preincubation-induced enhancement of this binding seen in control tissues containing endogenous dopamine. Previously, Schwartz and colleagues have demonstrated similar changes in [³H]-agonist/antagonist competition curves following 6-OHDA lesions (Sokoloff *et al.*, 1980a,b). They concluded that the lost "D-3" sites were presynaptic. However, the important dopamine depletion controls were not undertaken. The present results suggest that "D-3" binding sites are not presynaptic but are postsynaptic. This is reinforced by our preliminary findings that kainate lesion of the striatum, which destroys neuronal cell bodies, reduces both D-1 [^{3}H]-flupenthixol binding and "D-3" [^{3}H]-DA binding by more than 70% (Leff *et al.*, 1981; S. E. Leff and I. Creese, unpublished data).

In β-adrenergic systems associated with the stimulation of cAMP production, a high-affinity agonist-binding state of the receptor exists in membrane preparations that is guanine nucleotide sensitive (Lefkowitz and Williams, 1977; Williams and Lefkowitz, 1977). Our recent studies have indeed suggested that D-1 dopamine receptors labeled with [^{3}H]-flupenthixol demonstrate high- and low-affinity agonist binding states in much the same way D-2 receptors do that are modulated by guanine nucleotides. We suggest, therefore, that "D-3" binding may, at least in part, label the high-affinity agonist state of the D-1 receptor. This is reinforced by a series of corroborative findings. First, "D-3" binding is reduced by striatal kainic acid lesions that remove striatal intrinsic neurons that contain D-1 receptors. Secondly, agonist displacement of [^{3}H]-flupenthixol binding to D-1 receptors is biphasic, with the K_H of the high-affinity displacement phase matching the K_D of direct [^{3}H]-agonists' binding to "D-3" sites (Fig. 13). Thirdly, both types of agonist binding (displacement of [^{3}H]-flupenthixol binding to D-1 receptors of [^{3}H]-agonist binding to "D-3" sites) are equivalently sensitive to GTP. Fourthly, antagonist affinities at "D-3" sites correlate highly with antagonist affinities at D-1 receptors (Fig. 14).

4. Concluding Comments

The interpretation of early dopamine receptor binding studies with striatal membranes was difficult—the data did not describe a system containing a single set of homogeneous receptors. A number of approaches have now allowed the clear division of CNS dopamine receptors into subtypes. Among the most important advances have been the examination of binding characteristics in other tissues such as anterior pituitary and the use of discrete CNS lesions to remove particular presynaptic or postsynaptic cellular elements. Such studies have now characterized two dopamine receptor subtypes known as D-1 and D-2. Table III summarizes our current characterization of dopamine receptors by the radioligand binding technique and combines this information with what is known concerning these receptors' biochemical and pharmacological characteristics.

This classification is, as yet, preliminary; a number of questions remain. For instance, the possibility that a portion of the [^{3}H]-agonist "D-3" binding sites may label autoreceptors has not yet been rigorously ex-

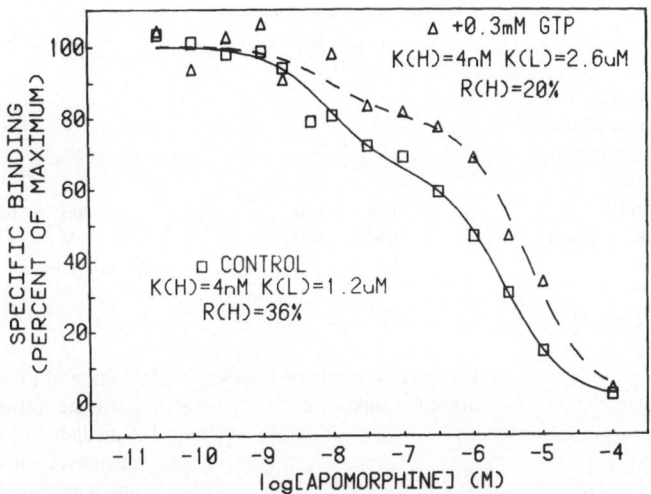

Figure 13. Apomorphine inhibition of [³H]-flupenthixol binding to rat striatal D-1 receptors demonstrating high- and low-affinity displacement in the absence and presence of GTP. GTP causes the proportions of R_H to decrease from 36% to 20% without significantly affecting affinities of the two components.

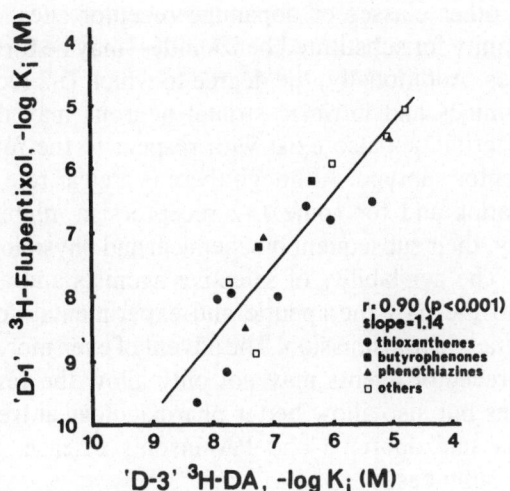

Figure 14. Correlation of antagonist K_is at D-1 receptors labeled by [³H]-flupenthixol and "D-3" sites labeled by [³H]-dopamine in rat striatum.

Table III. Characteristics of Dopaminergic Binding Sites

Receptor	D-1		D-2	
	$R_H \rightleftharpoons R_L$ ("D-3")		$R_H \rightleftharpoons R_L$	
Usable radioligands				
[^{3}H]-Thioxanthenes	+	+	+	+
[^{3}H]-Butyrophenones	–	–	+	+
[^{3}H]-Agonists	+	–	+	–
Agonist affinity	nM	μM	nM	μM
Butyrophenone affinity	μM	μM	nM	nM
Adenylate cyclase association	Stimulatory		Inhibitory or unassociated	
Guanine nucleotide sensitivity	+ +	–	+	–
Function	Parathyroid hormone release Striatum: unknown		Inhibition of pituitary hormone release DA mediated behavioral responses and their antagonism by neuroleptics	
Striatal location	Intrinsic neurons		Intrinsic neurons Corticostriate afferents	
Pituitary location	–		+	

cluded. Also, other classes of dopamine receptor sites, such as those having high affinity for substituted benzamides, may be further elucidated in future studies. Additionally, the degree to which D-2 receptors on corticostriate terminals and intrinsic striatal neurons may differ is as yet uncertain. Uncertainties also exist with respect to the function of each dopamine receptor subtype. Although there is a clear role for D-1 receptors in stimulating and for some D-2 receptors in inhibiting adenylate cyclase activity, their subsequent biochemical and physiological functions are unknown. The availability of selective agonists and antagonists has been central to the past therapeutic and experimental advances in the field of dopaminergic transmission. The advent of even more selective D-1, D-2, and autoreceptor agents may not only allow the resolution of the above questions but also allow better pharmacological treatment of disorders such as schizophrenia and Parkinson's disease, which involve these receptor subtypes.

ACKNOWLEDGMENTS. This work was supported by PHS MH32990. I. Creese is a recipient of a RCDA MH00316. We thank D. D. Taitano for manuscript typing.

References

Ahn, H. S., Gardner, E., and Makman, M. H., 1979, Anterior pituitary adenylate cyclase: Stimulation by dopamine and other monoamines, *Eur. J. Pharmacol.* **53**:313–317.

Bach, N. J., Kornfeld, E. C., Jones, N. D., Chaney, M. D., Dorman, D. E., Paschal, J. W., Clemens, J. A., and Smalstig, E. B., 1980, Bicyclic and tricyclic ergoline partial structures. Rigid 3-(2-aminoethyl) pyrazoles and 3- and 4-(2-aminoethyl) pyrazoles as dopamine agonists, *J. Med. Chem.* **23**:481–491.

Bacopolous, N. G., 1981, Acute changes in the state of dopamine receptors; *in vitro* monitoring with ^{3}H-dopamine, *Life Sci.* **29**:2407–2414.

Bannon, M. J., Grace, A. A., Bunney, B. S., and Roth, R. H., 1980, Evidence for an irreversible interaction of bromocryptine with central dopamine receptors, *Naunyn Schmiedebergs Arch. Pharmacol.* **312**:37–41.

Battaglia, G., and Titeler, M., 1981, Direct binding of ^{3}H-lisuride to adrenergic and serotonergic receptors, *Life Sci.* **29**:909–916.

Bennett, J. P., Jr., 1978, Methods in binding studies, in: *Neurotransmitter Receptor Binding* (H. I. Yamamura, S. J. Enna, and M. J. Kuhar, eds.), Raven Press, New York, pp. 57–90.

Bethea, C. L., Ramsdell, J. S., Jatte, R. B., Wilson, C. B., and Weiner, R. I., 1982, Characterization of the dopaminergic regulation of human prolactin-secreting cells cultured on extracellular matrix, *J. Clin. Endocrinol. Metab.* **54**:892–902.

Boeynaems, J. M., and Dumont, J. E., 1977, The two-step model of ligand–receptor interaction, *Mol. Cell. Endocrinol.* **7**:33–47.

Burt, D. R., 1978, Criteria for receptor identification, in: *Neurotransmitter Receptor Binding* (H. I. Yamamura, S. J. Enna, and M. J. Kuhar, eds.), Raven Press, New York, pp. 41–55.

Burt, D. R., Enna, S. J., Creese, I., and Snyder, S. H., 1975, Dopamine receptor binding in the corpus striatum of mammalian brain, *Proc. Natl. Acad. Sci. U.S.A.* **72**:4655–4659.

Burt, D. R., Creese, I., and Snyder, S. H., 1976, Properties of [^{3}H]haloperidol and [^{3}H]dopamine binding associated with dopamine receptors in calf brain membranes, *Mol. Pharmacol.* **12**:800–812.

Calabro, M. A., and MacLeod, R. M., 1978, Binding of dopamine to bovine anterior pituitary gland membranes, *Neuroendocrinology* **25**:32–46.

Camerman, N., and Camerman, A., 1981, On the stereochemistry of dopaminergic ergoline derivatives, *Mol. Pharmacol.* **19**:517–519.

Cannon, J. G., Demopoulos, B. J., Long, J. P., Flynn, J. R., and Sharabi, F. M., 1981, Proposed dopaminergic pharmacophore of lergotrile pergolide, and related ergot alkaloid derivatives, *J. Med. Chem.* **24**:238–240.

Caron, M. C., Beaulieu, M., Raymond, V., Gagne, B., Drouin, J., Lefkowitz, R. J., and Labrie, F., 1978, Dopaminergic receptors in the anterior pituitary gland: Correlation of [^{3}H]dihydroergocryptine binding with the dopaminergic control of prolactin release, *J. Biol. Chem.* **253**:2244–2253.

Cech, S. Y., Broaddus, W. C., and Maguire, M. E., 1980, Adenylate cyclase: The role of magnesium and other divalent cations, *Mol. Cell Biochem.* **33**:67–92.

Chang, R. S., and Snyder, S. H., 1980, Histamine H_1-receptor binding sites in guinea pig brain membranes: Regulation of agonist interactions by guanine nucleotides and cations, *J. Neurochem.* **34**:916–922.

Clement-Cormier, Y. C., Heindel, J. J., and Robison, G. A., 1977, Adenylyl cyclase from a prolactin producing tumour cell: The effect of phenothiazines, *Life Sci.* **21**:1357–1364.

Creese, I., and Sibley, D. R., 1979, Radioligand binding studies: Evidence for multiple dopamine receptors, *Commun. Psychopharmacol.* **3**:385–395.

Creese, I., and Sibley, D. R., 1981, Receptor adaptations to centrally acting drugs, *Annu. Rev. Pharmacol. Toxicol.* **21**:357–391.

Creese, I., and Snyder, S. H., 1977, Simple and sensitive radioreceptor assay for anti-schizophrenic drugs in blood, *Nature* **270**:180–182.

Creese, I., and Snyder, S. H., 1978, Dopamine receptor binding of ^{3}H-ADTN (2-amino-6,7-dihydroxy-1,2,3,4-tetrahydronaphthalene) regulated by guanyl nucleotides, *Eur. J. Pharmacol.* **50**:459–461.

Creese, I., Burt, D. R., and Snyder, S. H., 1975, Dopamine receptor binding: Differentiation of agonist and antagonist states with ^{3}H-dopamine and ^{3}H-haloperidol, *Life Sci.* **17**:993–1001.

Creese, I., Burt, D. R., and Snyder, S. H., 1976, Dopamine receptor binding predicts clinical and pharmacological potencies of antischizophrenic drugs, *Science* **192**:481–483.

Creese, I., Schneider, R., and Snyder, S. H., 1977a, ^{3}H-Spiroperidol labels dopamine receptors in pituitary and brain, *Eur. J. Pharmacol.* **46**:377–381.

Creese, I., Burt, D. R., and Snyder, S. H., 1977b, Dopamine receptor binding enhancement accompanies lesion-induced behavioral supersensitivity, *Science* **197**:596–598.

Creese, I., Burt, D. R., and Snyder, S. H., 1978a, Biochemical actions of neuroleptic drugs: focus on the dopamine receptor, in: *Handbook of Psychopharmacology*, Volume 10 (L. L. Iversen, S. D. Iversen, and S. H. Snyder, eds.), Plenum Press, New York, pp. 37–89.

Creese, I., Padgett, L., Fazzini, E., and Lopez, F., 1979a, ^{3}H-N-1-Propylnorapomorphine: A novel agonist ligand for central dopamine receptors, *Eur. J. Pharmacol.* **56**:411–412.

Creese, I., Usdin, T. B., and Snyder, S. H., 1979b, Guanine nucleotides distinguish between two dopamine receptors, *Nature* **278**:577–578.

Creese, I., Usdin, T. B. and Snyder, S. H., 1979c, Dopamine receptor binding regulated by guanine nucleotides, *Mol. Pharmacol.* **16**:69–76.

Creese, I., Stewart, K., and Snyder, S. H., 1979d, Species variations in dopamine receptor binding, *Eur. J. Pharmacol.* **60**:55–66.

Creese, I., Sibley, D. R., Hamblin, M. W., and Leff, S. E., 1983, The classification of dopamine receptors: Relationship to radioligand binding, *Annu. Rev. Neurosci.* **6**:43–71.

Cronin, M. J., and Weiner, R. I., 1979, [^{3}H]Spiroperidol (spiperone) binding to a putative dopamine receptor in sheep and steer pituitary and stalk median eminence, *Endocrinology* **104**:307–312.

Cronin, M. J., Roberts, J. M., and Weiner, R. I., 1978, Dopamine and dihydroergocryptine binding to the anterior pituitary and other brain areas of the rat and sheep, *Endocrinology* **103**:302–309.

Cross, A. J., and Owen, F., 1980, Characteristics of ^{3}H-*cis*-flupenthixol binding to calf brain membranes, *Eur. J. Pharmacol.* **65**:341–347.

Dannies, P. S., Gautvik, K. M., and Tashjian, A. H., 1976, A possible role of cyclic AMP in mediating the effects of thyrotropin-releasing hormone on prolactin release and on prolactin and growth hormone synthesis in pituitary cells in culture, *Endocrinology* **98**:1147–1159.

De Camilli, P., Macconi, D., and Sdada, A., 1979, Dopamine inhibits adenylate cyclase in human prolactin-secreting pituitary adenomas, *Nature* **278**:252–254.

De Lean, A., Stadel, J. M., and Lefkowitz, R. J., 1980, A ternary complex model explains the agonist-specific binding properties of the adenylate cyclase-coupled beta-adrenergic receptor, *J. Biol. Chem.* **255**:7108–7117.

Delitala, G., Yeo, T., Grossman, A., Hathway, N. R., and Besser, G. M., 1980, A comparison of the effects of four ergot derivatives on prolactin secretion by dispersed rat pituitary cells, *J. Endocrinol.* **87**:95–103.

Fields, J. Z., Reisine, T. D., and Yamamura, H. I., 1977, Biochemical demonstration of dopaminergic receptors in rat and human brain using [^{3}H]spiroperidol, *Brain Res.* **136**:578–584.

Fujita, N., Saito, K., Yonehara, N., Watanabe, Y., and Yoshida, H., 1979, Binding of ^{3}H-lisuride hydrogen maleate to striatal membranes of rat brain, *Life Sci.* **25**:969–973.

Furchgott, R. F., 1978, Pharmacological characterization of receptors: Its relation to radioligand-binding studies, *Fed. Proc.* **37**:115–120.

Fuxe, K., Currodi, H., Hokfelt, T., Lidbrink, P., and Ungerstedt, U., 1974, Ergocornine and 2 Br-α-ergocryptine. Evidence for prolonged dopamine receptor stimulation, *Med. Biol.* **52**:121–132.

Fuxe, K., Agnati, L. F., Kohler, C., Kuonen, D., Ogren, S. O., Anderson, K., and Hokfelt, T., 1981, Characterization of normal and supersensitive dopamine receptors: Effects of ergot drugs and neuropeptide, *J. Neural Transm.* **51**:3–37.

Garcia-Sainz, J. A., Li, S. Y., and Fain, J. N., 1981, Alpha$_2$ adrenergic amines, adenosine and prostaglandins inhibit lipolysis and cyclic AMP accumulation in hamster adipocytes in the absence of extracellular sodium, *Life Sci.* **28**:401–406.

Giannattasio, G., DeFerrari, M. E., and Spada, A., 1981, Dopamine-inhibited adenylate cyclase in female rat adenohypophysis, *Life Sci.* **28**:1605–1612.

Glossmann, H., and Hornung, R., 1980, Alpha-adrenoreceptors in rat brain: Sodium changes the affinity of agonists for prazosin sites, *Eur. J. Pharmacol.* **61**:407–408.

Goldsmith, P. C., Cronin, M. J., and Weiner, R. I., 1979, Dopamine receptor sites in the anterior pituitary, *J. Histochem. Cytochem.* **27**:1205–1207.

Gorissen, H., and Laduron, P., 1979, Solubilisation of high-affinity dopamine receptors, *Nature* **279**:72–74.

Gorissen, H., Ilien, B., Aerts, G., and Laduron, P., 1980, Differentiation of solubilized dopamine receptors from spirodecanone binding sites in rat striatum, *FEBS Lett.* **121**:133–138.

Hamblin, M., and Creese, I., 1982a, Phenoxybenzamine treatment differentiates dopaminergic ^{3}H-ligand binding sites in bovine caudata membranes, *Mol. Pharmacol.* **21**:44–51.

Hamblin, M. W., and Creese, I., 1982b, ^{3}H-Dopamine binding to rat striatal D-2 and D-3 sites: Enhancement by magnesium and inhibition by sodium, *Life Sci.* **30**:1587–1595.

Heidenreich, K. A., Weiland, G. A., and Molinoff, P. B., 1980, Characterization of radiolabeled agonist binding to β-adrenergic receptors in mammalian tissues, *J. Cyclic Nucleotide Res.* **6**:217–230.

Heidenreich, K. A., Weiland, G. A., and Molinoff, P. B., 1982, Effects of magnesium and N-ethylmaleimide on the binding of ^{3}H-hydroxybenzylisoproterenol to β-adrenergic receptors, *J. Biol. Chem.* **257**:804–810.

Hoffman, B. B., and Lefkowitz, R. J., 1980, Radioligand binding studies of adrenergic receptors: New insights into molecular and physiological regulation, *Annu. Rev. Pharmacol. Toxicol.* **20**:581–608.

Hoffman, B. B., Michel, T., Brenneman, T. B., and Lefkowitz, R. J., 1982, Interactions of agonists with platelet α$_2$-adrenergic receptors, *Endocrinology* **110**:926–932.

Howlett, D. R., and Nahorski, S. R., 1978, A comparative study of [^{3}H]haloperidol and [^{3}H]spiroperidol binding to receptors on rat cerebral membranes, *FEBS Lett.* **87**:152–156.

Hyttel, J., 1978a, A comparison of the effect of neuroleptic drugs on the binding of ^{3}H-haloperidol and ^{3}H-cis(Z)-flupenthixol and on adenylate cyclase activity in rat striatal tissue *in vitro*, *Prog. Neuropsychopharmacol.* **2**:329–335.

Hyttel, J., 1978b, Effects of neuroleptics on ^{3}H-haloperidol and ^{3}H-cis(Z)-flupenthixol binding and on adenylate cyclase activity *in vitro*, *Life Sci.* **23**:551–555.

Hyttel, J., 1980, Further evidence that ^{3}H-cis(Z)flupenthixol binds to the adenylate cyclase-associated dopamine receptor (D-1) in rat corpus striatum, *Psychopharmacology* **67**:107–109.

Hyttel, J., 1981, Similarities between the binding of ^{3}H-piflutixol and ^{3}H-flupentixol to rat striatal dopamine receptors *in vitro*, *Life Sci.* **28**:563–569.

Jacobs, S., and Cuatrecasas, P., 1976, The mobile receptor hypothesis and "cooperativity" of hormone binding application to insulin, *Biochim. Biophys. Acta* **433**:482–495.

Kebabian, J. W., and Calne, D. B., 1979, Multiple receptors for dopamine, *Nature* **277**:93–96.

Kent, R. S., De Lean, A., and Lefkowitz, R. J., 1980, A quantitative analysis of beta-adrenergic receptor interactions: Resolution of high and low affinity states of the receptor by computer modeling of ligand binding data, *Mol. Pharmacol.* **17**:14–23.

Komiskey, H. L., Bossart, J. F., Miller, D. D., and Patil, P. N., 1978, Conformation of dopamine at the dopamine receptor, *Proc. Natl. Acad. Sci. U.S.A.* **75**:2641–2643.

Korner, M., Gilon, C., and Schramm, M., 1982, Locking of hormone in the β-adrenergic receptor by attack on a sulfhydryl in an associated component, *J. Biol. Chem.* **257**:3389–3396.

LaBrie, F., Ferland, L., DiPaolo, T., and Veilleux, R., 1980, Modulation of prolactin secretion by sex steroids and thyroid hormones, in: *Central and Peripheral Regulation of Prolactin Function* (R. M. MacLeod and U. Scapagnini, eds.), Raven Press, New York, pp. 97–113.

Lad, P. M., Nielsen, T. B., Preston, M. S., and Rodbell, M., 1980, The role of the guanine nucleotide exchange reaction in the regulation of the beta-adrenergic receptor and in the actions of catecholamines and choleratoxin on adenylate cyclase in turkey erythrocyte membranes, *J. Biol. Chem.* **255**:988–995.

Larsen, N. E., Mullikin-Kilpatrick, K., and Blume, A. J., 1981, Two different modifications of the neuroblastoma × glioma hybrid opiate receptors induced by N-ethylmaleimide, *Mol. Pharmacol.* **20**:255–262.

Leff, S. E., and Creese, I., 1982, Solubilization of D-2 dopamine receptors from canine caudate: Agonist-occupation stabilizes guanine nucleotide sensitive receptor complexes, *Biochem. Biophys. Res. Commun.* **108**:1150–1157.

Leff, S. E., and Creese, I., 1983, Dopaminergic D-3 sites are postsynaptic, *Nature* **306**:586–589.

Leff, S., Adams, L., Hyttel, J., and Creese, I., 1981, Kainate lesion dissociates striatal dopamine receptor radioligand binding sites, *Eur. J. Pharmacol.* **70**:71–75.

Leff, S. E., Hamblin, M. W., and Creese, I., 1982, Acute reserpine mimics the effects of nigrostriatal 6-hydroxydopamine lesions on "D-3" specific ^{3}H-dopamine binding in rat striatum, *Soc. Neurosci. Abstr.* **8**:717.

Lefkowitz, R. J., 1980, Modification of adenylate cyclase activity by alpha and beta-adrenergic receptors: Insights from radioligand binding studies, in: *Psychopharmacology and Biochemistry of Neurotransmitter Receptors* (H. I. Yamamura, R. W. Olsen, and E. Usdin, eds.), Elsevier Press, New York, pp. 155–170.

Lefkowitz, R. J., and Williams, L. T., 1977, Catecholamine binding to the beta-adrenergic receptor, *Proc. Natl. Acad. Sci. U.S.A.* **74**:515–519.

Levitski, A., 1978, The mode of coupling of adenylate cyclase to hormone receptors and its modulation by GTP, *Biochem. Pharmacol.* **27**:2083–2088.

Leysen, J. E., Gommeren, W., and Laduron, P. M., 1978, Spiperone: A ligand of choice for neuroleptic receptors. I. Kinetics and characteristics of *in vitro* binding, *Biochem. Pharmacol.* **27**:307–316.

Limbird, L. E., 1981, Activation and attenuation of adenylate cyclase. The role of GTP-binding proteins as macromolecular messengers in receptor–cyclase coupling, *Biochem. J.* **195**:1–13.

Limbird, L. E., Gill, D. M., and Lefkowitz, R. J., 1980, Agonist-promoted coupling of the beta-adrenergic receptor with the guanine nucleotide regulatory protein of the adenylate cyclase system, *Proc. Natl. Acad. Sci. U.S.A.* **77**:775–779.

List, S., Titeler, M., and Seeman, P., 1980, High-affinity ^{3}H-dopamine receptors (D_3 sites) in human and rat brain, *Biochem. Pharmacol.* **29**:1621–1622.

MacLeod, R. M., Nagy, I., Login, I. S., Kimura, H., Valdenegro, C. A., and Thorner, M. O., 1980, The role of dopamine, cAMP, and calcium in prolactin secretion, in: *Central and Peripheral Regulation of Prolactin Function* (R. M. MacLeod and U. Scapaagnini, eds.), Raven Press, New York, pp. 27–41.

Madras, B. K., Davis, A., Kunashko, P., and Seeman, P., 1980, Solubilization of dopamine receptors from dog and human brains, in: *Psychopharmacology and Biochemistry of Neurotransmitter Receptors* (H. I., Yamamura, R. W. Olsen, and E. Usdin, eds.), Elsevier/North-Holland, New York, pp. 411–419.

Markstein, R., 1981, Neurochemical effects of some ergot derivatives: A basis for their antiparkinson action, *J. Neural Transm.* **51**:39–59.

Meunier, H., and Labrie, F., 1982, The dopamine receptor in the intermediate lobe of the rat pituitary gland is negatively coupled to adenylate cyclase, *Life Sci.* **30**:963–968.

Mowles, T. F., Burghardt, B., Burghardt, C., Charneki, A., and Sheppard, H., 1978, The dopamine receptor of the rat mammotroph in cell culture as a model for drug action, *Life Sci.* **22**:2103–2112.

Muller, E. E., Panerai, A. E., Cocchi, D., and Mantegazza, P., 1977, Endocrine profile of ergot alkaloids, *Life Sci.* **21**:1545–1558.

Munemura, M., Eskay, R. L., and Kebabian, J. W., 1980a, Release of α-melanocyte-stimulating hormone from dispersed cells of the intermediate lobe of the rat pituitary gland: Involvement of catecholamines and adenosine 3',5'-monophosphate, *Endocrinology* **106**:1795–1803.

Munemura, M., Cote, T. E., Tsuruta, K., Eskay, R. L., and Kebabian, J. W., 1980b, The dopamine receptor in the intermediate lobe of the rat pituitary gland: Pharmacological characterization *Endocrinology* **107**:1676–1683.

Munson, P. J., and Rodbard, D., 1980, Ligand: A versatile computerized approach for characterization of ligand-binding systems, *Anal. Biochem.* **107**:220–239.

Nagy, J. I., Lee, T., Seeman, P., and Fibiger, H. C., 1978, Direct evidence for presynaptic and postsynaptic dopamine receptors in brain, *Nature* **274**:278–281.

Naor, Z., Snyder, G., Fawcett, C. P., and McCann, S. M., 1980, Pituitary cyclic nucleotides and thyrotropin-releasing hormone action: The relationship of adenosine 3',5'-monophosphate and guanosine 3',5'-monophosphate to the release of thyrotropin and prolactin, *Endocrinology* **106**:1304–1310.

Onali, P., Schwartz, J. P., and Costa, E., 1981, Dopaminergic modulation of adenylate cyclase stimulation of vasoactive intestinal peptide (VIP) in anterior pituitary, *Proc. Natl. Acad. Sci. U.S.A.* **78**:6531–6534.

Pardo, J. V., Creese, I., Burt, D. R., and Snyder, S. H., 1977, Ontogenesis of dopamine receptor binding in the corpus striatum of the rat. *Brain Res.* **125**:376–382.

Pawlikowski, M., Karasek, E., Kunert-Radek, J., and Stepien, H., 1979, Dopamine blockade of the thyroliberin-induced cyclic AMP accumulation in rat anterior pituitary, *J. Neural Transm.* **45**:75–79.

Pawlikowski, M., Karasek, E., Kunert-Radek, J., and Jaranowska, M., 1981, Effects of dopamine on cyclic AMP concentration in the anterior pituitary gland *in vitro*, *J. Neural Transm.* **50**:179–184.

Pert, C. B., Pasternak, G., and Snyder, S. H., 1973, Opiate agonists and antagonists discriminated by receptor binding in brain, *Science* **182**:1359–1361.

Quik, M., and Iversen, L. L., 1979, Regional study of ³H-spiperone binding and the dopamine-sensitive adenylate cyclase in rat brain, *Eur. J. Pharmacol.* **56**:323–330.

Ray, K. P., and Wallis, M., 1980, Is cyclic adenosine 3':5'-monophosphate involved in the dopamine-mediated inhibition of prolactin secretion?, *J. Endocrinol.* **85**:59p.

Reynolds, G. P., and Riederer, P., 1981, The effects of lisuride and some other dopaminergic agonists on receptor binding in human brain, *J. Neural Transm.* **51**:107–111.

Rutschmann, J., and Stadler, P. A., 1978, Chemical background, in: *Ergot Alkaloids and Related Compounds* (B. Berde and H. O. Schild, eds.), Springer-Verlag, New York, pp. 29–78.

Schachter, M., Bedard, P., Debono, A. G., Jenner, P., Marsden, C. D., Price, P., Parkes, J. D., Keenan, J. Smith, B., Rosenthaler, J., Horowski, R., and Dorow, R., 1980, The role of D-1 and D-2 receptors, *Nature* **286**:157–159.

Schmidt, M. J., and Hill, L. E., 1977, Effects of ergots on adenylate cyclase activity in the corpus striatum and pituitary, *Life Sci.* **20**:789–798.

Schwarcz, R., Creese, I., Coyle, J. T., and Snyder, S. H., 1978, Dopamine receptors localized on cerebral cortical afferents to rat corpus striatum, *Nature* **271**:766–768.

Seeman, P., 1980, Brain dopamine receptors, *Pharmacol. Rev.* **32**:229–313.

Seeman, P., Chau-Wong, M., Tedesco, J., and Wong, K., 1975, Brain receptors for antipsychotic drugs and dopamine: Direct binding assays, *Proc. Natl. Acad. Sci. U.S.A.* **72**:4376–4380.

Seeman, P., Lee, T., Chau-Wong, M., Tedesco, J., and Wong, K., 1976a, Dopamine receptors in human and calf brains, using [³H]apomorphine and an antipsychotic drug, *Proc. Natl. Acad. Sci. U.S.A.* **73**:4354–4358.

Seeman, P., Lee, T., Chau-wong, M., and Wong, K., 1976b, Antipsychotic drug doses and neuroleptic/dopamine receptors, *Nature* **261**:717–719.

Seeman, P., Woodruff, G. N., and Poat, J. A., 1979, Similar binding of ³H-ADTN and ³H-apomorphine to calf brain dopamine receptors, *Eur. J. Pharmacol.* **55**:137–142.

Shaar, C. J., and Clemens, J. A., Inhibition of lactation and prolactin secretion in rats by ergot alkaloids, 1972, *Endocrinology* **90**:285–288.

Shane, E., Gammon, D. E., and Bilezikian, J. P., 1981, Guanine nucleotide-induced shift in binding affinity for beta-adrenergic agonists in rat reticulocyte and turkey erythrocyte membranes, *Biochem. Pharmacol.* **30**:531–535.

Sibley, D. R., and Creese, I., 1979, Multiple pituitary dopamine receptors: Effects of guanine nucleotides, *Soc. Neurosci. Abstr.* **5**:352.

Sibley, D. R., and Creese, I., 1982, Anterior pituitary dopamine receptors: Demonstration of interconvertible high and low affinity states of D-2 dopamine receptor, *J. Biol. Chem.* **257**:6351–6361.

Sibley, D. R., and Creese, I., 1983a, Regulation of ligand binding to pituitary D-2 dopaminergic receptors: Effects of divalent cations and functional group modification, *J. Biol. Chem.* **258**:4957–4965.

Sibley, D. R., and Creese, I., 1983b, Interactions of ergot alkaloids with anterior pituitary D-2 dopamine receptors, *Mol. Pharmacol.* **23**:585–593.

Sibley, D. R., Leff, S. E., and Creese, I., 1982, Interactions of novel dopaminergic ligands with D-1 and D-2 dopamine receptors, *Life Sci.* **31**:637–645.

Sibley, D. R., Mahan, L. C., and Creese, I., 1983, Dopamine receptor binding on intact cells: Absence of high affinity agonist–receptor binding state, *Mol. Pharmacol.* **23:**295–302.

Smith, S. K., and Limbird, L. E., 1982, Apparent independence of the alpha-adrenergic receptor (α-AR) of the human platelet from the adpribosylated 42,000 M_r subunit of the adenylate cyclase system, *Fed. Proc.* **41:**899.

Sokoloff, P., Martres, M.-P., and Schwartz, J.-C., 1980a, ^{3}H-Apomorphine labels both dopamine postsynaptic receptors and autoreceptors, *Nature* **288:**283–286.

Sokoloff, P., Martres, M. P., and Schwartz, J. C., 1980b, Three classes of dopamine receptor (D-2, D-3, D-4) identified by binding studies with ^{3}H-apomorphine and ^{3}H-domperidone, *Naunyn Schmiedebergs Arch. Pharmacol.* **315:**89–102.

Stefanini, E., Dejoto, P., Marchisio, A., Vernaleone, F., and Collu, R., 1980, [^{3}H]Spiroperidol binding to a putative dopaminergic receptor in rat pituitary gland, *Life Sci.* **26:**583–587.

Tamminga, C. A., and Schaffer, M. H., 1979, Treatment of schizophrenia with ergot derivatives, *Psychopharmacology* **66:**239–242.

Thal, L., Creese, I., and Snyder, S. H., 1978, ^{3}H-Apomorphine interactions with dopamine receptors in calf brain, *Eur. J. Pharmacol.* **49:**295–299.

Titeler, M., and Seeman, P., 1978, Antiparkinsonian drug doses and neuroleptic **34:**1490–1492.

Titeler, M., and Seeman, P., 1979, Selective labeling of different dopamine receptors by a new agonist ^{3}H-ligand: ^{3}H-N-propylnorapomorphine, *Eur. J. Pharmacol.* **56:**291–292.

Titeler, M., Weinreich, P., Sinclair, D., and Seeman, P., 1978, Multiple receptors for brain dopamine, *Proc. Natl. Acad. Sci. U.S.A.* **75:**1153–1156.

Titeler, M., List, S., and Seeman, P., 1979, High affinity dopamine receptors (D₃) in rat brain, *Commun. Psychopharmacol.* **3:**411–420.

Tsai, B. S., and Lefkowitz, R. J., 1978, Agonist-specific effects of monovalent and divalent cations on adenylate cyclase-coupled alpha adrenergic receptors in rabbit platelets, *Mol. Pharmacol.* **14:**540–548.

Tsurata, K., Frey, E. A., Grewe, C. W., Cote, T. E., Eskay, R. L., and Kebabian, J. W., 1981, Evidence that LY-141865 specifically stimulates the D-2 dopamine receptor, *Nature* **292:**463–465.

Usdin, T. B., Creese, I., and Snyder, S. H., 1980, Regulation by cations of ^{3}H-spiroperidol binding associated with dopamine receptors of rat brain, *J. Neurochem.* **34:**669–676.

Vauquelin, G., and Maguire, M. E., 1980, *Mol. Pharmacol.* **18:**362–369.

Vauquelin, G., Bottari, S., Kanarek, L., and Strosberg, A. D., 1979, Evidence for essential disulfide bonds in β₁-adrenergic receptors of turkey erythrocyte membranes, *J. Biol. Chem.* **254:**4462–4469.

Vauquelin, G., Bottari, S., and Strosberg, A. D., 1980a, Inactivation of β-adrenergic receptors by N-ethylmaleimide: Permissive role of β-adrenergic agents in relation to adenylate cyclase activation, *Mol. Pharmacol.* **17:**163–171.

Vauquelin, G., Bottari, S., Andre, C., Jacobson, B., and Strosberg, A. D., 1980b, Interaction between β-adrenergic receptors and guanine nucleotide sites in turkey erythrocyte membranes, *Proc. Natl. Acad. Sci. U.S.A.* **77:**3801–3805.

Weber, H. P., 1980, The molecular architecture of ergopeptines: A basis for biological interaction, in: *Ergot Compounds and Brain Function: Neuroendocrine and Neuropsychiatric Aspects* (M. Goldstein, D. B. Calne, A. Lieberman, and M. Thorner, eds.), Raven Press, New York, pp. 25–34.

Weiner, W. J., Goetz, C. G., Nausieda, P. A., and Klawans, H. L., 1979, Amphetamine-induced hypersensitivity in guinea pigs, *Neurology (N.Y.)* **29:**1054–1057.

Williams, L. T., and Lefkowitz, R. J., 1977, Slowly reversible binding of catecholamine to a nucleotide-sensitive state of the beta-adrenergic receptor, *J. Biol. Chem.* **252:**7207–7213.

Yeo, T., Thorner, M. O., Jones, A., Lowry, P. J., and Besser, G. M., 1979, The effects of dopamine, bromocriptine, lergotrile and metoclopramide on prolactin release from continuously perfused columns of isolated rat pituitary cells, *Clin. Endocrinol.* **10:**123–130.

Zahniser, N. R., and Molinoff, P. B., 1978, Effect of guanine nucleotides on striatal dopamine receptors, *Nature* **275:**453–455.

Quantitative Assay of Dopamine Receptor Subtypes

RITA M. HUFF and PERRY B. MOLINOFF

1. Introduction

Dopamine, acting as a neurotransmitter in the central nervous system, is involved in the regulation of a variety of behaviors in man and animals. Studies carried out over the last decade have shown that not all of the responses attributed to the release of dopamine are mediated through the same kind of receptor. Cools and Van Rossum (1976) first proposed the existence of two types of receptors for dopamine in an attempt to explain results obtained in studies of the effects of dopamine and apomorphine on stereotypy and locomotor activity. However, precise pharmacological characterization of receptors is difficult if only behavioral models are utilized. Biochemical studies have shown that stimulation of dopamine receptors can result, in some tissues, in an increase in the accumulation of cyclic AMP through activation of dopamine-sensitive adenylate cyclase (Kebabian and Greengard, 1971). Not all dopamine receptors, however, appear to act through increases in cyclic AMP levels.

Based on these observations, Kebabian and Calne (1979) provided the most widely accepted classification scheme for subtypes of dopamine receptors. Dopamine receptors that activate adenylate cyclase were termed D-1 receptors. Prototype D-1 receptors are found in the parathyroid gland, where dopamine causes release of parathyroid hormone through an increase in cyclic AMP levels (Brown *et al.*, 1977). D-2 receptors, as defined by Kebabian and Calne (1979), do not mediate re-

RITA M. HUFF and PERRY B. MOLINOFF • Department of Pharmacology, University of Pennsylvania School of Medicine, Philadelphia, Pennsylvania 19104. *Present address of R.M.H.:* Division of Cardiology, Brigham and Women's Hospital, Boston, Massachusetts 02115.

sponses through activation of adenylate cyclase. Prototype D-2 receptors are found in the anterior pituitary, where dopamine-mediated inhibition of prolactin secretion does not follow an increase in adenylate cyclase activity (Rappaport and Grant, 1974). Both D-1 and D-2 receptors are thought to be present in the caudate nucleus (Kebabian et al., 1972; Krueger et al., 1976; Zahniser and Molinoff, 1978).

[^{3}H]-Spiroperidol is widely used as a radioligand for the study of dopamine receptors. The sites labeled by this compound have the pharmacological specificity expected of a dopamine receptor (Leysen et al., 1978a). The affinities of these receptors for a wide variety of antipsychotic agents correlated well with the clinical potencies of these agents in treating schizophrenia (Seeman, 1977), suggesting that these sites are important clinically. [^{3}H]-Spiroperidol appeared to label D-2 receptors, since the pharmacological specificity of the binding sites in the anterior pituitary was similar to that determined in studies of dopamine-mediated inhibition of prolactin secretion. Whether or not [^{3}H]-spiroperidol also labeled D-1 receptors was a source of controversy for many years.

Dopamine-sensitive adenylate cyclase activity was abolished following the intrastriatal administration of kainic acid (Schwarcz et al., 1978). A marked decrease in the density of binding sites for [^{3}H]-spiroperidol was also observed following the administration of kainic acid. It was suggested that at least some of the receptors labeled by [^{3}H]-spiroperidol might be D-1 receptors (Schwarcz et al., 1978). Zahniser and Molinoff (1978) showed that receptors labeled with [^{3}H]-spiroperidol have a decreased affinity for agonists when assays are carried out in the presence of guanine nucleotides such as GTP. Similar findings have been obtained in studies of the interactions of agonists with glucagon and β-adrenergic receptors as well as other receptors that function through activation of adenylate cyclase (Maguire et al., 1976; Rodbell et al., 1971; Lefkowitz et al., 1977). Thus, the findings of Zahniser and Molinoff (1978) also suggested that some of the binding sites for [^{3}H]-spiroperidol were linked to dopamine-sensitive adenylate cyclase.

Marchais and Bockaert (1980), however, found that phenoxybenzamine completely abolished the binding of [^{3}H]-spiroperidol in the striatum without diminishing dopamine-stimulated adenylate cyclase activity, implying that the binding sites for [^{3}H]-spiroperidol are not related to the sites through which dopamine mediates activation of the enzyme. In addition, spiroperidol inhibits dopamine-stimulated adenylate cyclase activity only at concentrations at least 200 times greater than those used in binding assays employing [^{3}H]-spiroperidol as a radioligand (Miller et al., 1974; Creese et al., 1979; Zahniser et al., 1981). Under the conditions used in binding assays, [^{3}H]-spiroperidol is labeling at most 1% of the receptors that are linked to activation of adenylate cyclase. The guanine nucleotide-induced decrease in the affinity of these sites for agonists may be related to the recently discovered dopamine-mediated inhibition of adenylate cyclase activity (Munemura *et al.*, 1980). These considerations lead to the conclusion that [^{3}H]-spiroperidol does not label D-1 receptors. It should therefore be thought of as a selective radioligand for the study of D-2 receptors.

Several investigators have proposed expanding the classification scheme of Kebabian and Calne (1979). It has been suggested that as many as four types of dopamine receptors exist (Seeman, 1980; Sokoloff *et al.*, 1980). Most of these suggested classifications were based on results obtained in studies of the binding of radiolabeled agonists and/or inhibition of the binding of radiolabeled antagonists by agonists. For example, List and Seeman (1982) have suggested that [^{3}H]-dopamine labels a subclass of dopamine receptors termed D-3 receptors. Sokoloff *et al.* (1980) classified dopamine receptors as D-2, D-3, and D-4 based on studies of the inhibition by dopamine and apomorphine of the binding of [^{3}H]-domperidone. As is discussed below, agonist interactions with receptors often involve multistep, multicomponent binding reactions that can resemble reactions observed in the presence of multiple classes of receptors even if there is only a single, homogeneous population of receptors in the tissue (Boeynaems and Dumont, 1977). These complications can be avoided by the use of radiolabeled antagonists and by studying agonist inhibition of the binding of radioligands only in the presence of GTP (Minneman *et al.*, 1981).

Since most evidence indicates that [^{3}H]-spiroperidol does not label D-1 receptors, an appropriate ligand for labeling these sites was needed. Clement-Cormier *et al.* (1974) showed that low concentrations of phenothiazines and thioxanthenes are potent inhibitors of dopamine-stimulated adenylate cyclase activity. Hyttel (1978) proposed that [^{3}H]-α-flupenthixol, a thioxanthene, was an appropriate radioligand with which to study D-1 receptors. He demonstrated that the pharmacological specificity of the binding sites labeled by [^{3}H]-α-flupenthixol in the striatum resembled that of dopamine-stimulated adenylate cyclase activity. On the other hand, Cross and Owen (1980) found that inhibition of the binding of [^{3}H]-α-flupenthixol by spiroperidol resulted in a biphasic plot, suggesting that the radioligand might not be a specific ligand for the study of D-1 receptors.

2. Interactions of Agonists with Dopamine Receptors

The interactions of agonists with receptors are often more complex than simple bimolecular reactions. In many receptor systems, inhibition of the binding of a radiolabeled antagonist by an agonist results in dose–response curves with shallow slopes (Maguire et al., 1976; Hegstrand et al., 1979). The low Hill coefficients of such curves may be erroneously interpreted as reflecting the existence of multiple subtypes of receptor (see Molinoff et al., 1981). De Lean et al. (1980) reported that the interactions of agonists with β-adrenergic receptors can be described by a two-step/three-component binding reaction involving the agonist, the receptor, and a guanine nucleotide-binding protein. In this reaction sequence, the agonist binds to the receptor in the first step. The agonist-bound receptor then binds to a guanine nucleotide-binding protein, forming a ternary complex. Ternary complex formation is thought to precede activation of adenylate cyclase by catecholamines (Maguire et al., 1977). In the presence of GTP, the ternary complex is destabilized so that only the first step in the reaction sequence is detected. When inhibition of the binding of a radiolabeled antagonist by an agonist is studied in the presence of GTP, the affinity of the receptor for the agonist is decreased, and the curves become steeper (Maguire et al., 1976). Hegstrand et al. (1979) studied the effects of guanine nucleotides on the inhibition of the binding of a radiolabeled antagonist by agonists in tissues known to contain only a single class of receptors. Under these conditions, Hill coefficients were 0.7–0.8 in the absence of guanine nucleotides and approximately 1.0 in the presence of guanine nucleotides. Therefore, agonist interactions with receptors studied in the presence of GTP may follow simple principles of mass action.

Inhibition of the binding of [^{3}H]-spiroperidol by dopamine results in shallow displacement curves (Zahniser and Molinoff, 1978). The affinity of the sites labeled by [^{3}H]-spiroperidol for dopamine is decreased in the presence of GTP (Zahniser and Molinoff, 1978). Inhibition of the binding of [^{3}H]-spiroperidol by two agonists, dopamine and N-propylnorapomorphine, in the presence and absence of GTP is shown in Fig. 1. The displacement curves were shifted to the right, and the Hill coefficients were increased when assays were carried out in the presence of GTP. The effects of GTP appeared to be specific for agonists, since the dose–response curves of the antagonists domperidone and sulpiride were not affected by the presence of GTP (Fig. 1).

In recent experiments, guanine nucleotides have been shown to alter the interactions of antagonists with some receptors. Wolfe and Harden (1981) demonstrated a GTP-induced increase in the binding of a radiolabeled antagonist to β-adrenergic receptors. De Lean et al. (1982) have reported a GTP-induced change in the binding of [^{3}H]-spiroperidol to dopamine receptors in the porcine anterior pituitary. The effects of guanine nucleotides on the interactions of antagonists with receptors could

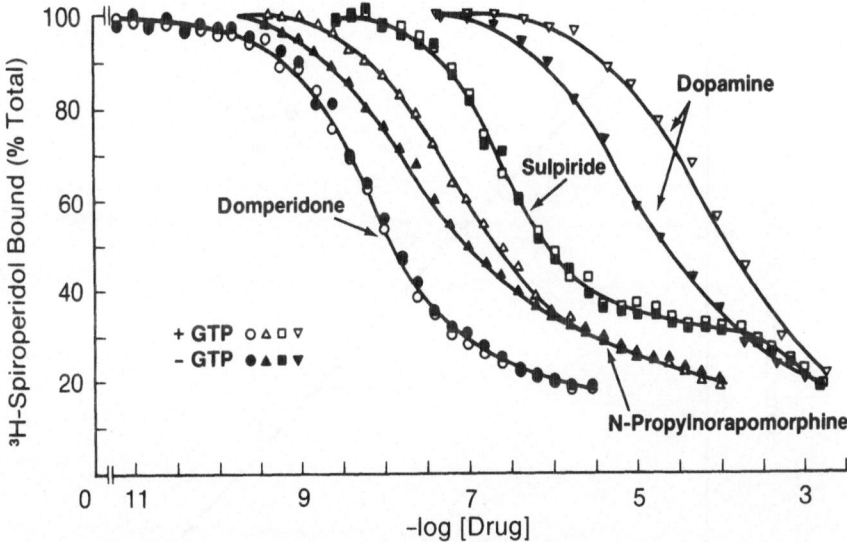

Figure 1. The effects of GTP on inhibition of the binding of [³H]-spiroperidol by agonists and antagonists. Rat striatal membranes (0.04 mg protein/ml) were incubated for 45 min at 37°C with [³H]-spiroperidol (500–700 pM) and increasing concentrations of competing drugs. The dose–response curve of each drug for inhibition of the binding of [³H]-spiroperidol was generated in the absence (closed symbols) and presence (open symbols) of 300 μM GTP. The results shown are mean values obtained in 3–7 experiments performed in duplicate.

suggest that some of the receptors are precoupled to a guanine nucleotide-binding protein (Wolfe and Harden, 1981). Complicated kinetics resulting from precoupled receptors might also be interpreted incorrectly as providing evidence for the existence of multiple subtypes of receptors. As noted above, GTP did not change the affinity of the antagonists sulpiride and domperidone for the binding sites labeled with [³H]-spiroperidol (Fig. 1). Significant effects could have been masked, however, by a concomitant change in the affinity of the receptor for the radioligand, since EC₅₀ values of competing drugs are dependent on the affinity of the receptor for the radioligand (Cheng and Prusoff, 1973). The binding of [³H]-spiroperidol in the rat striatum is not, however, changed by the presence of GTP (Fig. 2). It appears, at least in the rat striatum, that the effects of guanine nucleotides are specific for the interactions of agonists with the receptors.

Determination of the properties of receptor subtypes is difficult when radiolabeled agonists are used. In the absence of GTP, the high-affinity form of the receptor may represent only the receptors that are involved in ternary complex formation rather than providing a measure of the total

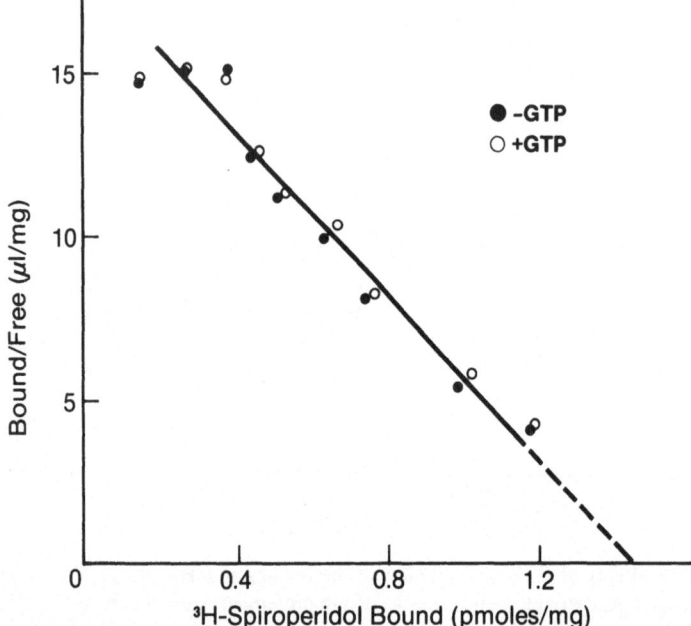

Figure 2. The effects of GTP on the binding of [^{3}H]-spiroperidol. Rat striatal membranes were incubated with increasing concentrations of [^{3}H]-spiroperidol (10–300 pM) for 45 min at 37°C. Specific binding was defined as the amount of radioligand binding inhibited by 2 μM (+)-butaclamol. The experiments were carried out in the absence (●) and presence (○) of 300 μM GTP. The data, transformed by the method of Scatchard (1949), represent the mean of three experiments performed in duplicate. The K_d values of the receptors for [^{3}H]-spiroperidol were 82 ± 6.2 pM in the absence of GTP and 84 ± 7.1 pM in the presence of GTP. The B_{max} values were 1470 ± 150 fmole/mg protein without GTP and 1530 ± 56 fmole/mg protein with GTP.

population of receptors. The affinity of receptors for agonists in the presence of GTP is often too low to be detected in radioligand binding studies using labeled agonists. Therefore, accurate estimates of the density of receptors cannot be obtained by this method. In studies designed to subclassify receptors, one must be able to determine the numbers and characteristics of receptors. For these types of measurements it is best to use radiolabeled antagonists.

3. Assay of D-2A and D-2B Receptors

[^{3}H]-Spiroperidol appears to label D-2 receptors in the caudate. As discussed above, the concentrations of radioligand used in binding assays

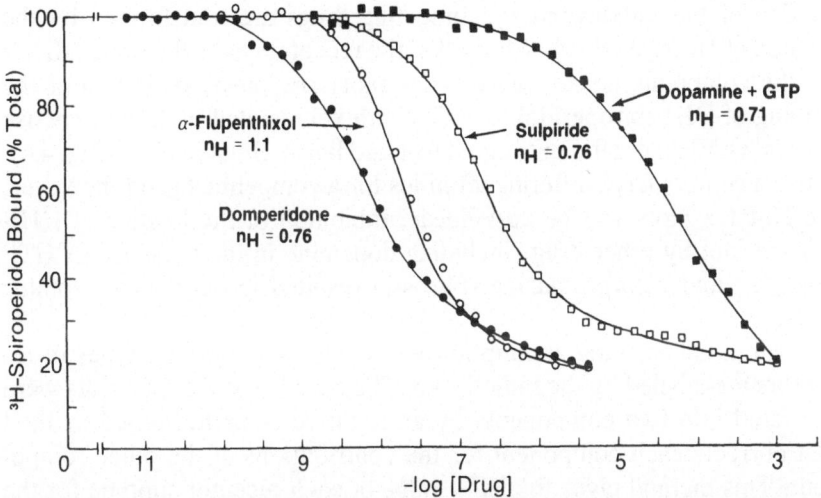

Figure 3. Inhibition of the binding of [^{3}H]-spiroperidol by agonists and antagonists. Rat striatal membranes were incubated as described in the legend to Fig. 1 with [^{3}H]-spiroperidol and increasing concentrations of competing drugs. The data represent the mean of 3–8 experiments performed in duplicate. The Hill coefficient (n_H) for each inhibition curve is shown.

are too low to allow detection of D-1 receptors. Scatchard analysis of the binding of [^{3}H]-spiroperidol to receptors in homogenates of rat striatum results in linear plots over a broad concentration range when (+)-buta-clamol is used to define specific binding (Fig. 2), indicating that all of the labeled sites have the same high affinity for spiroperidol. The dose–response curves of a number of competing ligands, however, did not appear to follow simple Michaelis–Menten kinetics. Inhibition of the binding of [^{3}H]-spiroperidol by the antagonists domperidone and sulpiride resulted in curves with Hill coefficients less than 1 (Fig. 3). The agonists dopamine (Fig. 3) and N-propylnorapomorphine, even when studied in the presence of maximally effective concentrations of GTP, also resulted in shallow curves with Hill coefficients less than 1. Since these results were obtained in studies with antagonists and studies with agonists even in the presence of guanine nucleotides, we suggested that more than one type of receptor was labeled by [^{3}H]-spiroperidol (Huff and Molinoff, 1982).

There are several means of measuring multiple receptor subtypes present in a single tissue. One method involves labeling the sites with a nonselective radioligand that has equal affinity for all the sites. This appeared to be the case for sites labeled by [^{3}H]-spiroperidol since Scatchard plots were linear (Fig. 2). Data obtained in studies of the inhibition of the binding of the radioligand by competing drugs are transformed by the method of Hofstee (1952). When all of the receptors have the same affinity for the competing ligand, the Hofstee plots are linear. Inhibition of the binding of [^{3}H]-spiroperidol by α-flupenthixol resulted in dose–response curves with Hill coefficients equal to 1 and linear Hofstee plots (Fig. 4A). If the receptors have differing affinities for a competing ligand, however, the Hofstee plots will be curvilinear. Inhibition of the binding of [^{3}H]-spiroperidol by other drugs including dopamine in the presence of GTP (Fig. 4B) and chlorpromazine (Fig. 4C) resulted in curvilinear Hofstee plots.

An initial working assumption was made that only two types of receptors are labeled by the radioligand. The curvilinear Hofstee plots were dissected into two components by an iterative computer-based method that corrects each component for the contributions of the other component. This method gives the EC$_{50}$ value of each receptor subtype for the drugs studied and the relative proportions of each subtype as determined by that drug. This type of analysis has been used successfully for the quantitative determination of β_1- and β_2-adrenergic receptor subtypes in tissues that contain both populations of receptors (Minneman et al., 1979). The initial assumption of the presence of only two subtypes labeled by the radioligand was tested in studies using a variety of competing ligands. If only two classes of receptors are present, the relative proportions of the two classes of receptors should be the same regardless of the agent used for the determination. Since [^{3}H]-spiroperidol was shown to be nonselective for the sites that it labels, and studies with several competing ligands resulted in curvilinear Hofstee plots, this method of analysis was utilized to quantitate dopamine receptor subtypes in rat striatum.

Experiments carried out with several antagonists and two agonists in the presence of GTP revealed that the binding sites for [^{3}H]-spiroperidol could be separated into two populations of receptors. In each case, the results were consistent with the existence of two populations of receptors present in a ratio of approximately 3 to 1. Thus, our assumption that only two classes of receptors are present appears to be valid (Table I). Two drugs, α-flupenthixol and spiroperidol, were shown to be nonselective for either class of receptor. The smaller class of receptors, called D-2A receptors, had a higher affinity for the antagonists domperidone and bromocriptine and the agonist dopamine than the larger class of sites, called D-2B. On the other hand, D-2B receptors had a higher affinity than D-2A receptors for the antagonists sulpiride, fluphenazine, chlorpromazine, and (+)-butaclamol and for the agonist N-propylnorapomorphine.

A second method of measuring multiple receptor subtypes involves choosing a radioligand for which the putative populations of receptors

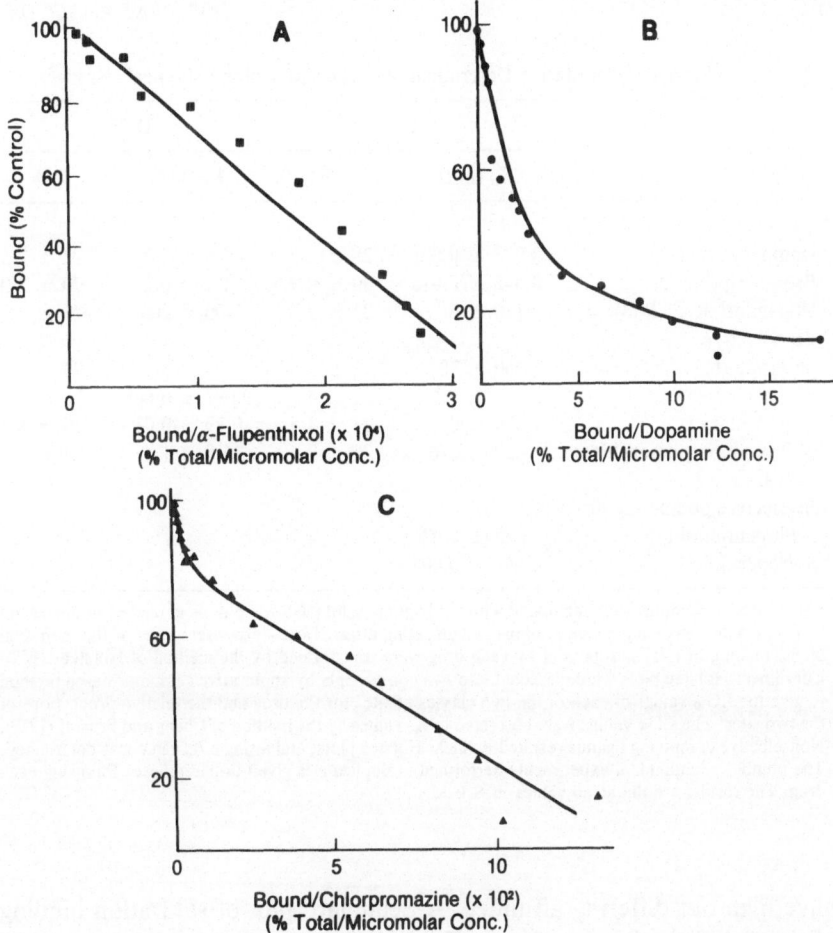

Figure 4. Hofstee plots of the inhibition of the binding of [³H]-spiroperidol by competing drugs. Rat striatal membranes were incubated as described in the legend to Fig. 1 with [³H]-spiroperidol and increasing concentrations of competing drugs. The data, mean values determined in duplicate in three experiments, were transformed by the method of Hofstee (1952). The amount of drug bound (% control) is plotted against the amount bound divided by the concentration of competing drug. The concentration of competing drug is micromoles per liter. A: Hofstee transformation of data obtained in studies of the inhibition of the binding of [³H]-spiroperidol by α-flupenthixol. B: Hofstee transformation of data obtained in studies of the inhibition of the binding of [³H]-spiroperidol by dopamine in the presence of 300 μM GTP. The data were dissected into two components of binding sites by an iterative computer-based method; 17% of the receptors had an EC_{50} value for dopamine of 0.52 μM, and 83% of the receptors had an EC_{50} value for dopamine of 33 μM. The curve represents the theoretical Hofstee plot for the two-site model that best fits the experimental data. C: Hofstee transformation of data obtained in studies of the inhibition of the binding of [³H]-spiroperidol by chlorpromazine. The data were dissected into two components of binding sites; 80% of the sites had an affinity for chlorpromazine of 0.058 μM, and 20% of the sites had an affinity for chlorpromazine of 5.8 μM. The curve represents the theoretical Hofstee plot for a two-site model with affinities and proportions of each class as determined from the experimental data.

Table I. Quantitative Determination of D-2 Receptor Subtypes[a]

	D-2A		D-2B	
	K_d (nM)	%	K_d (nM)	%
D-2A selective				
Domperidone (7)	0.093 ± 0.001	28 ± 2.5	1.8 ± 0.2	72 ± 2.5
Bromocriptine (3)	0.042 ± 0.018	30 ± 2.9	1.1 ± 0.2	70 ± 2.9
Dopamine + GTP (3)	130 ± 6	23 ± 2.7	5300 ± 200	77 ± 2.7
D-2B selective				
Sulpiride (6)	450 ± 70	20 ± 3.3	16 ± 3	80 ± 3.3
Fluphenazine (5)	1.4 ± 0.4	25 ± 4.5	0.097 ± 0.008	75 ± 4.5
Butaclamol (5)	8.0 ± 0.3	21 ± 4.5	0.29 ± 0.03	79 ± 4.5
N-Propylnorapomorphine + GTP (7)	420 ± 210	26 ± 2.4	6.5 ± 1.4	74 ± 2.4
Nonselective competing drugs				
α-Flupenthixol (3)	0.25 ± 0.02			
Spiroperidol (4)	0.047 ± 0.005			

[a] Rat striatal membranes were incubated with [³H]-spiroperidol (500–700 pM) as described in the legend to Fig. 1 with increasing concentrations of competing drugs. Dose–response curves of the inhibition of the binding of [³H]-spiroperidol by each drug were transformed by the method of Hofstee (1952). Curvilinear Hofstee plots were dissected into two components by an iterative computer-based method to give the EC_{50} values of each of the two classes of sites for the drug and the relative proportions of the two sites. The EC_{50} values were corrected to K_d values by the method of Cheng and Prusoff (1973). Nonselective competing ligands resulted in linear Hofstee plots, and a single K_d value was determined. The number of individual experiments performed in duplicate is given in parentheses following each drug. The results are the mean values ± S.E.M.

have high but differing affinities. A Scatchard plot of saturation binding of the radioligand is curvilinear if the tissue contains multiple classes of receptors. Such curves can be dissected into two components by an iterative computer-assisted method. [³H]-Domperidone, an antagonist that gives curvilinear Hofstee plots for inhibition of the binding of [³H]-spiroperidol, was recently introduced as a radioligand (Martres *et al.*, 1978). Like spiroperidol, domperidone is a weak inhibitor of dopamine-stimulated adenylate cyclase activity (Laduron and Leysen, 1979) and therefore probably does not label D-1 receptors. Scatchard analysis of the binding of [³H]-domperidone resulted in curvilinear plots in the striatum (Fig. 5; Rzezniczak *et al.*, 1982; Huff and Molinoff, 1982). Studies of the binding of [³H]-domperidone showed that the radioligand binds to two components with the same densities and having the same affinities for domperidone as the D-2A and D-2B receptors described in studies of the inhibition of the binding of [³H]-spiroperidol by nonradioactive domperidone. We therefore concluded that [³H]-spiroperidol and [³H]-domperidone were labeling the same two classes of receptors.

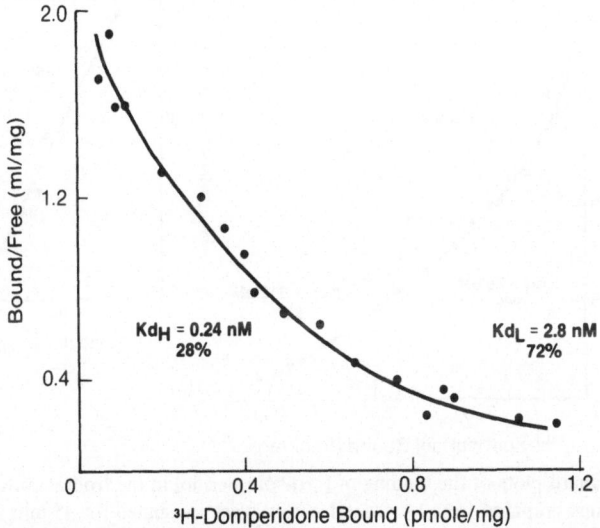

Figure 5. Scatchard plot of the binding of [³H]-domperidone. Rat striatal membranes (160 μg protein/ml) were incubated for 30 min at 37°C with increasing concentrations of [³H]-domperidone (40 pM–6 nM). Nonspecific binding of the radioligand was defined in the presence of 2 μM (+)-butaclamol. Assays were carried out in triplicate, and results transformed as described by Scatchard (1949). The curvilinear Scatchard plot was dissected into two components by an iterative computer-based method, which showed that 28% of the sites had an affinity for [³H]-domperidone of 0.24 nM and 72% of the sites had an affinity of 2.8 nM. The curved line represents the theoretical Scatchard plot that would be observed for two populations of receptors having affinities and proportions as determined from the experimental data.

The studies with [³H]-domperidone were used to provide an additional test of the original assumption that only two populations of receptors were being labeled by [³H]-spiroperidol and [³H]-domperidone in the striatum. The saturation curve of the binding of [³H]-domperidone was analyzed by nonlinear regression analysis, which determines how well the data fit model curves describing the binding of a ligand to one, two, or three types of binding sites. The goodness of fit of the binding data obtained with [³H]-domperidone assuming only one type of receptor site was significantly improved by fitting the data to a model curve for two sites, whereas postulating the presence of a third site did not improve the goodness of fit (Huff and Molinoff, 1982).

4. Serotonin Receptors in the Striatum

[³H]-Spiroperidol has been used by many investigators for the study of putative 5-HT₂ receptors in the frontal cortex (Pedigo *et al.*, 1978;

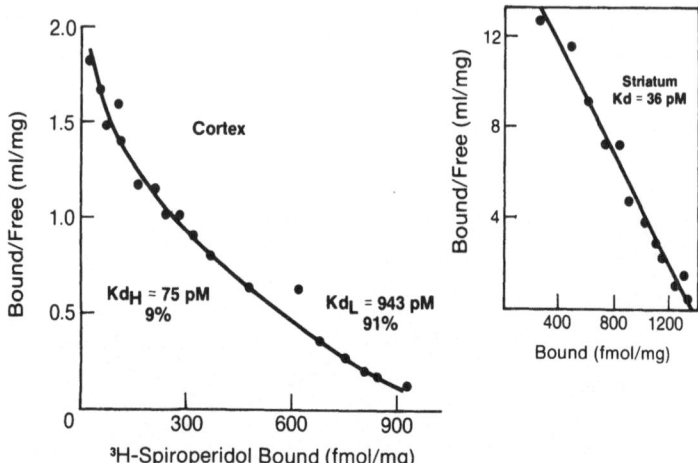

Figure 6. Scatchard plots of the binding of [³H]-spiroperidol in the frontal cortex and striatum. Membranes prepared from rat frontal cortex were incubated for 45 min at 37°C with
increasing concentrations of [³H]-spiroperidol (20 pM–7.5 nM). Nonspecific binding was
determined as the amount of radioligand bound in the presence of 2 μM (+)-butaclamol.
The data shown are from a representative experiment determined in duplicate and transformed into a Scatchard plot. The curvilinear Scatchard plot, dissected into two components
by an iterative computer-based method, gave the affinities and proportions of two classes
of sites shown in the figure. Inset: Rat striatal membranes were incubated with varying
concentrations of [³H]-spiroperidol (10 pM–1 nM) with and without 2 μM (+)-butaclamol.
The data determined in duplicate were transformed as described by Scatchard (1949). The
K_d value obtained by linear regression analysis is given.

Leysen *et al.,* 1978b). Studies of these sites show that serotonin is more
potent than dopamine in inhibiting the binding of [³H]-spiroperidol. Although the majority of the receptors labeled by [³H]-spiroperidol in the
striatum are clearly dopaminergic, it has been suggested that the radioligand may also label a small population of 5-HT₂ receptors (Pedigo *et
al.,* 1978). List and Seeman (1981) showed that inhibition of the binding
of [³H]-spiroperidol by sulpiride resulted in a shallow displacement curve.
It was suggested that the receptors with a low affinity for sulpiride were
5-HT₂ receptors. We found that this small population of receptors with
a low affinity for sulpiride, the D-2A receptors, had a higher affinity for
dopamine than the larger population of receptors (Table I). It is thus
unlikely that these sites represent receptors for serotonin.

The properties of the binding of [³H]-spiroperidol in the frontal cortex
and the striatum were compared. Scatchard analysis of the binding of
[³H]-spiroperidol in the frontal cortex resulted in a curvilinear plot (Fig.
6). Other investigators have shown that [³H]-spiroperidol labels a small

population of dopamine receptors in the frontal cortex in addition to labeling 5-HT$_2$ receptors (Marchais *et al.*, 1980). Dissection of the curvilinear Scatchard plot of [^{3}H]-spiroperidol binding showed that approximately 10% of the sites had approximately the same affinity for the radioligand as did D-2A and D-2B receptors in the striatum (Inset, Fig. 6). The majority of the sites, however, had a 20-fold lower affinity for the radioligand. Therefore, the affinities of dopamine receptors in the caudate and 5-HT$_2$ receptors in the cortex for [^{3}H]-spiroperidol differ by more than an order of magnitude. Inhibition of the binding of [^{3}H]-spiroperidol by ketanserin, a compound reported to be selective for serotonergic receptors (Leysen *et al.*, 1981), was examined in both the striatum and frontal cortex (Fig. 7). The majority of the [^{3}H]-spiroperidol receptors in the frontal cortex had a high affinity for ketanserin (see Leysen *et al.*, 1981). Inhibition of the binding of [^{3}H]-spiroperidol in the striatum by ketanserin resulted in a dose–response curve with a Hill coefficient less than 1, consistent with the existence of multiple classes of receptors. Neither population of receptors, however, had the same high affinity for ketanserin associated with 5-HT$_2$ receptors in the frontal cortex. Inhibition of the binding of [^{3}H]-spiroperidol by domperidone was also studied in both the striatum and frontal cortex. The 5-HT$_2$ receptors in the frontal cortex had a 60-fold lower affinity for domperidone than either of the populations of receptors labeled by [^{3}H]-spiroperidol in the striatum (Fig. 7). We have thus shown that the affinity of the D-2A and D-2B receptors for [^{3}H]-spiroperidol, ketanserin, and domperidone are not similar to the affinities of 5-HT$_2$ receptors for these compounds.

The most compelling evidence that the D-2A or D-2B receptors are not serotonergic comes from examination of the inhibition of the binding of [^{3}H]-spiroperidol by dopamine and serotonin in the striatum (Fig. 8). These studies were carried out in the presence of GTP so that the affinities of the receptors for both compounds could be determined without the complications caused by a multistep binding reaction and the accumulation of a ternary complex. Hofstee analysis of the curves showed that the K_d values of each population of receptors for 5-HT were lower than those of the corresponding population of receptors for dopamine. Therefore, dopamine is more potent than serotonin at both D-2A and D-2B receptors. According to classical methods of receptor classification, the D-2A and D-2B receptors cannot be considered serotonergic.

5. D-1 Receptors

To complete the study of dopamine receptor subtypes, a method of measuring D-1 receptors by means of radioligand binding assays is re-

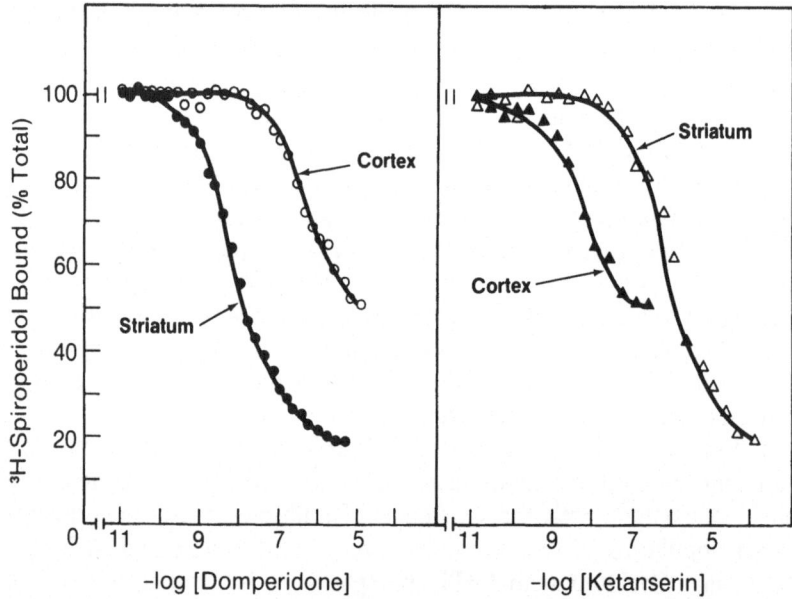

Figure 7. Inhibition of the binding of [³H]-spiroperidol by domperidone and ketanserin in the striatum and frontal cortex. Membranes prepared from rat striatum or frontal cortex were incubated with [³H]-spiroperidol (500–700 pM in the striatum and 2 nM in the frontal cortex) and increasing concentrations of domperidone or ketanserin. Hofstee plots of the data obtained in studies with striatal membranes were dissected into two components by an iterative computer-based method. When domperidone was used to inhibit the binding of [³H]-spiroperidol to receptors in the striatum, 28% of the sites had a K_d value of 0.093 nM, and 72% of the sites had a K_d value of 1.8 nM. The K_d value for inhibition of [³H]-spiroperidol binding by domperidone in the frontal cortex was 300 nM. When ketanserin was used to inhibit the binding of [³H]-spiroperidol in the striatum, 16% of the sites had a K_d value of 7.5 nM, and 84% of the sites had a K_d value of 340 nM. The K_d value for the inhibition of [³H]-spiroperidol binding by ketanserin in the frontal cortex was 2 nM.

quired. Hyttel (1978) suggested that [³H]-α-flupenthixol was an appropriate ligand for the study of D-1 receptors. However, experiments carried out in our laboratory have shown that D-2 receptors also have a high affinity for α-flupenthixol. α-Flupenthixol is one of the two compounds thus far identified that does not discriminate between D-2A and D-2B receptors. Dose–response curves of the inhibition of the binding of [³H]-spiroperidol by α-flupenthixol resulted in Hill coefficients of 1 and linear Hofstee plots (Fig. 4). Scatchard analysis of the binding of [³H]-α-flupenthixol in the striatum also resulted in linear plots (Fig. 9). The affinity of the sites labeled by [³H]-α-flupenthixol for the radioligand was similar to the affinity of D-2A and D-2B receptors for α-flupenthixol. Thus, [³H]-

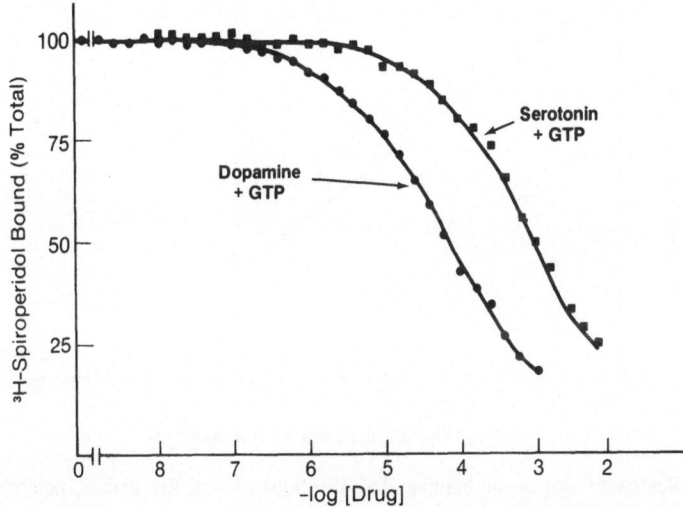

Figure 8. Inhibition of the binding of [³H]-spiroperidol by dopamine and serotonin. Rat stria-tal membranes were incubated with [³H]-spiroperidol (500–700 pM) and increasing concen-trations of dopamine or serotonin in the presence of 300 μM GTP. The data are mean values obtained from three experiments performed in duplicate. Hofstee plots of the data were dissected into two components by an iterative computer-based method. When inhibition of the binding of [³H]-spiroperidol by dopamine was studied, 23% of the sites had a K_d value of 130 nM, and 77% of the sites had a K_d value of 5.3 μM. When inhibition of the binding of [³H]-spiroperidol by serotonin was studied, 15% of the sites had a K_d value of 21 μM, and 85% of the sites had a K_d value of 920 μM.

α-flupenthixol appears to label at least three classes of receptors. To fur-ther investigate this possibility, the inhibition of the binding of [³H]-α-flupenthixol by spiroperidol was studied. A biphasic dose–response curve was obtained, consistent with the existence of multiple classes of recep-tors. A 10,000-fold difference was observed in the affinity of D-1 and D-2 receptors for spiroperidol. Therefore, nanomolar concentrations of spi-roperidol were used to block the binding of [³H]-α-flupenthixol to D-2A and D-2B receptors without interfering with the binding of the radioligand to D-1 receptors.

Studies of the receptors labeled with [³H]-α-flupenthixol in the pres-ence of spiroperidol showed that these sites resemble D-1 receptors. As described earlier, receptors linked to stimulation of adenylate cyclase activity have a decreased affinity for agonists when assays are carried out in the presence of guanine nucleotides. Receptors labeled with [³H]-α-flupenthixol in the presence of spiroperidol had a decreased affinity for dopamine when assays were carried out in the presence of GTP. These

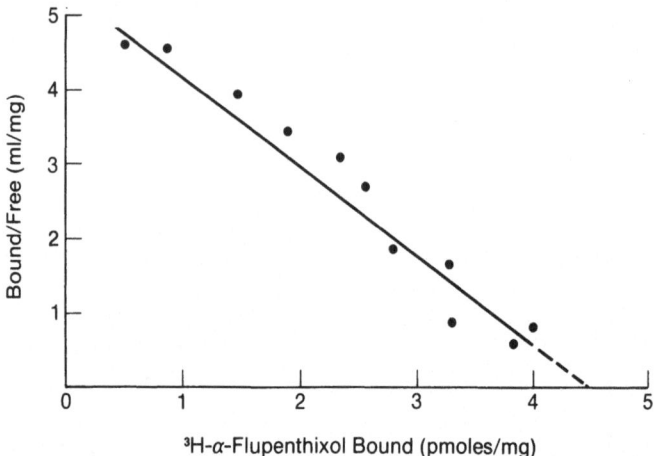

Figure 9. Scatchard plot of the binding of [³H]-α-flupenthixol. Rat striatal membranes (70 μg protein in 2 ml) were incubated with increasing concentrations of [³H]-α-flupenthixol (0.13–7 nM) for 30 min at 37°C. Nonspecific binding was defined in the presence of 2 μM (+)-butaclamol. The data shown were obtained from a representative experiment performed in triplicate. Scatchard analysis of the data gave a K_d value of 790 pM and a B_{max} of 4.5 pmole/mg protein.

findings support the possibility that these receptors are linked to activation of adenylate cyclase.

The pharmacological specificity of these sites, as defined using a variety of antagonists, still resembled the specificity determined by Hyttel (1978). These findings were not surprising since the sites labeled by [³H]-α-flupenthixol in the presence of spiroperidol represent approximately 80% of the total number of dopamine receptors in the tissue. In spite of the fact that dose–response curves obtained with the various agents for inhibition of the binding of [³H]-α-flupenthixol will be influenced by the affinities of D-2A and D-2B receptors for the competing agent, the predominant influence will be that of the D-1 receptors. Hyttel (1978) demonstrated that these affinities correlated well with the potencies of the drugs for inhibition of dopamine-stimulated adenylate cyclase activity, and therefore the receptors resembled the so-called D-1 receptors. We have found that the receptors labeled with [³H]-α-flupenthixol in the presence of spiroperidol represent a homogeneous population of receptors. The Hill coefficients determined for all of the competing antagonists (Fig. 10) and for dopamine in the presence of GTP are close to 1. Thus, D-1 receptors can be selectively studied with [³H]-α-flupenthixol and an appropriate concentration of spiroperidol.

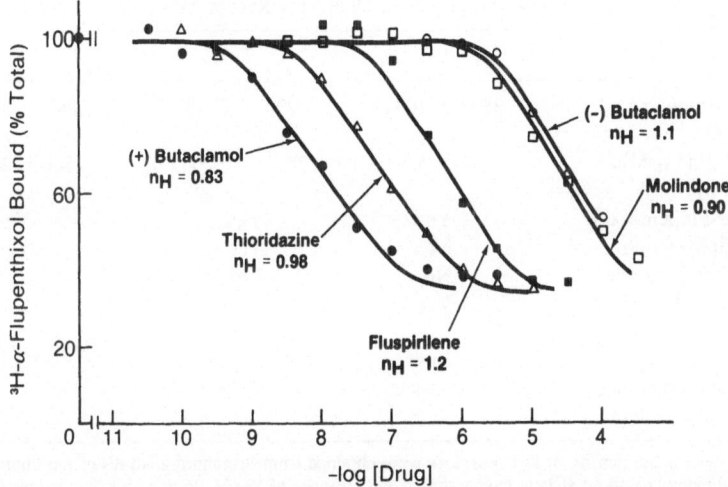

Figure 10. Inhibition of the binding of [³H]-α-flupenthixol by antagonists. Rat striatal membranes were incubated with [³H]-α-flupenthixol (500–800 pM) and increasing concentrations of competing drugs for 30 min at 37°C in the presence of 10 nM spiroperidol. The results shown are the mean values obtained from three experiments performed in duplicate. The Hill coefficients for the dose–response curve of each competing drug are shown. The K_d values are as follows: (+)-butaclamol, 8.4 ± 1.1 nM; thioridazine, 51 ± 5.5 nM; fluspirilene, 450 ± 90 nM; molindone, 13 ± 2.2 μM; (−)-butaclamol, 12.3 ± 0.6 μM.

6. Conclusions

Through the use of radiolabeled antagonists, three subtypes of receptors for dopamine have been identified. The presence of these populations of receptors was suggested by the existence of anomalous kinetics for the interactions of various compounds with the receptors. The interactions of several antagonists with the receptors labeled by [³H]-spiroperidol and [³H]-α-flupenthixol did not obey simple laws of mass action for a single class of receptors. The binding of the radioligand [³H]-domperidone also did not follow Michaelis—Menten kinetics. Complications arising from the existence of a multistep/multicomponent reaction sequence similar to those described for agonist interactions with β-adrenergic receptors were eliminated by the inclusion of GTP. The complicated kinetics are best explained by postulating heterogeneous receptor populations labeled by the radioligands. Using several techniques for the study of multiple receptors labeled by a radioligand, we have been able to characterize three subtypes of dopamine receptors. Dissection of the curvilinear Hofstee plots resulting from inhibition of the binding of [³H]-spiroperidol by several competing ligands enabled us to determine the

Table II. Properties of Dopamine Receptors[a]

	D-1	D-2A	D-2B
Density (fmole/mg protein)	3800 ± 100 (3)	290 ± 70 (8)	1040 ± 80 (8)
K_d dopamine (μM)	24 ± 5.1 (3)	0.13 ± 0.006 (3)	5.3 ± 2 (3)
Labeled by			
[³H]-α-Flupenthixol	Yes	Yes	Yes
[³H]-Spiroperidol	No	Yes	Yes
[³H]-Domperidone	No	Yes (H)	Yes (L)
Linked to activation of adenylate cyclase	Yes	No	No
Linked to a guanine nucleotide-binding regulatory protein	Yes	?	?

[a] The values for the density of D-1 receptors were obtained from Scatchard analyses of the binding of [³H]-α-flupenthixol to rat striatal membranes in the presence of 10 nM spiroperidol. The values of the densities of the D-2A and D-2B receptor populations were obtained from computer-assisted iterative analyses of curvilinear Scatchard plots obtained in studies of the binding of [³H]-domperidone to rat striatal membranes. The K_d values of the D-1 receptors for dopamine were determined from dose–response curves of the inhibition of binding of [³H]-α-flupenthixol by dopamine in the presence of 10 nM spiroperidol and 300 μM GTP. The K_d values of the D-2A and D-2B receptors for dopamine were determined from dose–response curves of the inhibition of binding of [³H]-spiroperidol by dopamine in the presence of 300 μM GTP. Curvilinear Hofstee plots were dissected into two components by an iterative computer-based method. The EC_{50} values in all cases were corrected to K_d values by the Cheng–Prusoff (1973) equation.

densities of the D-2A and D-2B receptors. In addition, we were able to demonstrate that the affinities of the D-2A and D-2B receptors for the competing ligands differed. Dissection of curvilinear Scatchard plots of the binding of [³H]-domperidone, a radioligand that has a tenfold greater affinity for D-2A receptors than for D-2B receptors, provided another means of determining the densities of the two populations of receptors. Both methods revealed that there are approximately three times as many D-2B receptors as D-2A receptors in the rat striatum. Studies with [³H]-α-flupenthixol showed that this radioligand labels the D-2A and D-2B receptors and a third population of sites, which resemble D-1 receptors. Spiroperidol can be used to block the binding of [³H]-α-flupenthixol to D-2A and D-2B receptors, allowing selective study of D-1 receptors.

Table II provides a summary of some of the characteristics of the three subtypes of dopamine receptors. In the rat striatum there are approximately four times as many D-1 receptors as D-2 receptors. Since 75% of the D-2 receptors are D-2B receptors, the D-2A receptors represent a very small portion of the total number of dopamine receptors in the striatum. However, this population of receptors has the highest affinity for the endogenous neurotransmitter dopamine. D-1 receptors appear to be linked to a guanine nucleotide-binding protein, since GTP causes a decrease in the affinity of these receptors for agonists. Since these receptors are thought to mediate activation of adenylate cyclase, these findings are not surprising. At least one of the subtypes of D-2 receptors is also linked to a guanine nucleotide-binding regulatory protein, since GTP affects the interactions of agonists with receptors labeled with [³H]-spiroperidol (Zahniser and Molinoff, 1978). An examination of the inhibition of the binding of [³H]-spiroperidol by N-propylnorapomorphine in the presence and absence of GTP (Fig. 1) suggests that only the D-2B receptor population is affected. The D-2B receptors have a higher affinity for N-propylnorapomorphine than the D-2A receptors, and the high-affinity portion of this curve appears to be selectively decreased in the presence of GTP. However, it has not been possible to test this hypothesis in a quantitative way. Present models are not adequate to describe binding reactions involving two receptor populations with differing affinities for agonists if one of the subtypes is involved in a multistep reaction sequence. To investigate the effects of guanine nucleotides in a quantitative way, it will be necessary to selectively study tissues containing only D-2A or D-2B receptors.

Munemura *et al.* (1980) have described dopamine-mediated inhibition of adenylate cyclase activity in the intermediate lobe of the pituitary. Although butyrophenones are weak inhibitors of dopamine-stimulated adenylate cyclase, they are very potent inhibitors of the inhibitory response measured in the intermediate lobe. Receptors for [³H]-spiroperidol have also been demonstrated in this tissue (Sibley and Creese, 1980). It is possible that these binding sites are dopamine receptors that are linked to inhibition of adenylate cyclase activity. If so, [³H]-spiroperidol binding sites in other tissues may also mediate the same response. It is possible that one of the D-2 receptors characterized with *in vitro* radioligand binding studies in the striatum will be linked to this response. The physiological response of the other class of D-2 receptors cannot be surmised at this time, but studies using selective drugs may reveal that one or several of the many known dopamine-mediated responses involves activation of this population of receptors. The ultimate goal of these investigations is to identify subclasses of dopamine receptors that are selectively associated with specific therapeutic effects of agonists or antagonists thought to act through dopamine receptors.

ACKNOWLEDGMENT. This work was supported by the U.S. Public Health Service (Grant NS 18591).

References

Boeynaems, J. M., and Dumont, J. E., 1977, The two-step model of ligand-receptor interaction, *Mol. Cell. Endocrinol.* **7**:33–47.

Brown, E. M., Carroll, R. J., and Aurbach, G. D., 1977, Dopaminergic stimulation of cyclic AMP accumulation and parathyroid hormone release from dispersed bovine parathyroid cells, *Proc. Natl. Acad. Sci. U.S.A.* **74**:4210–4213.

Cheng, Y-C., and Prusoff, W. H., 1973, Relationship between the inhibition constant (K_I) and the concentration of inhibitor which causes 50 percent inhibition (I_{50}) of an enzymatic reaction, *Biochem. Pharmacol.* **22**:3099–3108.

Clement-Cormier, Y. C., Kebabian, J. W., Petzold, G. L., and Greengard, P., 1974, Dopamine-sensitive adenylate cyclase in mammalian brain: A possible site of action of antipsychotic drugs, *Proc. Natl. Acad. Sci. U.S.A.* **71**:1113–1117.

Cools, A. R., and Van Rossam, J. M., 1976, Excitation-mediating and inhibition-mediating dopamine-receptors: A new concept towards a better understanding of electrophysiological, biochemical, pharmacological, functional, and clinical data, *Psychopharmacologia* **45**:243–254.

Creese, I., Stewart, K., and Snyder, S. H., 1979, Species variations in dopamine receptor binding, *Eur. J. Pharmacol.* **60**:55–66.

Cross, A. J., and Owen, F., 1980, Characteristics of ^{3}H-*cis*-flupenthixol binding to calf brain membranes, *Eur. J. Pharmacol.* **65**:341–347.

De Lean, A., Stadel, J. M., and Lefkowitz, R. J., 1980, A ternary complex model explains the agonist-specific binding properties of the adenylate cyclase-coupled β-adrenergic receptor, *J. Biol. Chem.* **255**:7108–7117.

De Lean, A., Kilpatrick, B. F., and Caron, M. G., 1982, Guanine nucleotides regulate both dopaminergic agonist and antagonist binding in porcine anterior pituitary, *Endocrinology* **110**:1064–1066.

Hegstrand, L. R., Minneman, K. P., and Molinoff, P. B., 1979, Multiple effects of guanosine triphosphate on *beta* adrenergic receptors and adenylate cyclase activity in rat heart, lung and brain, *J. Pharmacol. Exp. Ther.* **210**:215–221.

Hofstee, B. H. J., 1952, On the evaluation of the constants V_m and K_m in enzyme reactions, *Science* **116**:329–331.

Huff, R. M., and Molinoff, P. B., 1982, Quantitative determination of dopamine receptor subtypes not linked to activation of adenylate cyclase in rat striatum, *Proc. Natl. Acad. Sci. U.S.A.* **79**:7561–7565.

Hyttel, J., 1978, Effects of neuroleptics on ^{3}H-haloperidol and ^{3}H-*cis*(Z)-flupenthixol binding and on adenylate cyclase activity *in vitro*, *Life Sci.* **23**:551–556.

Kebabian, J. W., and Calne, D. B., 1979, Multiple receptors for dopamine, *Nature* **277**:93–96.

Kebabian, J. W., and Greengard, P., 1971, Dopamine-sensitive adenyl cyclase: Possible role in synaptic transmission, *Science* **174**:1346–1349.

Kebabian, J. W., Petzold, G. L., and Greengard, P., 1972, Dopamine-sensitive adenylate cyclase in caudate nucleus of rat brain, and its similarity to the "dopamine receptor," *Proc. Natl. Acad. Sci. U.S.A.* **69**:2145–2149.

Krueger, B. K., Forn, J., Walters, J. R., Roth, R. H., and Greengard, P., 1976, Stimulation by dopamine of adenosine cyclic 3′,5′-monophosphate formation in rat caudate nucleus: Effect of lesions of the nigro-neostriatal pathway, *Mol. Pharmacol.* **12**:639–648.

Laduron, P. M., and Leysen, J. E., 1979, Domperidone, a specific *in vitro* dopamine antagonist, devoid of *in vivo* central dopaminergic activity, *Biochem. Pharmacol.* **28**:2161–2165.

Lefkowitz, R. J., Mullikin, D., Wood, C. L., Gore, T. B., and Mukherjee, C., 1977, Regulation of prostaglandin receptors by prostaglandins and guanine nucleotides in frog erythrocytes, *J. Biol. Chem.* **252**:5295–5303.

Leysen, J. E., Gommeren, W., and Laduron, P. M., 1978a, Spiperone: A ligand of choice for neuroleptic receptors. I. Kinetics and characteristics of *in vitro* binding, *Biochem. Pharmacol.* **27**:307–316.

Leysen, J. E., Niemegeers, C. J. E., Tollenaere, J. P., and Laduron, P. M., 1978b, Serotonergic component of neuroleptic receptors, *Nature* **272**:168–171.

Leysen, J. E., Awouters, F., Kennis, L., Laduron, P. M., Vandenberk, J., and Janssen, P. A. J., 1981, Receptor binding profile of R 41 468, a novel antagonist at 5-HT$_2$ receptors, *Life Sci.* **28**:1015–1022.

List, S. J., and Seeman, P., 1981, Resolution of dopamine and serotonin receptor components of [^{3}H]spiperone binding to rat brain regions, *Proc. Natl. Acad. Sci. U.S.A.* **78**:2620–2624.

List, S. J., and Seeman, P., 1982, [^{3}H]-Dopamine labeling of D$_3$ dopaminergic sites in human, rat, and calf brain, *J. Neurochem.* **39**:1363–1373.

Maguire, M. E., Van Arsdale, P. M., and Gilman, A. G., 1976, An agonist-specific effect of guanine nucleotides on binding to the *beta* adrenergic receptor, *Mol. Pharmacol.* **12**:335–339.

Maguire, M. E., Ross, E. M., and Gilman, A. G., 1977, β-Adrenergic receptor: Ligand binding properties and the interaction with adenylyl cyclase, *Adv. Cyclic Nucleotide Res.* **8**:1–83.

Marchais, D., and Bockaert, J., 1980, Is there a connection between high affinity [^{3}H]-spiperone binding sites and DA-sensitive adenylate cyclase in corpus striatum?, *Biochem. Pharmacol.* **29**:1331–1336.

Marchais, D., Tassin, J. P., and Bockaert, J., 1980, Dopaminergic component of [^{3}H]spiroperidol binding in the rat anterior cerebral cortex, *Brain Res.* **183**:235–240.

Martres, M.-P., Baudry, M., and Schwartz, J.-C., 1978, Characterization of ^{3}H-domperidone binding on striatal dopamine receptors, *Life Sci.* **23**:1781–1784.

Miller, R. J., Horn, A. S., and Iversen, L. L., 1974, The action of neuroleptic drugs on dopamine-stimulated adenosine cyclic 3′,5′-monophosphate production in rat neostriatum and limbic forebrain, *Mol. Pharmacol.* **10**:759–766.

Minneman, K. P., Hegstrand, L. R., and Molinoff, P. B., 1979, Simultaneous determination of *beta*-1 and *beta*-2-adrenergic receptors in tissues containing both receptor subtypes, *Mol. Pharmacol.* **16**:34–46.

Minneman, K. P., Pittman, R. N., and Molinoff, P. B., 1981, β-Adrenergic receptor subtypes: Properties, distribution, and regulation, *Annu. Rev. Neurosci.* **4**:419–461.

Molinoff, P. B., Wolfe, B. B., and Weiland, G. A., 1981, Quantitative analysis of drug–receptor interactions. II. Determination of the properties of receptor subtypes, *Life Sci.* **29**:427–443.

Munemura, M., Cote, T. E., Tsuruta, K., Eskay, R. L., and Kebabian, J. W., 1980, The dopamine receptor in the intermediate lobe of the rat pituitary gland: Pharmacological characterization, *Endocrinology* **107**:1676–1683.

Pedigo, N. W., Reisine, T. K., Fields, J. Z., and Yamamura, H. I., 1978, ^{3}H-Spiroperidol binding to two receptor sites in both the corpus striatum and frontal cortex, *Eur. J. Pharmacol.* **50**:451–453.

Rappaport, R. S., and Grant, N. H., 1974, Growth hormone releasing factor of microbial origin, *Nature* **248**:73–75.

Rodbell, M., Krans, H. M. J., Pohl, S. L., and Birnbaumer, L., 1971, The glucagon-sensitive adenyl cyclase system in plasma membranes of rat liver. IV. Effects of guanyl nucleotides on binding of (^{125}I)-glucagon, *J. Biol. Chem.* **246**:1872–1876.

Rzezniczak, H. W., Gundlach, A. L., and Beart, P. M., 1982, Labelling of high (D-2 receptor) and low affinity sites by [³H]domperidone in homogenates of the corpus striatum of the rat, *Neurosci. Lett.* **30**:63–68.

Scatchard, G., 1949, The attractions of proteins for small molecules and ions, *Ann. N.Y. Acad. Sci.* **51**:660–671.

Schwarcz, R., Creese, I., Coyle, J. T., and Snyder, S. H., 1978, Dopamine receptors localised on cerebral cortical afferents to rat corpus striatum, *Nature* **271**:766–768.

Seeman, P., 1977, Anti-schizophrenic drugs—membrane receptor sites of action, *Biochem. Pharmacol.* **26**:1741–1748.

Seeman, P., 1980, Brain dopamine receptors, *Pharmacol. Rev.* **32**:229–313.

Sibley, D. R., and Creese, I., 1980, Dopamine receptor binding in bovine intermediate lobe pituitary membranes, *Endocrinology* **107**:1405–1409.

Sokoloff, P., Martres, M. P., and Schwartz, J. C., 1980, Three classes of dopamine receptor (D-2, D-3, D-4) identified by binding studies with ³H-apomorphine and ³H-domperidone, *Naunyn Schmiedebergs Arch. Pharmacol.* **315**:89–102.

Wolfe, B. B., and Harden, T. K., 1981, Guanine nucleotides modulate the affinity of antagonists at β-adrenergic receptors, *J. Cyclic Nucleotide Res.* **7**:303–312.

Zahniser, N. R., and Molinoff, P. B., 1978, Effect of guanine nucleotides on striatal dopamine receptors, *Nature* **275**:453–455.

Zahniser, N. R., Heidenreich, K. A., and Molinoff, P. B., 1981, Binding of [³H]amino-6,7-dihydroxy-1,2,3,4-tetrahydronaphthalene to rat striatal membranes. Effects of purine nucleotides and ultraviolet irradiation, *Mol. Pharmacol.* **19**:372–378.

4

Structure–Activity Relationships of Dopamine Receptor Agonists

CARL KAISER

1. Introduction

Dopamine (DA*), which is chemically defined as β-(3,4-dihydroxy-phenyl)ethylamine, 3-hydroxytyramine, or 5-(2-aminoethyl)-1,2-benze-nediol, was first synthesized in 1910 (Mannich and Jacobsohn, 1910). At that time it was classified as a sympathomimetic amine because only its epinephrinelike actions were known (Barger and Dale, 1910). Although its formation from L-Tyr via L-DOPA was recognized (Blaschko, 1939; Holtz, 1939), DA was not identified in the mammalian organism and shown to have pharmacological actions differing from those of epineph-rine until 1942 (Holtz *et al.*, 1942). It was first shown to be present in mammalian tissue by Goodall (1950a,b, 1951). Blaschko (1957) first sug-gested an independent physiological role for DA in the periphery. More recently, DA has been identified as a neurotransmitter in the CNS (Carls-son *et al.*, 1958; Carlsson, 1959; Goodall and Alton, 1968; Hornykiewicz, 1971).

In the relatively short time since its identification as a neurotrans-mitter, DA has surpassed acetylcholine and norepinephrine as the most extensively investigated neurotransmitter in the nervous system. Dopa-mine has also been shown to have hormonal functions. As a consequence,

---

* The abbreviations used are: DA, dopamine; DOPA, 3,4-dihydroxyphenylalanine; SAR, structure–activity relationships; ADTN, 2-amino-6,7-dihydroxy-1,2,3-4-tetrahydrona-phthalene; A-5,6-DTN, 2-amino-5,6-dihydroxy-1,2,3,4-tetrahydronaphthalene.

CARL KAISER • Smith Kline & French Laboratories, Research and Development Di-vision, Philadelphia, Pennsylvania 19101.

DA and various DA receptor agonists have been utilized clinically for the treatment of certain neurological, endocrinologic, and a variety of other disorders (Calne and Larsen, 1983). Studies on new classes of dopaminergic agents, their mode of interaction with DA receptor(s), and SAR have paralleled the dramatic increase in DA-related research, which has escalated from about 50 publications in 1967 to nearly 2000 or more yearly since 1976.

In this chapter attention is focused on the development of new classes of DA receptor agonists, SAR within some of these classes as well as among different classes, and the implications of these findings relative to the mode of interaction of these agents with the DA receptor(s). Although a great many different subpopulations of DA receptors have been proposed on the basis of anatomic location, pharmacological actions, and biochemical and binding studies (e.g., Cools and Van Rossum, 1976; Goldberg et al., 1977; Kebabian, 1978; Creese and Sibley, 1979; Kebabian and Calne, 1979; Seeman, 1980; Creese and Leff, 1982; Goldberg and Kohli, 1983; for reviews see Seeman et al., 1978a; Sokoloff et al., 1980a; Cavero et al., 1982a,b; Creese, 1982; Gower and Marriott, 1982; Offermeier and van Rouyen, 1982; Seeman, 1982), no attempt is made here to distinguish among the actions of DA agonists on the different receptor(s).

Some rationale for this approach is provided by the observation (Nichols, 1983) that the different subtypes must have originated from a common DA receptor with evolution leading primarily to modifications involving the immediate environment around the active site and in auxiliary binding loci. It is important to recognize, however, that the primary test systems utilized in this review to evaluate DA receptor agonist potency are likely reflective of action on different subtypes, e.g., those classed as D-1 or D-2 (Kebabian and Calne, 1979). Thus, the test for stimulation of central DA-sensitive adenylate cyclase (e.g., Setler et al., 1978a) is indicative of interaction with D-1 receptors, whereas displacement of spiroperidol binding (Fujita et al., 1978) is more suggestive of D-2 DA receptor modulation (Frey et al., 1982). Activation of D-2 receptors seems important for induction of contralateral rotations in rats with unilateral lesions of the substantia nigra (Corrodi et al., 1972; Setler et al., 1978b; Gershanik et al., 1983).

2. Derivation and General Classification of Dopamine Receptor Agonists

As has been noted previously (Nichols, 1983), the design of receptor modulators in general, and those of DA specifically, follows several pathways. These involve systematic structural modifications of the agonist, including derivatives that rigidly fix the conformation and configuration to fit the receptor(s), and, secondly, systematic fragmentation of agonist molecules discovered in the course of screening procedures. The derivation of agonists is usually more difficult than for antagonists because, as noted by Gund (1982), receptor accommodation of agonists requires the delicate balance of a membrane-recycling process, whereas antagonists have the option of binding to any accessible conformation of the receptor.

The fundamental approaches to the derivation of agonists of DA receptor(s) thus may follow three paths, i.e., modifications that leave the side chain intact, incorporation of the ethylamine side chain into a cyclic moiety, and discovery of novel agonists by a program of random screening.

2.1. Acyclic Dopamine Derivatives

In this general class are included compounds that retain the ethylamine side chain of DA. It is generally observed that substitution of the α or β positions of the side chain, as well as shortening the chain, e.g., to give a benzylamine, or lengthening it to give a phenylpropylamine, results in a striking decrease of DA receptor agonist potency (Goldberg *et al.*, 1968; Woodruff, 1971; Costall *et al.*, 1974; Sheppard and Burghardt, 1974). Even incorporation of the α and β positions into a strained ring system, such as either the *E*- or *Z*-2-(3,4-dihydroxyphenyl)cyclopropylamine (Borgman *et al.*, 1978; Erhardt *et al.*, 1979; Gorczynski *et al.*, 1979) and the geometric isomers of 2-(3,4-dihydroxyphenyl)cyclobutylamine (Miller, 1978), results in loss or a marked decrease of dopaminergic activity.

Several exceptions to these structure–activity generalizations are notable. For example, the α-methylated phenethylamine, amphetamine, appears to produce DA-like effects via indirect mechanisms involving release of endogenous DA and inhibition of reuptake (Carlsson *et al.*, 1966; McKenzie and Szerb, 1968; Besson *et al.*, 1969). Also, the α-carboxylated derivative L-DOPA is a dopaminergic as a result of its rapid and efficient decarboxylation to DA (Holtz, 1959). As described in greater detail in the following section, α or β substitution of the ethylamine side chain to form cyclic structures, e.g., aminoindans, aminotetralins, octahydrobenzoquinolines, and 3-phenylpiperidines, frequently results in compounds with significant DA-like activity.

Interpretation of SAR data relating to N-substitution is complicated by the many different pharmacological and biochemical test systems em-

Table I. Dopaminergic Actions of N-Substituted DA Derivatives[a]

R_1	R_2	Rats, unilateral striatal lesions, dose (mg/kg i.p.)	Rotations (min)	Net cAMP[b]	Dog, renal vascular relaxation[c]
H	H	—	—	21.0	1
CH_3	CH_3	10	0	—	—
H	CH_3	10	0	24.3	1
CH_3	$n\text{-}C_3H_7$	10	161 (30)	5.1	—
CH_3	$n\text{-}C_4H_9$	10	295 (30)	14.4	—
$n\text{-}C_3H_7$	$n\text{-}C_3H_7$	—	—	—	0.03
$n\text{-}C_3H_7$	$n\text{-}C_4H_9$	3	234 (30)	18.8	0.04
$n\text{-}C_3H_7$	$n\text{-}C_5H_{11}$	—	—	—	0.04
$n\text{-}C_3H_7$	$Ph(CH_2)_2$	—	—	—	0.007
$n\text{-}C_3H_7$	C_2H_5	—	—	—	0.007
$n\text{-}C_4H_9$	C_2H_5	—	—	—	0.04
$\text{-}(CH_2)_5\text{-}$		—	—	0	—

[a] Data from Ginos et al. (1975) and Goldberg and Kohli (1983).
[b] In vitro stimulation of adenylate cyclase of mouse caudate nucleus using 10 μM compound.
[c] Approximate potency relative to DA (McNay and Goldberg, 1966).

ployed to measure dopaminergic activity. Many of these tests are indirect and complex. Thus, the actions measured may actually be manifested by α- or β-adrenergic mechanisms. As a general rule, mono- or dialkylation of DA markedly reduces or abolishes dopaminergic activity. The only exception among monoalkylated derivatives is N-methyl-DA, epinine, which retains a high order of potency in stimulating cAMP production (Sheppard and Burghardt, 1974; Ginos et al., 1975) and in inducing relaxation of renal vasculature (Goldberg et al., 1968; Goldberg and Kohli, 1983), and N-γ-glutamyl-DOPA, which is specifically metabolized in the kidney to release DA (Wilk et al., 1978). A rather remarkable effect, which has been referred to as the "n-propyl phenomenon," is noted among N,N-disubstituted DA derivatives. This is the observation (Ginos et al., 1975; Kohli et al., 1980) that if one of the substituents is an n-propyl or perhaps an n-butyl group, then, as illustrated in Table I, significant dopaminergic activity is retained. The explanation for this phenomenon is not obvious. It is not simply a result of increased lipophilicity, as activity through the series methyl–ethyl–propyl is not continuous. Apparently a specific interaction with a hydrophobic binding site perhaps having the unique geometry to accommodate an *n*-propyl group is involved (Seiler and Markstein, 1982). As noted in Table I, it is remarkable that if one of the substituents on the tertiary amine is *n*-propyl, groups as large as phenethyl retain some, albeit weak, activity in causing renal vascular relaxation on intraarterial administration to phenoxybenzamine-treated dogs (McNay and Goldberg, 1966).

2.2. Dopamine Analogues Incorporating the Side Chain in a Cyclic System

Incorporation of the DA side chain into a ring may be achieved so that the nitrogen is part of the ring or exocyclic to it, as illustrated in Fig. 1.

2.2.1. Incorporation of the Dopamine Side Chain into a Heterocyclic Ring

Bridging the nitrogen to the ethylamine chain of DA into the catechol ring via a methylene bridge affords *tetrahydroisoquinoline derivatives*, e.g., **1a**, which has weak activity as a stimulant of rat caudate adenylate cyclase (Miller *et al.*, 1974; Horn, 1974) but is inactive in relaxing the dog renal vasculature (Volkman *et al.*, 1977). Both enantiomers of salsolinol (**1b**), as well as their N-methylated derivatives, were inactive as stimulants of DA-sensitive adenylate cyclase (Sheppard and Burghardt, 1974) but showed weak activity (1/300–1/2250 that of DA) in inhibiting [^{3}H]-apomorphine binding to rat brain striatum (Seeman, 1980). Conversely, bridging the nitrogen into the catechol ring of DA via an ethylene bridge affords the tetrahydro-3-benzazepine **2a**, which is a modest stimulant of DA-sensitive adenylate cyclase (EC$_{50}$ = 5.2 µM) and causes contralateral rotations in rats having lesions in the substantia nigra (RD$_{500}$ = 0.5 µg/rat, intracaudal administration). The 1-phenyl derivative (**2b**, SK&F 38393) is even more potent (EC$_{50}$ = 71 nM; RD$_{500}$ = 0.18 µg/rat); it is of special interest because of its selectivity for the D-1 subpopulation of DA receptors (Pendleton *et al.*, 1978; Setler *et al.*, 1978a; Kaiser *et al.*, 1982).

An alternative means for incorporating the ethylamine side chain into a ring involves connection of the terminal nitrogen to the α or β carbon of the side chain. Such an incorporation into the α position via a tetramethylene bridge affords *2-(3,4-dihydroxybenzyl)piperidine* (**3**). Behavioral effects of **3**, as well as those of its N-methyl and N-propyl derivatives, in a test for induction of body curving in mice with a partially ablated right caudate nucleus indicated a lack of DA-like activity (Ginos *et al.*,

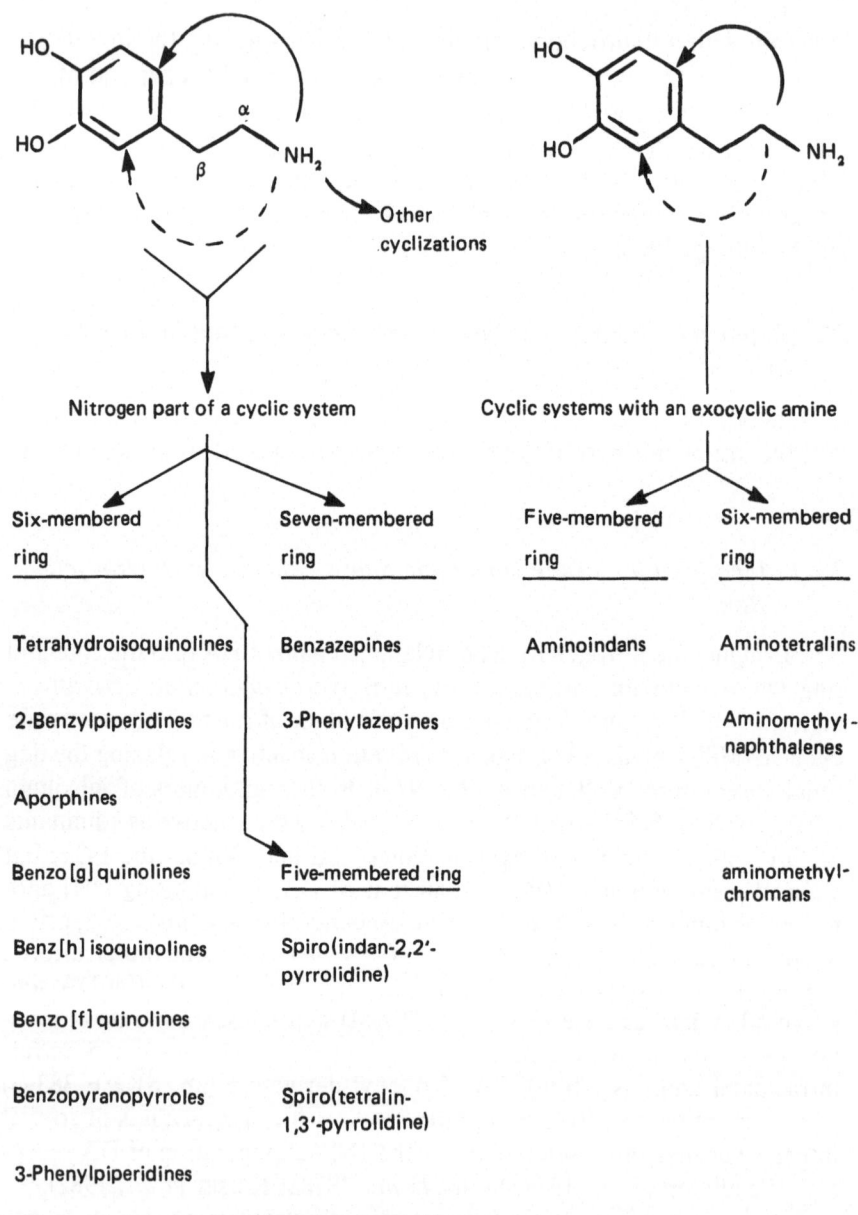

Figure 1. Dopamine analogues incorporating the side chain in a cyclic system.

1975) in contrast to the efficacy that had been anticipated for these compounds (Cotzias *et al.*, 1970).

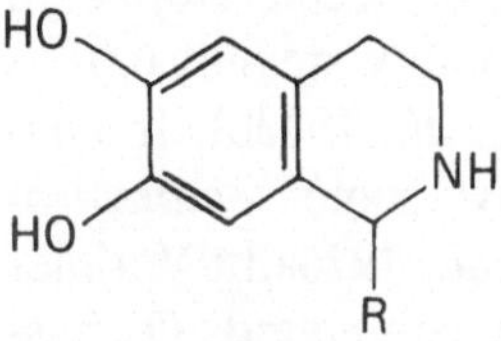

1a, R = H
b, R = CH$_3$

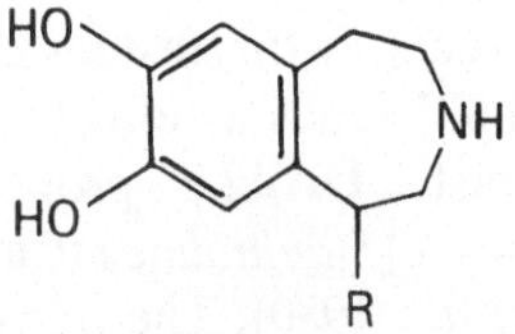

2a, R = H
b, R = C$_6$H$_5$

A more complex bridging of the nitrogen into the α position of the ethylamine side chain is observed in the alkaloid apomorphine (**4**). This aporphine derivative was first noted to have a structural similarity to DA in the early 1960s (Ernst and Smilek, 1966; Ernst, 1967; Neumeyer *et al.*, 1981a). This observation has led to an exhaustive study of dopaminergic, as well as antidopaminergic, effects of many aporphines (cf. Burkman and Cannon, 1972; Tolosa *et al.*, 1977) and apomorphine fragments (cf. Pinder *et al.*, 1971, 1972; Lal *et al.*, 1972; Dandiya *et al.*, 1975; Cheng *et al.*, 1976; DiChiara and Gessa, 1978; Sheppard and Burghardt, 1978). The SAR among aporphines related to apomorphine have been studied most extensively by Neumeyer and his colleagues (cf. Arana *et al.*, 1983; Neumeyer *et al.*, 1981a–c, 1983). Some of the compounds deriving from structural dissection of apomorphine retain a bridge between the nitrogen and the α position of the DA side chain. An example of this is provided by *trans*-7,8-dihydroxy-1,2,3,4,5,5a,10,10a-octahydrobenzo[*g*]quinoline (**5**), and some of its derivatives. These linear *benzo[g]quinolines* are noteworthy because of their near inactivity in a renal blood flow assay, lowering blood pressure, slowing resting heart rate, inhibiting the cardioaccelerator nerve, or inducing stereotyped behavior in animals (Cannon *et al.*, 1980a).

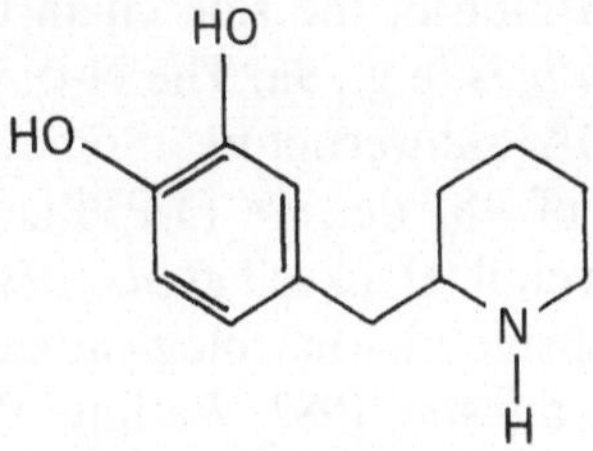

3

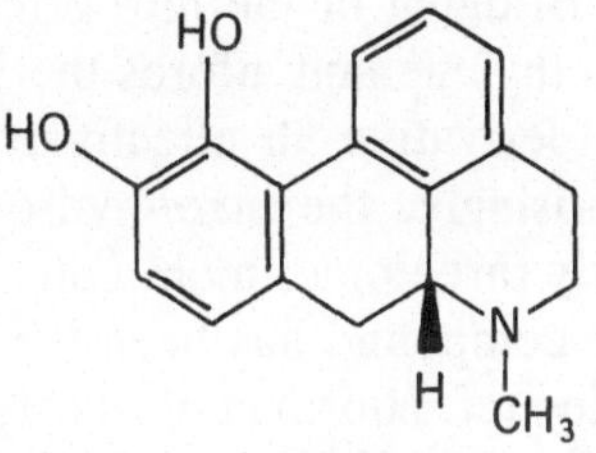

4

A similar class of compounds, in which, however, the nitrogen is bridged to the β position of the DA side chain is exemplified by

cis- and trans-8,9-dihydroxy-1,2,3,4,4a,5,6,10b-octahydrobenz[h]iso-
quinolines (6). These benz[h]isoquinolines had low potency in antagonizing the effect of stimulation of the postganglionic cardioaccelerator nerve
in cats. In this test for DA-like activity, these compounds were only 0.027–
0.073 times as effective as apomorphine (Cannon et al., 1980b). In contrast, DA-like properties are demonstrated by some octahydrobenzo[f]quinolines (Cannon et al., 1976; Sharabi et al., 1976a,b; Verimer
et al., 1980). The trans isomers of a series of these compounds (7) possessed a high level of central and peripheral effects, whereas the cis series
had only weak DA-like activity or was ineffective (Cannon et al., 1979).
In a series of monophenolic octahydrobenzo[f]quinolines, several trans
derivatives showed marked postsynaptic DA-like activity (Wikström et
al., 1982). Still another method of tying the nitrogen of DA into the β
position of the side chain is exemplified by compounds with potential DA-
like activity, i.e., some benzopyrano[3,4-c]pyrroles (8) (Loozen et al.,
1982).

Bridging of the nitrogen into the β position of the side chain by a
trimethylene unit affords the 3-phenylpiperidines, e.g., 9a. The N-(n-propyl) derivative 9b effectively stimulates DA autoreceptors. Somewhat
surprisingly, the meta-hydroxyl analogue of 9b, i.e., 9c (3-PPP), was
nearly three times more potent than the catechol (Hacksell et al., 1981b).
This compound has been the focus of extensive pharmacological examination (cf. Hjorth et al., 1981; Nilsson and Carlsson, 1982; Watling, 1982;
Watling and Williams, 1982). The exo and endo isomers of 9d have little
or no activity on the uptake of DA by rat brain synaptosomes, in displacing
apomorphine binding, or as stimulants of DA-sensitive adenylate cyclase
(Law et al., 1982), as was also the observation with various 1,4-ethylene-

bridged piperidines related to **9c** (Hacksell *et al.*, 1981b). Incorporating the nitrogen of the DA side chain into the β position of the *meta*-hydroxyl derivatives via an ethylene or tetramethylene bridge, i.e., the *3-phenyl-pyrrolidine* **10** and the *3-phenylazepine* **11**, respectively, likewise resulted in an almost total loss of presynaptic DA receptor agonist activity (Hacksell *et al.*, 1981b).

Another class of compounds in which the nitrogen of DA is bridged to the β position of the side chain is exemplified by analogues of nomifensine (**12a**), an antidepressant that inhibits presynaptic uptake of DA (Hoffmann *et al.*, 1971) with weak direct DA receptor agonist properties (Gianutsos *et al.*, 1982). *3′,4′-Dihydroxynomifensine* (**12b**) has DA-like activity in stimulating adenylate cyclase (Poat *et al.*, 1978), relaxing renal vasculature (Kohli and Goldberg, 1980), and in behavioral tests (Costall and Naylor, 1978). Apparently the aniline nitrogen in position 8 does not contribute to activity. Thus, **12c** has dopaminergic activity similar to that of **12b** (Jacob *et al.*, 1981).

Two other complex systems that incorporate the nitrogen into the α and β positions of the side chain are the spiro compounds *5,6-dihydrox-yspiro[indan-2,2′-pyrrolidine]* (**13**) (Crooks and Rosenberg, 1979) and the related *6,7-dihydroxyspiro[tetralin-1,3′-pyrrolidine]* (**14**) (Crooks *et al.*, 1980). Some of the compounds in which the nitrogen is part of a five-membered ring have weak DA agonist–antagonist activity.

12a, $R^1 = R^2 = H$; $X = NH_2$
b, $R^1 = R^2 = OH$; $X = NH_2$
c, $R^1 = R^2 = OH$; $X = H$

2.2.2. Side-Chain-Modified Dopamine Derivatives Having an Exocyclic Amino Group

Incorporation of the α carbon of the ethylamine side chain into the catechol ring of DA via a methylene unit as illustrated in Fig. 1 affords *2-aminoindans*. The resulting 4,5-dihydroxy-2-aminoindan (**15a**), as well as its 5,6-isomer **15b**, only weakly displaced agonists and antagonists from calf brain striatal tissue. The N,N-diethyl and N,N-dipropyl derivatives of **15**, however, were potent emetics in dogs and were very effective in blocking the effect of stimulation of the cardioaccelerator nerve of cats (Cannon *et al.*, 1972, 1982). Interestingly, the 4-monohydroxylated 2-(dipropylamino)indan **15c** had extremely potent DA-like activity (Hacksell *et al.*, 1981a). Further, it has been observed that the nonhydroxylated 2-(dipropylamino)-4,7-dimethoxyindan (**15d**) was equipotent with apomorphine in various tests for central and peripheral dopaminergic activity (Sindelar *et al.*, 1982; Clark *et al.*, 1982).

15a, X=4, 5-(OH)$_2$; R=H
  b, X=5, 6-(OH)$_2$; R=H
  c, X=4-OH; R=n-C$_3$H$_7$
  d, X=4, 7-(OCH$_3$)$_2$; R=n-C$_3$H$_7$

16a, X=5, 6-(OH)$_2$; R=H
  b, X=6, 7-(OH)$_2$; R=H
  c, X=5, 6-(OH)$_2$; R=n-C$_3$H$_7$
  d, X=5, 6-(OH)$_2$; R=CH$_3$
  e, X=6, 7-(OH)$_2$; R=CH$_3$
  f, X=5-OH; R=n-C$_3$H$_7$
  g, X=6-OH; R=n-C$_3$H$_7$
  h, X=7-OH; R=n-C$_3$H$_7$
  i, X=8-OH; R=n-C$_3$H$_7$
  j, X=H; R=n-C$_3$H$_7$

Joining of the α carbon to the catecholic ring of DA by an ethylene bridge via the two routes indicated in Fig. 1 affords *2-amino-5,6-dihydroxytetralin* (A-5,6-DTN, **16a**) and *2-amino-6,7-dihydroxytetralin* (ADTN, **16b**). These two compounds, both of which display striking DA-like activity, as well as various N-substituted derivatives, have been the basis of extensive research. The synthesis and pharmacology of **16a** and some of its N-substituted derivatives have been described (Cannon *et al.*, 1972; McDermed *et al.*, 1975; Volkman *et al.*, 1977; Cannon *et al.*, 1978; Sheppard *et al.*, 1978). Although minimal DA-like activity was observed for the primary amine **16a**, the N,N-dipropyl derivative **16c** was extremely effective in various tests, including relaxation of renal vasculature in dogs (Kohli *et al.*, 1982). This interesting observation of relative lack of DA-like activity for **16a**, whereas **16c** is very potent, has also been noted in a test for stimulation of adenylate cyclase (Schorderet *et al.*, 1978). Both pre- and postsynaptic DA receptors are activated by **16a** (Hoffmann *et al.*, 1980) and **16c** (Hicks and Cannon, 1979; Stoof *et al.*, 1980). The N,N-dimethyl derivative of **16a**, i.e., **16d** (M-7), is a potent emetic in dogs

(Burkman, 1973); however, its antihypertensive actions apparently involve stimulation of presynaptic DA receptors (Clapham and Hamilton, 1982). Adrenergic effects have been attributed to a number of N-monoalkylated derivatives of **16a** (Ilhan *et al.*, 1976; Maixner *et al.*, 1981).

The 6,7-dihydroxyaminotetralin **16b** is more potent in certain tests for DA-like activity; however, potency of the isomeric **16a** and **16b** clearly depends on the test system that is used (Costall *et al.*, 1982). The DA receptor agonist properties of ADTN (**16b**) have been reviewed (Pinder *et al.*, 1972; Woodruff *et al.*, 1974; Davis *et al.*, 1978; Freedman *et al.*, 1981; Woodruff, 1982); it is more potent than **16a** as a stimulant of adenylate cyclase (EC$_{50}$ = 2.63 μM *vs.* 52.4 μM) and in inhibiting haloperidol binding (IC$_{50}$ = 0.26 μM *vs.* 1.9 μM); however, it is less effective in inducing stereotypy (minimal intrastriatal dose = 36 nM *vs.* 8.9 nM) (Cannon *et al.*, 1978). Like **16a**, **16b** has marked presynaptic effects on rat striatal DA-containing neurons (Hoffmann *et al.*, 1980). The N,N-dimethyl derivative of **16b**, i.e., **16e** (TL-99), is a selective presynaptic DA receptor agonist (Goodale *et al.*, 1980; Martin *et al.*, 1982a).

Various monohydroxylated derivatives of 2-amino- and 2-(dipropylamino)tetralins have been studied (Seiler and Markstein, 1982). In various binding studies the potency was in the order: **16f** > **16h** > **16g** (McDermed *et al.*, 1976; Tedesco *et al.*, 1979; Feenstra *et al.*, 1980). In some tests, the 8-monohydroxyl derivative **16i** is devoid of DA receptor-stimulating activity; however, it acts as a central agonist of serotonin receptors (Arvidsson *et al.*, 1981). The nonhydroxylated 2-dipropylaminoindan has DA-like activity in certain tests (Rusterholz *et al.*, 1979); however, it is ineffective in others (Costall *et al.*, 1977; Sheppard *et al.*, 1978).

Two bridged tricyclic analogues of ADTN (**16b**), namely, *exo-* and *endo*-2-amino-6,7-dihydroxybenzonorbornene (**17**), had IC$_{50}$ values greater than 2000 nM for displacing various ligands from calf and rat striatal homogenates (Schuster *et al.*, 1982). Expansion of the bridge between the α carbon and the aromatic ring of DA also appears to result in a loss of dopaminergic activity. The 2-aminobenzocycloheptene derivatives **18** were devoid of DA-like activity in several tests (Rusterholz *et al.*, 1979; Hacksell *et al.*, 1981a).

17   **18**   (X=H, OH)

There are two reported examples of exocyclic amino analogues of DA in which the β position of the side chain is bridged to the catechol ring. 1-Aminomethyl-7,8-dihydroxy-1,2,3,4-tetrahydronaphthalene (**19**) is claimed (Bailey, 1982) to have cardiotonic activity. The *1-aminomethylisochromans* (**20**) were examined for DA vascular agonist activity in anesthetized dogs (Kohli *et al.*, 1979). Interestingly, the 5,6-dihydroxylated derivative **20a**, as well as its N-methylated derivative, was equipotent with DA and four- to tenfold less potent than norepinephrine as an α-adrenergic agonist. In contrast, the 6,7-dihydroxylated isomer **20b** and its N-methylated derivative were virtually inactive on either DA vascular or α-adrenergic receptors.

19

20a, X=5, 6-(OH)$_2$
b, X=6, 7-(OH)$_2$

2.3. Miscellaneous Dopamine Receptor Agonists

Among the "miscellaneous" class of DA receptor agonists are included those compounds whose structural similarity to the naturally occurring catecholamine is not overtly apparent. These have been divided into two categories, namely, those related to the ergot alkaloids and synthetic compounds of diverse chemical structure.

2.3.1. Ergotlike Compounds

The central and peripheral dopaminergic properties of certain *derivatives of ergot alkaloids*, e.g., lergotrile (**21a**) (Fuxe *et al.*, 1978; Goldstein *et al.*, 1978; McDermed and Miller, 1979; Marek and Roth, 1980; Cannon *et al.*, 1981), pergolide (**21b**) (Lemberger and Crabtree, 1979; Goldstein *et al.*, 1980; Hahn, 1981; Liebowitz *et al.*, 1981; Fuller *et al.*, 1982), lisuride (**22a**) (Horowski and Wachtel, 1976; Kehr, 1977), and bromocriptine (**22b**) (Corrodi *et al.*, 1973; DiChiara *et al.*, 1978; Markstein *et al.*, 1978; Lew *et al.*, 1979; Bannon *et al.*, 1980; Montastruc and Montastruc, 1981; Weir *et al.*, 1981), are well documented (Clark, 1979).

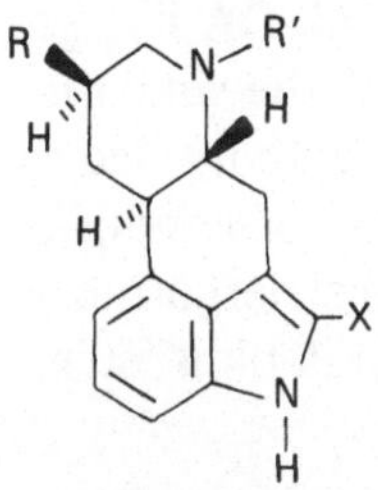

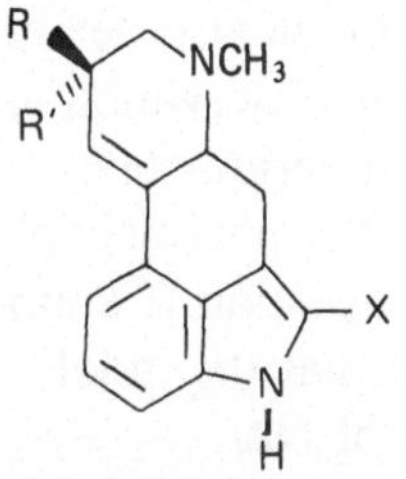

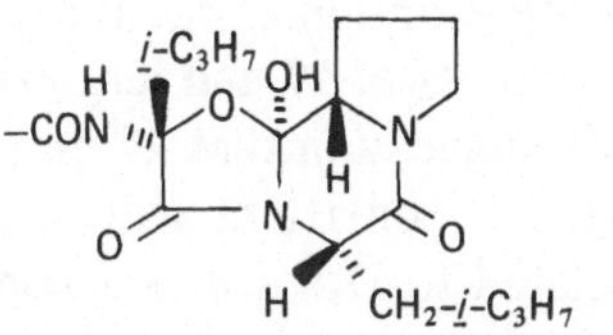

21a, R=CH₂CN; R'=CH₃; X=Cl
b, R=CH₂SCH₃; R'=n-C₃H₇;
X=H

22a, X = R = H
R' = NHCON(C₂H₅)₂

22b, R= as above; R'=H; X = Br

Like other dopaminergic agents, these ergot derivatives inhibit prolactin secretion, decrease DA turnover in the CNS, stimulate DA-sensitive adenylate cyclase, and stimulate presynaptic DA receptors. Bromocriptine and lergotrile are D-1 receptor antagonists but D-2 receptor agonists, whereas pergolide is a stimulant of both D-1 and D-2 receptors (Gershanik *et al.*, 1983). Some related 8α-aminoergolines, CH 29-717 (**23a**), CQ 32-084 (**23b**), and CU 32-085 (**23c**) have similarly been characterized as DA receptor agonists (Enz, 1981; Flueckiger *et al.*, 1978, 1979). A related compound, Sandoz CM 29-712 (6-methyl-8α-cyanomethylergoline-1) was as effective as apomorphine in four different turning models in the rat (Jaton *et al.*, 1978).

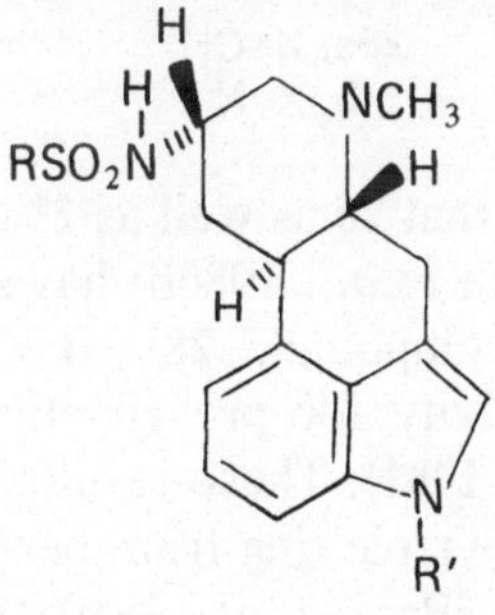

23a, R=N(CH₃)₂; R'=H
b, R=N(C₂H₅)₂; R'=H
c, R=N(CH₃)₂; R'=CH₃

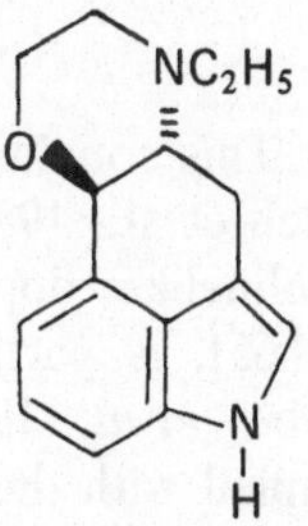

24

Another ergoline derivative, 6-ethyl-9-oxaergoline (EOE, **24**), especially the (−) enantiomer, was equipotent to or more potent than apomorphine in most tests for DA-like activity (Martin *et al.*, 1982b) and lowered blood pressure in rats by a complex mechanism likely involving presynaptic DA receptors (Sweet *et al.*, 1982).

Some simpler derivatives of the ergot-type compounds also demonstrate significant DA-like activity. Such compounds include the ergoline fragment **25** (RU 28251) (Euvrard *et al.*, 1981), which has been claimed (Bach and Kornfeld, 1978) to have DA-like properties, e.g., inhibition of prolactin secretion and displacement of DA from binding sites. The BC bicyclic partial ergoline structure **26** also demonstrates weak DA-like activity (Cannon *et al.*, 1981). This observation, coupled with the similarity of effects of **27** and lergotrile in various tests for DA-like activity, led to the suggestion that **27** may be the pharmacophoric portion of lergotrile. This is consistent with the suggestion (Cannon, 1979) that lergotrile is related to DA if it is accepted that the indolic NH group is bioisosteric with the *meta*-hydroxyl group of DA.

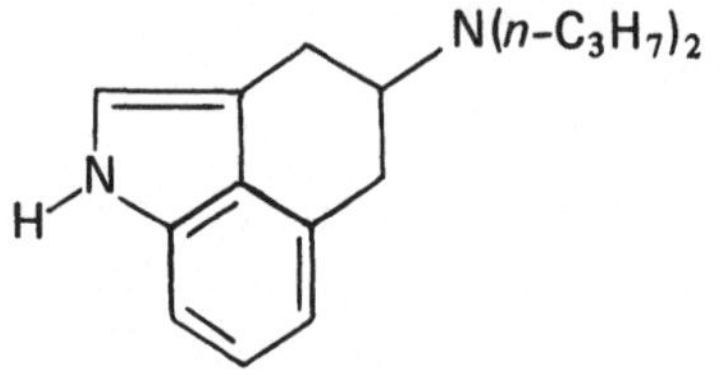

25

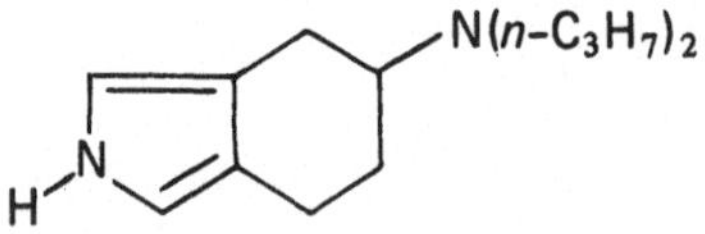

26

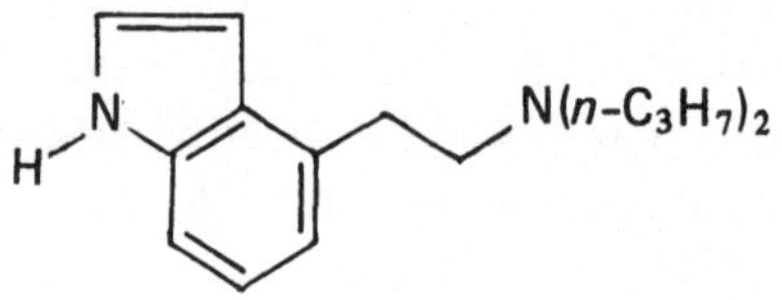

27

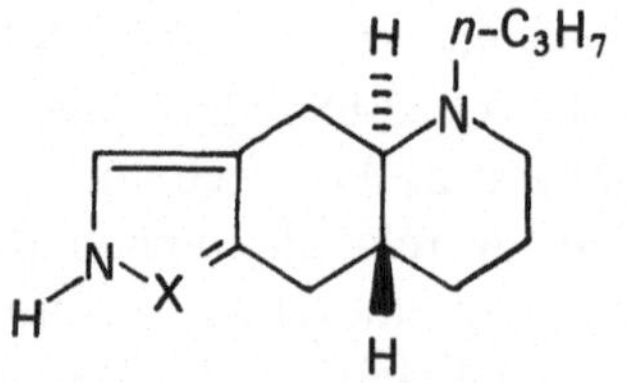

**28a, X=CH
b, X=N**

This conclusion conflicts with the observation that **26** as well as **28a** (Bach et al., 1980a) and its aza analogue **28b** (Bach *et al.*, 1980b) have ergolinelike dopaminergic activity. The latter compound, **28b** (LY 141865), is particularly noteworthy for its selectivity for presynaptic (Rabey *et al.*, 1981) D-2 receptors (Tsuruta *et al.*, 1981). These results, coupled with the observation that removal of the pyrrole ring from pergolide results in greatly decreased DA-like activity (Bach *et al.*, 1980c), suggest that the pharmacophoric constituent of the ergolines may be the pyrroleethylamine moiety. A possible explanation may be found in the slow onset on the DA-like activity of **27**. Perhaps **27** is metabolically activated by hydroxylation at the 6 position. Lergotrile is hydroxylated at the corresponding 13 position to give a metabolite that is an order of magnitude more potent than the parent (Parli *et al.*, 1978; Nichols, 1983).

2.3.2. Other Miscellaneous Structures

Several compounds of widely differing structures that are not clearly related to that of DA are capable of producing dopaminergic actions. One of the first of these agents to be recognized was the piperazine derivative ET 495 (piribedil, **29a**). It produced a long duration of contralateral rotations in the lesioned rat model in a dose-dependent fashion, and, as with direct-acting DA receptor agonists, it decreased DA turnover in rat brain (Corrodi *et al.*, 1971, 1972). Behavioral evidence in rats suggested that the activity of piribedil might derive from its metabolism to a catecholic metabolite, S584 (**29b**) (Creese, 1974). Although initial studies (Miller and Iversen, 1974) indicated that the metabolite (Jenner *et al.*, 1973) produced a dose-dependent increase in cAMP in rat striatal homogenates, later attempts to reproduce this were unsuccessful (Bockaert, 1978). Further, **29b** was ineffective on dopaminergic receptors in the renal vascular bed of dogs (Goldberg *et al.*, 1977). Also, in a lesioned rat rotational model, **29a** was more potent than **29b**, but it had only a short duration of activity at high doses (Setler *et al.*, 1978b).

Additional suggestive evidence that the catecholic metabolite **29b** may not be required for DA-like activity is provided by the direct dopaminergic stimulant activity of compounds such as 1-(coumaran-5-yl-methyl)-4-(2-thiazolyl)piperazine (S3608, **30**) (Poignant *et al.*, 1975) and 1-(2-naphthylmethyl)-4-(2-pyridyl)piperazine (SK&F 64961, **31**) (Hill and Lafferty, 1975) as well as many similar piperazines (Lafferty *et al.*, 1983) that could not be expected to be metabolized to a catecholic product. In a series of piribedil-related compounds, N-substituted 2-aminopyrimidines, e.g., **32**, showed modest apomorphinelike activity in producing stereotyped behavior in rats (Moragues *et al.*, 1980).

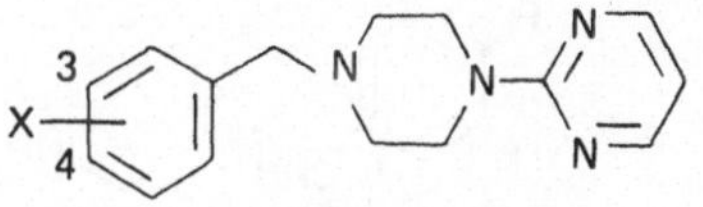

29a, X=3,4-OCH$_2$O
b, X=3,4-(OH)$_2$

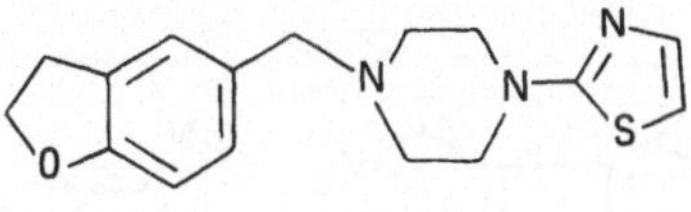

30

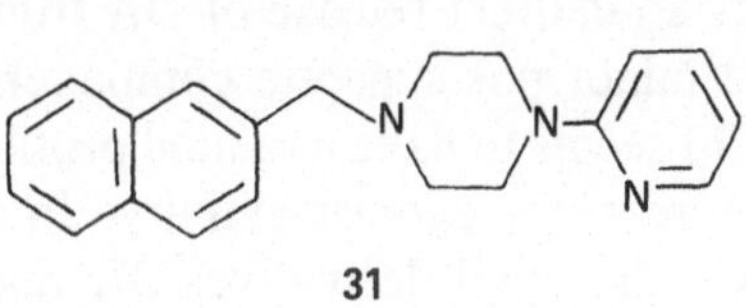

31

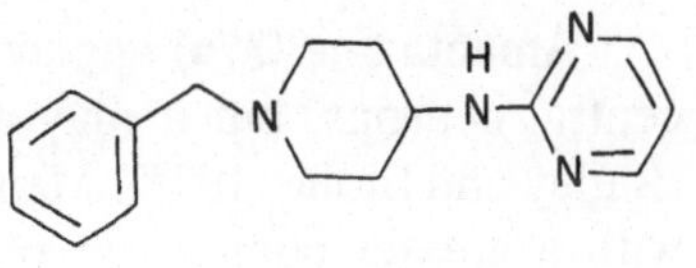

32

Another compound, 2-(3,4-dihydroxyphenylimino)imidazolidine (DPI, **33**), has been described as a potent agonist at DA receptors mediating neuronal inhibition (Struyker-Boudier *et al.*, 1975). Other studies indicated that it was a selective agonist for DA receptors in the coronary, but not renal, vasculature (Woodman *et al.*, 1981); however, recent studies suggest that **33** acts mainly as a nonselective α-adrenoceptor agonist (Baggio and Ferrari, 1981; Van Oene *et al.*, 1982a,b). An analogue of **33**, i.e., 2-(3,4-dihydroxybenzyl)-2-imidazoline (**34**), had DA-like effects in relaxing both the rabbit isolated renal and ear arteries (O'Donnell *et al.*, 1979). Perhaps significantly, the aralkylamine moiety of this molecule can be superimposed on the trans conformation of DA.

Recently, an indole derivative EMD 23 448 (**35**) that has been characterized as a nonrigid ergoline type has been shown to have DA-like activity in a lesioned rat rotational model and in displacement of ADTN and spiroperidol binding (IC_{50} = 10 and 80 nM, respectively) (Seyfried and Fuxe, 1982). Dopaminelike peripheral actions other than emesis have been described for the benzhydryl ether **36** (van Beek and Timmerman, 1974), whereas some related piperazine derivatives act as potent and selective inhibitors of DA uptake (van der Zee *et al.*, 1980).

Amantadine (**37a**) apparently causes an indirect release of DA from central neurons, but it may also have a minor postsynaptic component (Bailey and Stone, 1975). Memantine (**37b**) seems to have a related profile with a greater component of direct DA receptor agonist activity. In a series of related adamantane derivatives, the ethyl derivatives **37c** and **37d** showed weak but reproducible direct DA agonist activity in the lesioned rat model (Henkel *et al.*, 1982). Diprobutine (**38**), another compound that presents a sterically hindered amine, resembles amantadine in some of its pharmacological actions (Broll *et al.*, 1978). Dopaminergic properties have also been described for Ro 8-4650 (**39**); however, it was of little benefit in parkinsonian patients (Birket-Smith *et al.*, 1978).

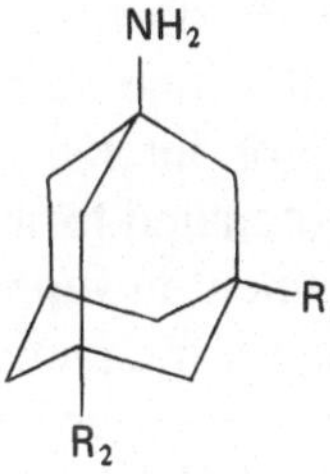

37a, $R_1 = R_2 = H$
 b, $R_1 = R_2 = CH_3$
 c, $R_1 = R_2 = C_2H_5$
 d, $R_1 = C_2H_5$; $R_2 = H$

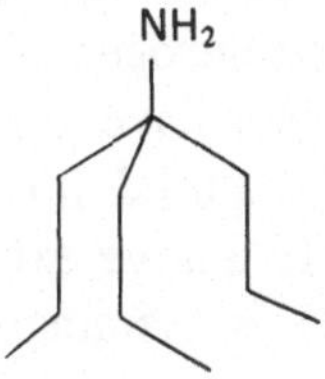

Several other compounds that lack a structural relationship to DA have been reported to have dopaminergic activity. These include quipazine (Schechter and Concannon, 1982), B-HT 920, an azepine with α_2-adrenoreceptor activity (Andén *et al.*, 1982), and nicotine (Lichtensteiger *et al.*, 1982).

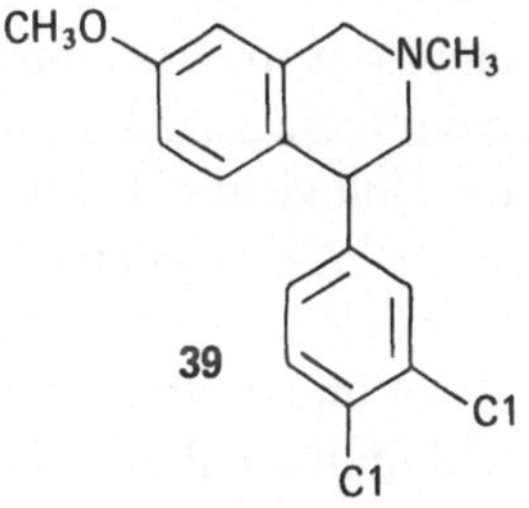

3. Structure–Activity Considerations

In order to understand the mode of interaction of DA and its various simulators with the DA receptor(s), it is important to evaluate SAR among the different classes of agonists. A primary consideration is definition of the dopaminergic pharmacophore, i.e., the essential structural features needed for interaction with the receptor(s). Many of the rigid analogues that simulate DA's activity provide information relating to the conformation that must be assumed by the naturally occurring catecholamine and other agonists in order to act on the receptor(s). A great deal of information relative to the mode of interaction of agonists with the DA receptor(s) may also be garnered from a study of enantiomers. These are particularly important because they have identical physical properties. Thus, unless they are metabolized differently, pharmacological differences between optical antipodes can be associated with receptor-related events. Another factor that may influence the potency of DA receptor agonists is biomembrane solubility, which is related to lipophilicity.

3.1. Dopaminergic Pharmacophore

Studies with acyclic DA derivatives (Section 2.1) suggest that a two-carbon spacing between the aromatic ring and the nitrogen is important for dopaminergic activity. The precise mode of binding of the nitrogen with the receptor, or if indeed a nitrogen is required, is a matter for conjecture. It has been suggested that the active form of apomorphine at DA receptor(s) is the uncharged nitrogen (Armstrong and Barlow, 1976). Others (Remy and Martin, 1980) have suggested that the lone pair of electrons on the nitrogen is required for ligand–receptor interaction. Nonetheless, DA would exist to a large extent in the protonated form at physiological pH (Miller, 1978). A seemingly strong argument in support of the latter notion, i.e., that the cation is involved in receptor interaction, is provided by the observation that the dimethylsulfonium analogue **40** is about one-tenth as potent as DA in causing contralateral rotations in rats with unilateral lesions of the substantia nigra as well as in displacing DA from crude membrane fractions prepared from the striatum (Anderson *et al.*, 1981).

40

41a, R=*n*-C₃H₇

  b, R=CH₂CH₂C₆H₄-3-OH

  c, R=CH₂CH₂C₆H₅

The requirement of catecholic nucleus for activation of DA receptor(s) is likewise not entirely clear. In nearly all instances, both of the catecholic hydroxyls are required for stimulation of DA-sensitive adenylate cyclase, a D-1 response (Kebabian and Calne, 1979), and for the receptors subserving smooth muscle relaxation, i.e., DA_1 receptors (Goldberg and Kohli, 1983). It is essential in the D-1-selective benzazepine class of DA receptor agonists (Kaiser *et al.*, 1983); however, there are notable exceptions, particularly in a series of monohydroxyaminotetralins (Seiler and Markstein, 1982).

The requirements for D-2 or DA_2 receptor stimulation, however, appear much less stringent. Thus, various ergot derivatives and even the "miscellaneous" DA receptor agonist piribedil (**29a**) are agonists of these DA receptor subtypes. For stimulation of this subpopulation of DA receptors, presence of an aromatic hydroxyl group in a position meta to the ethylamine side chain is apparently sufficient to confer activity. Although *meta*-tyramine itself is ineffective or only weakly active (Seeman *et al.*, 1978a) as a DA receptor agonist (Goldberg *et al.*, 1968; Costall *et al.*, 1974), its N,N-dipropyl derivative **41a** has DA agonist actions (Geissler,

1977). Additionally, the *meta*-tyramine derivatives RU 24926 (**41b**) and RU 24213 (**41c**) (Nédélec *et al.*, 1978) appear to be selective D-2 receptor agonists (Euvrard *et al.*, 1980).

Additional examples of adequacy of a single hydroxyl group meta to the ethylamine side chain for activation of DA receptors are found in the 3-phenylpiperidine series, where 3-PPP (**9c**) has potent autoreceptor activity (Hacksell *et al.*, 1981b), in the 2-aminoindan class (e.g., **15c**), where striking potency is noted for the 4-hydroxylated derivative (Hacksell *et al.*, 1981a), for various monohydroxylated 2-aminotetralins, e.g., **16f–16i**, (cf. Seiler and Markstein, 1982) as well as 5-hydroxy-6-methyl-2-amino-tetralins, e.g., DK-118 (**42**) (Verimer *et al.*, 1980), and in the aporphine group of DA receptor agonists, where an 11-monohydroxylated analogue **43** of N-(*n*-propyl)norapomorphine, but not its 8- and 10-monohydroxyl congeners (the hydroxyl is not meta to the ethylamine moiety), has DA-receptor agonist activity *in vivo* and *in vitro* (Neumeyer *et al.*, 1974, 1981b, 1981c, 1983; Saari *et al.*, 1974; Schoenfeld *et al.*, 1975).

It has been suggested that the weakly acidic indole NH group is bioisosteric with the meta hydroxyl in the ergot-type DA receptor agonists (Cannon *et al.*, 1981). This notion appears to be supported by the activity of the indole derivatives **25** (Euvrard *et al.*, 1981), **27**, and **44** (Nédélec *et al.*, 1980), a bioisostere of 3-PPP (**9c**).

These observations lead to the tentative conclusion that the *meta*-hydroxyphenethylamine moiety may be the *dopaminergic pharmaco-*

phore, with the recognition that appropriate simulators of the hydroxyl or the amine may suffice for receptor interaction. A further note of caution in acceptance of this pharmacophoric unit is provided by the striking DA-like actions of certain nonhydroxylated relatives of various classes of DA receptor agonists. For example, DA-like properties have been noted for 2-(N,N-di-*n*-propylamino)-4,7-dimethoxyindan **(15d)** (Clark *et al.,* 1982; Sindelar *et al.,* 1982) and its 5,8-dimethoxytetralin derivatives **16** [X = 5,8-$(OCH_3)_2$; R = H, alkyl] (Dryer *et al.,* 1980; Arnerić *et al.,* 1982). Even some ring-unsubstituted 2-aminoindans and -tetralins, namely, N-methyl-N-propyl-2-aminotetralin, N,N-dipropyl-2-aminotetralin, and N,N-dipropyl-2-aminoindan, cause various DA-like actions, e.g., emesis, inhibition of prolactin release, and contralateral circling in unilaterally lesioned animals (Rusterholz *et al.,* 1979). In addition, as noted previously, the pyrrole ring of ergolines has been suggested to simulate the catecholic moiety of DA (Nichols, 1976; Bach *et al.,* 1980a). The recent observation (Berney and Schuh, 1982) that the catecholic A ring of apomorphine may be replaced by a pyrrole **(45a)** or pyrazole system **(45b)** with retention of DA-like activity is also intriguing.

3.2. Conformational Considerations

Knowledge of the conformation(s) of DA or the tentatively identified pharmacophore that interact(s) with the DA receptor(s) is critical to understanding of the binding of these agents. Various methods have been employed in an effort to learn more about the conformational requirements of dopaminergic agents. In the solid state, DA exists in a trans conformation (see Fig. 2) (Bergin and Carlström, 1968). Single-crystal X-ray diffractometric analysis of the hydrochloride also shows that the side chain is almost fully extended, forming a plane that is nearly orthogonal to the plane of the catecholic ring (Giesecke, 1980). Nuclear magnetic resonance studies and quantum chemical calculations indicate that in aqueous solution at room temperature the trans conformation is of lowest energy, but appreciable amounts of the gauche conformations are also present (Bustard and Egan, 1971) (see Fig. 2). It seems unlikely that partially (θ = 120°) or fully eclipsed (θ = 0°) conformers are present under these conditions. Also, it should be emphasized that a preferred conformation need not be the one that binds with the receptor (Scharfenberg and Sauer, 1980). Even the orthogonal relationship seen in the X-ray is of minor consequence. It is perfectly reasonable that the side chain and the catechol ring interact with the receptor in a rotameric conformation of the ring that places it in a plane with the side chain. If this is the case,

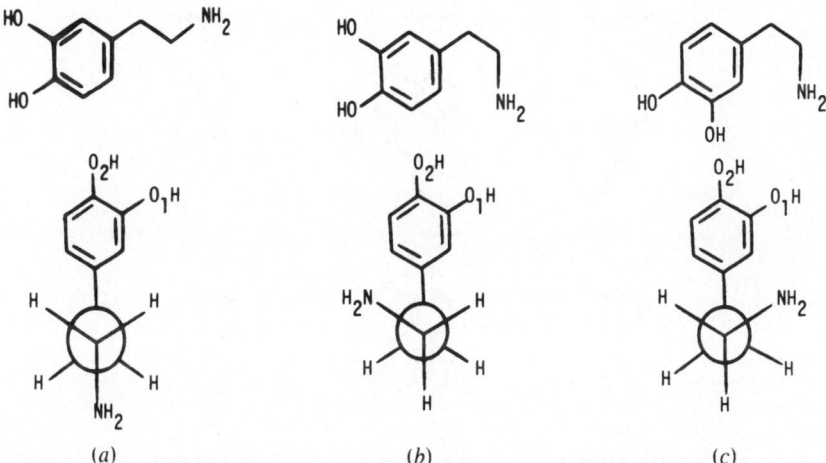

Figure 2. Structure, Newman projections, bond angles, and O–N distances for trans (*a*) and gauche (*b* and *c*) conformations of dopamine: (*a*) $\theta = 180°$. $O_1N = 6.83$ Å, $O_2N = 7.83$ Å; (*b*) $\theta = 300°$, $O_1N = 6.02$ Å. $O_2N = 6.21$ Å; (*c*) $\theta = 60°$, $O_1N = 4.97$ Å, $O_2N = 6.21$ Å.

then two rotameric extremes, the so-called α and β rotamers illustrated in Fig. 3, must be considered.

In this section, conformational requirements, including (1) aromatic ring-to-side chain orientation, (2) rotameric significance, (3) hydroxyl-to-nitrogen distance, and (4) directionality of the lone pair of *p*-orbital electrons on the nitrogen, as they influence DA-like activity are examined. This is best accomplished by analysis of rigid molecules possessing a fixed DA segment in the structure. A number of such compounds are available

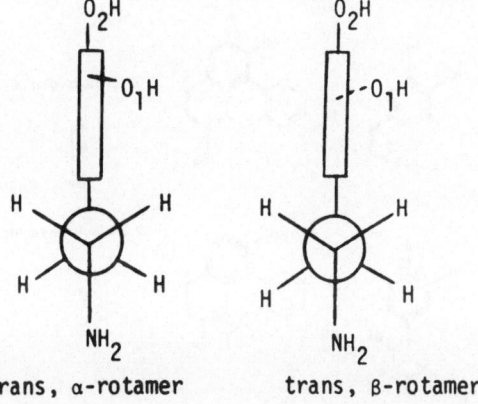

Figure 3. Newman projections of the α and β rotameric conformations of *trans*-dopamine.

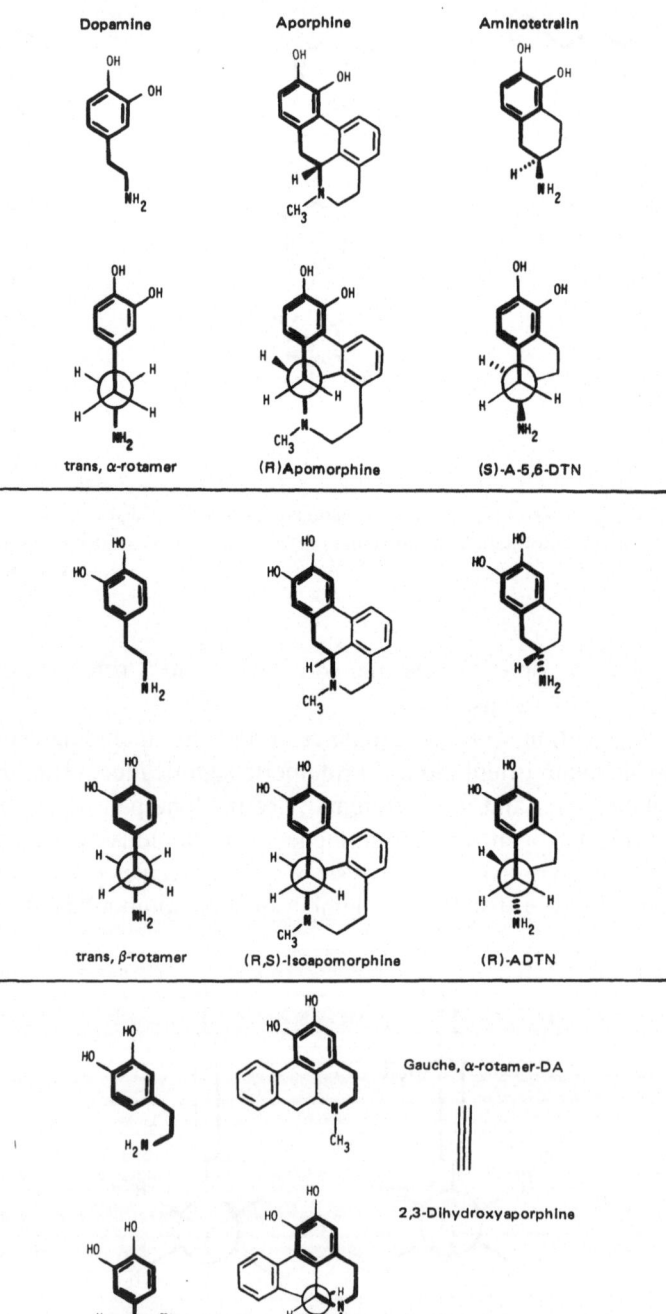

Dopamine   Aporphine   Aminotetralin

trans, α-rotamer   (R)Apomorphine   (S)-A-5,6-DTN

trans, β-rotamer   (R,S)-Isoapomorphine   (R)-ADTN

Gauche, α-rotamer-DA

2,3-Dihydroxyaporphine

Gauche, β-rotamer   1,2-Dihydroxyaporphine

in the various classes of dopaminergic agents outlined in Section 2. Here, the various conformational factors are treated generally; no attempt is made to address these subjects exhaustively.

3.2.1. Aromatic Ring-to-Side Chain Orientation

3.2.1a. Side Chain Conformation. Information concerning various conformational requirements for interaction of DA with its receptor(s) may be derived from analysis of the relationship of DA to rigid analogues, particularly those of the aporphine, 2-aminotetralin, and benzoquinoline type. Thus, as illustrated in Fig. 4, rigid aporphine derivatives, as well as the semirigid aminotetralins, simulate different rotameric conformations in a rigid, or at least semi-rigid, conformation (Neumeyer *et al.*, 1981b).

The trans α-rotameric conformation of DA is rigidified in 6aR-apomorphine, which has potent dopaminergic activity in the CNS (Ernst and Smelik, 1966), in producing DA-like renal vasodilation in dogs (Goldberg *et al.*, 1968), in causing a hypotensive effect in cats (Barnett and Fiove, 1971), in displacing DA receptor agonists and antagonists from their binding sites (Seeman, 1980), and in stimulating DA-sensitive (rat striatal) adenylate cyclase (EC_{50} = 2 μM) (Miller *et al.*, 1976). Apomorphine labels both DA postsynaptic receptors and autoreceptors (Sokoloff *et al.*, 1980b). The trans α-rotameric form of DA is also solidified in the dopaminergic (*S*)-**16a** (2-amino-5,6-dihydroxy-1,2,3,4-tetrahydronaphthalene, A-5,6-DTN), a moderately effective stimulant of DA-sensitive adenylate cyclase (EC_{50} = 52.4 μM), displacer of DA agonist and antagonist binding, and producer of DA-like behavioral effects (Cannon *et al.*, 1978; Seiler and Markstein, 1982), although it fails to produce DA-like renal vasodilation in dogs (Volkman *et al.*, 1977). These observations suggest that the trans α rotamer of DA is effective in binding with at least certain DA receptor sites.

The trans β rotameric conformation of DA is incorporated in isoapomorphine and in (*R*)-**16b** (2-amino-6,7-dihydroxy-1,2,3,4,-tetrahydronaphthalene, ADTN). (*R,S*)-Isoapomorphine (Fig. 4) lacks DA-like activity in causing postural asymmetries in caudate-lesioned mice (Saari *et al.*, 1974). Also, it does not cause stereotyped behavior in mice (Pinder *et al.*, 1972); it is relatively ineffective in displacement of DA receptor agonists and antagonists from binding sites (Seeman, 1980); it fails to activate DA

Figure 4. Comparison of conformational structures and Newman projections for trans and gauche rotamers of dopamine with rigid aporphine and aminotetralin analogues (Neumeyer *et al.*, 1981b).

receptors (Neumeyer *et al.*, 1973a); it does not induce DA-like renal vasodilation in dogs (Goldberg *et al.*, 1978a,b); nor does it stimulate rat striatal adenylate cyclase. In fact, it is a weak antagonist of DA-stimulated adenylate cyclase (Miller *et al.*, 1976). In contrast, **16b** (ADTN) is a potent DA receptor agonist (Woodruff, 1982); it is very effective in various neuronal, behavioral, biochemical, and pharmacological tests for DA-like activity. For example, it causes potent and long-lasting stimulation of motor activity (Woodruff *et al.*, 1974), it causes rotation in rats with unilateral lesions of the substantia nigra, it produces renal vasodilation in dogs (Goldberg *et al.*, 1978a), it stimulates DA-sensitive adenylate cyclase (Sheppard *et al.*, 1978), and it is effective in radioligand binding studies (Seiler and Markstein, 1982). In many of these tests, it is more potent than its 5,6-dihydroxy isomer **16a**.

As illustrated in Fig. 4 the cis, or gauche, conformation of DA is rigidified in 1,2-dihydroxyaporphine. This compound does not cause emesis in dogs at a dose ten times higher than that of apomorphine (Neumeyer *et al.*, 1973a) and does not stimulate rat striatal adenylate cyclase but instead weakly antagonizes the action of DA (Miller *et al.*, 1976). These observations, coupled with the lack of activity of tetrahydroisoquinolines, e.g., **1**, as DA receptor agonists, provide convincing evidence that the gauche conformation of DA is not involved in receptor interaction. It may be concluded that *DA interacts with its receptor(s) in a trans (fully extended, antiperiplanar) orientation.*

The lack of activity of (*R,S*)-isoapomorphine has been attributed to the presence of steric boundaries on the DA receptor that are exceeded by the unsubstituted benzo-fused ring of isoapomorphine, thus prohibiting its interaction with the primary binding sites (Goldberg *et al.*, 1978b; Grol and Rollema, 1977; McDermed *et al.*, 1979; Erhardt, 1980; Seeman, 1980; Neumeyer *et al.*, 1981b; Freeman and McDermed, 1982). This has been questioned by Cannon *et al.* (1980a) on observation that linear *trans*-octahydro-7,8-dihydroxybenzo[*g*]quinoline (**5**), i.e., an isoapomorphine congener lacking the unsubstituted benzo-fused ring, lacks DA-like activity. It is possible that in the case of the benzo[*g*]quinolines the vectorial direction of. the lone pair of electrons on the nitrogen may be improper for receptor interaction.

3.2.1b. Coplanarity of the Aromatic Ring with the Side Chain. In view of the conclusion that the trans conformation of DA is preferred for receptor interaction (Horn and Rodgers, 1980), a second conformational question that requires resolution is the rotameric orientation of the catechol ring relative to the ethylamine side chain. Crystallographic analysis, as well as NMR and molecular orbital studies, suggests that the ring

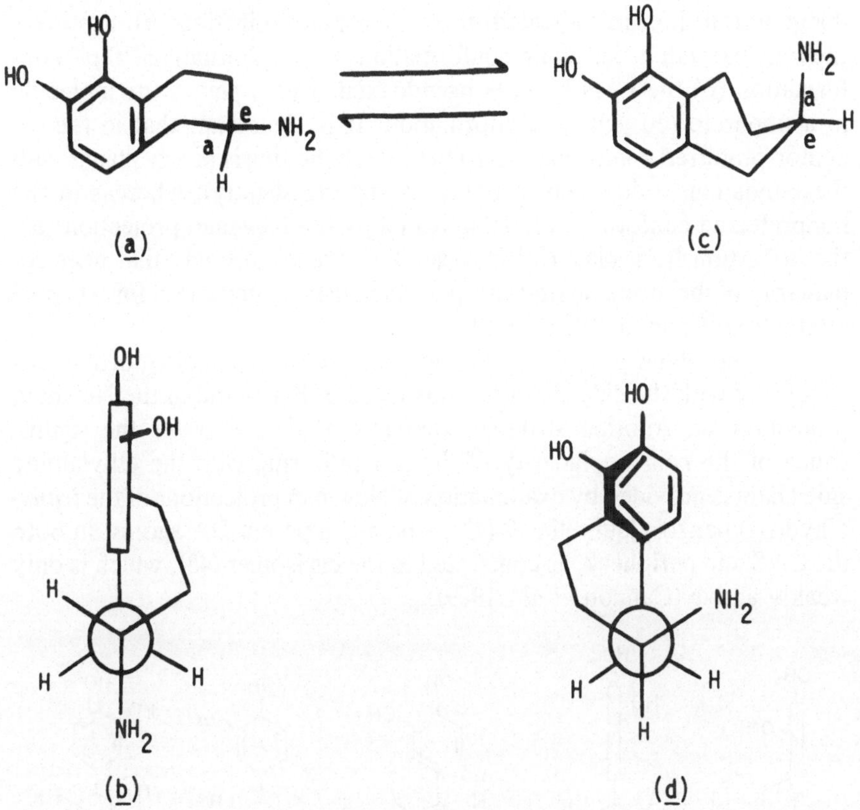

Figure 5. Comformational analysis of 2-aminotetralins (16) as illustrated by A-5,6-DTN (16a) (Cannon, 1979).

is perpendicular to the $CH_2CH_2NH_2$ unit (Bergin and Carlström, 1968; Geissner-Prettre and Pullman, 1975); however, potential energy differences among such rotameric forms are very small. More importantly, rigid DA receptor agonists from various classes, e.g., aporphines, 2-aminotetralins, octahydrobenzoquinolines, and ergolines, provide evidence concerning the relationship of the aromatic ring to the side chain that is required for binding to DA receptors.

The conformation of the aminotetralins 16 has been the subject of considerable study (Cannon *et al.*, 1972, 1977; McDermed *et al.*, 1975, 1976; Seiler and Markstein, 1982). These compounds are only semirigid; they can undergo conformational "flips." In one instance, as indicated in Fig. 5, **16a** is used as an example; however, the conformational analysis also pertains for **16b**. As indicated in structure *a*, the C–N bond is pseudoequatorial; i.e., as indicated in the Newman projection (*b*), it prefers the fully extended side chain conformation. In the alternative "flip" conformation (*c*) the C–N bond is pseudoaxial, which places the molecule in a nonpreferred gauche conformation. It is significant that in the receptor-preferred conformation (*b*) the catecholic ring is nearly planar with the ethylamine side chain (actually, it distorts slightly), whereas in the nonpreferred conformer (*c*), as indicated by the Newman projection (*d*), the distortion from planarity is large. This argues strongly that near coplanarity of the aromatic ring and side chain may be important for receptor interaction (Cannon, 1975, 1979).

Apomorphine provides a classic example of coplanarity of the catechol ring with the side chain, as illustrated in Fig. 4 and in the Newman projection **46**. Another striking example that demonstrates the significance of the near coplanarity of the aromatic ring with the ethylamine side chain is provided by examination of Newman projections of the *trans*-dihydroxybenzo[*f*]quinoline **7** (**47**), which is a potent DA agonist in both the CNS and periphery, as contrasted to the cis isomer (**48**), which is only weakly active (Cannon *et al.*, 1979).

A similar conformational argument can be advanced for the linear *trans*-benzo[*g*]quinoline **5**, which lacks significant DA-like activity (Cannon *et al.*, 1980a). As in the case of the cis isomer of **7**, which can attain several conformations, the preferred one illustrated by the Newman projection (**49**) of **5** suggests an orthogonal relationship of the catechol ring to the ethylamine side chain. A similar analysis may be made to rationalize the relative inactivity of the octahydrobenz[*h*]isoquinoline **6**. Inspection of a Dreiding model of **6**, as shown in the Newman projection **50**, indicates that the catechol ring deviates from coplanarity with the side chain by about 15°, although the large side chain bulk of this molecule might also rationalize its ineffectiveness (Cannon *et al.*, 1980b). These results offer compelling evidence that *near coplanarity of the aromatic ring and the ethylamine side chain of DA is required for agonist activity.* In these classes of DA receptor agonists, as well as in the ergot derivatives with DA-like potency, it has been noted that there is a slight deviation from coplanarity. Thus, if these molecules in a preferred conformation are viewed from the aromatic end toward the nitrogen, the nitrogen lies about 0.6 Å above the plane of the aromatic ring (Seeman, 1980).

3.2.2. Rotameric Conformation

Since the coplanar arrangement of the aromatic ring and the ethyl-amine side chain is important for interaction of DA with its receptors, determination of which of the two rotameric forms, i.e., α or β (see Fig. 3), is involved in the binding becomes significant. Initially, on the basis of the consistently more potent DA-like activity of ADTN (**16b**), a rigid analogue of the β rotamer, than that of the α rotamer analogue A-5,6-DTN (**16a**), it was rationalized that the β rotamer was involved in receptor binding (Horn and Rodgers, 1980, and references cited therein). Several more recent observations have brought this conclusion into doubt. Of particular note is the finding that 2-dipropylamino-5,6-dihydroxytetra-hydronaphthalene (**16c**), which simulates the α rotameric form of DA, was considerably more potent than its 6,7-dihydroxy counterpart in inhibiting spontaneous motor activity in mice (Costall *et al.*, 1982), relaxing renal vasculature (Kohli *et al.*, 1982), and stimulating adenylate cyclase activity (Seiler and Markstein, 1982). In the test for inhibition of spontaneous locomotion in rats, **16c** was 339 times more potent than its β rotameric counterpart **16** [X = 6,7-$(OH)_2$; R = n-C_3H_7]. Additionally, the mono-propyl relative of **16c** was 79 times and 179 times more potent than its 6,7- and 7,8-dihydroxy isomers, respectively. It was also noted that the *trans*-7,8-dihydroxy-N-propyloctahydrobenzo[*f*]quinoline [*trans*-N-(n-C_3H_7)-**7**] was 11 times more potent than the β rotameric 6,7-dihydroxy isomer. Further, in the octahydrobenzo[*g*]quinoline series **5**, which is generally considered to be relatively inactive (Cannon *et al.*, 1980a), the α rotameric N-propyl derivative was 467 times more potent than the β rotamer, and the α rotameric NH analogue was 46 times more effective than its β rotameric counterpart.

These data emphasize the extreme importance of N-propyl substi-tution on DA receptor activity. The inversion of activity so clearly noted on N-propylation and in different testing paradigms has led to the sug-gestion that definition of the rotameric form of DA that interacts with its receptor(s) may be an "illusory quest" (Costall *et al.*, 1982).

An extensive study of monohydroxyaminotetralins has resulted in comparable findings, i.e., N-propylation can invert the α or β rotameric preference of the DA receptor as measured in a test for stimulation of

Table II. Approximate Hydroxyl-to-Nitrogen Distances for Some Dopamine Derivatives

Compound	Distance (Å)		Dopaminelike activity (references)
	N to p-OH	N to m-OH	
DA (trans)[a]	7.8	7.3	Active
DA (partially eclipsed) (3-Benzazepines)	7.0	7.0	Active (Kaiser et al., 1982)
A-5,6-DTN (16a)	7.8	6.5	Inactive (Volkman et al., 1977)
N,N-Pr₂-16a (16c)	7.8	6.5	Active (Kohli et al., 1982)
ADTN (16b)	7.8	7.3	Active (Volkman et al., 1977)
Apomorphine (4)	7.8	6.5	Partial agonist (Goldberg et al., 1978a)
Isoapomorphine	7.8	7.3	Inactive (Goldberg et al., 1978b)
Tetrahydroisoquinolines	6.0	6.4	Inactive (Volkman et al., 1977)
16 (X = 5-OH, R = n-C₃H₇) (16f)	—	6.2	Active (Seiler and Markstein, 1982)
16 (X = 7-OH, R = H) (16h)	—	7.3	Active (Seiler and Markstein, 1982)
15c	—	5.5	Active (Hacksell et al., 1981a)

[a] For more precise distances, see Grol and Rollema (1977).

DA-sensitive adenylate cyclase. Thus, 7-hydroxy-2-aminotetralin was the most potent of the monohydroxylated primary amines, but the 5-hydroxyl derivative was the most potent in the N,N-dipropyl series. Further, in the 7-hydroxylated series, activity resided in the (2R) enantiomers, whereas in the 5-hydroxylated series the (2S) antipodes were more potent. These results, together with a lack of synergism with 5,7-dihydroxyaminotetralins, have been rationalized with a D-1 receptor model that contains two major binding sites and an accessory binding site to which the N,N-di-n-propyl substituents of the 5-hydroxylated series, but not those of the 7-hydroxylated series, have access. This model suggests that DA binds with its receptor in the β rotameric conformation; however, N,N-dipropylation causes a change in conformation at the receptor to favor the α rotameric form (Seiler and Markstein, 1982).

3.2.3. Hydroxyl-to-Nitrogen Distance

Various conformational analyses of DA receptor agonists have considered the O-to-N distance in these molecules (Grol and Rollema, 1977; Erhardt, 1980). Some of these distances are tabulated in Table II.

Comparison of the data shown here illustrates quite clearly that the hydroxyl-to-nitrogen distance is of little importance in determining DA-like activity. Any distance between the *meta*-hydroxyl and nitrogen that is less than that of DA in its fully extended form may be acceptable.

3.2.4. Directionality of the Nitrogen Lone Pair Electrons

The vectorial direction of the lone pair of electrons in the nitrogen *p* orbital has been suggested to be of importance in several conceptual models of the DA receptor (Goldberg *et al.*, 1978b; Nichols, 1983). It is particularly noteworthy that on N-propylation of the 3-benzazepine derivative **2b** (Wilson, 1978) and of the nomifensine analogue **12c** (Jacob *et al.*, 1981), DA-like activity is essentially lost. An obvious explanation for this effect is that in these compounds the N-*n*-propyl group can affect the conformation of the ring. It would be expected that the N-propyl group would assume a pseudoequatorial position. This, in turn, influences the vectorial direction of the nitrogen unshared electron pair, regardless of whether it is free or in a protonated form. Thus, if the electron pair must reside in a pseudoequatorial position and away from the meta hydroxyl group, a conformational change induced by N-propylation might account for the resultant inactivation caused by such modification in **2b** and **12c**. This is consistent with arguments for the importance of electron pair directionality of DA receptor agonists as proposed by Goldberg *et al.* (1978b).

Directionality of the nitrogen electron lone pair might also account for the inactivity of the benzo[*g*]quinoline **5**, which seems to have all other requisites for DA-like activity (Cannon *et al.*, 1980a). With no N-substituent, the electron pair could orient pseudoaxially, whereas on N-propylation, which confers DA-like activity in a behavioral model (Costall *et al.*, 1982), conformational changes induced in the molecule could force the free electron pair into a pseudoequatorial orientation to confer activity. It has been suggested (Nichols, 1983) that when agonists with an α rotameric conformation bind to the D-2 (or DA_2) receptor, they may possess steric bulk in the plane of the hydroxylated ring in a region corresponding to the unsubstituted benzo-fused ring of apomorphine. The orientation of the nitrogen electrons at this receptor is not critical. However, for β rotameric agonists, such steric bulk is not tolerated unless it can reside above the plane of the molecule. To be active at the D-1 (or DA_1) receptor, the nitrogen electrons must be oriented in an approximately pseudoequatorial orientation directed away from the meta hydroxyl group. These suggestions that the vectorial direction of the lone pair of nitrogen electrons might particularly influence heterocyclic DA analogues' ability to interact with the receptor(s) seem imminently reasonable.

3.3. Lipophilicity

Although lipophilicity is not essential for dopaminergic activity, increased lipophilicity generally appears to enhance DA-like activity. Thus, in a test for displacement of $[^3H]$-spiroperidol from binding sites of calf brain striatum the order of potency was: (R)-n-propylnorapomorphine (IC_{50} = 160 nM) > (R)-apomorphine (IC_{50} = 650 nM) > ($\pm$)-A-5,6-DTN (IC_{50} = 9000 nM); i.e., potency paralleled their lipophilicity (Seeman, 1980). In the same test, potency of a series of A-5,6-DTN derivatives also paralleled their lipophilicity: N,N-(n-C_3H_7)$_2$ (IC_{50} = 49 nM) > N,N-(C_2H_5)$_2$ (IC_{50} = 2100 nM) > N,N-(CH_3)$_2$ (IC_{50} = 3600 nM) > A-5,6-DTN (IC_{50} = 9000 nM) (Seeman, 1980). Comparable results were observed in the ability of these compounds to stimulate DA-sensitive adenylate cyclase; i.e., N,N-(n-C_3H_7)$_2$ (EC_{50} = 3.31 μM) > N,N-(C_2H_5)$_2$ (EC_{50} = 4.36 μM) > A-5,6-DTN (52.4 μM) (Cannon et al., 1978).

3.4. Enantioselectivity

Enantiomers of DA receptor agonists (e.g., Neumeyer et al., 1973a,b; Saari et al., 1973; Schoenfeld et al., 1975; Andrews et al., 1978; McDermed et al., 1979; Tedesco et al., 1979; Neumeyer et al., 1981b; McDermed and Freeman, 1982; Dandridge et al., 1984; Kaiser, 1983; Kaiser et al., 1982, 1983) and antagonists (Seidlova and Protiva, 1967; Humber et al., 1975, 1979; Metysova and Protiva, 1975; Petcher et al., 1975; Bird et al., 1976; Jaunin et al., 1977; Phillipp et al., 1979; Jenner et al., 1980; Kaiser and Zirkle, 1983) have consistently demonstrated enantioselectivity.

In virtually every general class of DA receptor agonist, enantioselectivity is displayed. Enantioselectivity has been convincingly demonstrated in a series of 1-substituted 3-benzazepines with DA-like activity; the 1R isomers of 2b and related compounds are strikingly more potent in various tests (Kaiser et al., 1982, 1983). Similarly, in the 3-phenylpiperidine series, 3-PPP (9c) has been resolved, and its enantiomers show strikingly different (agonist/antagonist) actions (Hjorth et al., 1982). In the aporphine series, it is not generally emphasized that absolute configuration is so critically important. Thus, (+)-6aS-bulbocapnine (51) is a DA receptor antagonist of the aporphine group whose absolute configuration is opposite to that of the DA agonist 6aR-apomorphine (4) (Wardell *et al.*, 1979). In addition, 6aS-apomorphine is an effective, albeit weak, DA receptor antagonist (Riffee *et al.*, 1982). Also, the alkaloid stephanine (**52**), which has the (−)-6aR stereochemistry, was one of the most potent members of a series of aporphine derivatives examined for DA receptor antagonist activity in several testing protocols (Ku *et al.*, 1983). The implications of these reversals of activity on inversion of the absolute configurations are confusing and remain to be explained.

51   52

Recently, *3',4'-dihydroxynomifensine* (**12b**) has been resolved, and the absolute configuration of its isomers has been determined. Enantioselective DA-like properties reside in the isomer with the *S* stereochemistry (Dandridge *et al.*, 1984). The enantioselectivity of mono- and dihydroxylated derivatives of *2-aminotetralins* (**16**) has been thoroughly documented, and the absolute configuration required for dopaminergic activity has clearly been shown to depend on the pattern of hydroxyl substitution (cf. McDermed *et al.*, 1976, 1979; McDermed and Freeman, 1982; Seiler and Markstein, 1982). Also, among the ergot derivatives, there is a clear requirement of a 5R absolute stereochemistry (Bach *et al.*, 1980a). Comparison of the dopaminergic ergolines with DA-like aporphines has been of particular interest. Several groups (Cannon, 1979; Camerman *et al.*, 1979; Camerman and Camerman, 1981) have suggested that the benzo-fused ring of the ergolines corresponds to the catecholic ring of apomorphine. This, however, places the asymmetric centers of these molecules in the opposite absolute configuration (compare **53** *vs.* **54a**). Conversely, if the NH of the ergoline pyrrole ring is approximately superimposed on the most important 11-hydroxyl group of the aporphine (compare **53** *vs.* **54b**), then the stereochemistry at position 5 of the ergoline is identical to that in position 6a of the aporphine, as suggested earlier (Nichols, 1976).

Exploration of the stereochemical relationship between DA-like aporphines and ergolines has resulted in the identification of novel dopaminergic agents, e.g., **26** and **28** (Bach and Kornfeld, 1978; Bach *et al.*, 1980a–c).

4. Summary of Structural Requirements for Dopamine Receptor Agonist Activity

The SAR studies with various classes of dopaminergic agents considered in Section 3 lead to some generalizations relating to structural requirements for interaction of DA and related agonists with the receptor(s). Although there are notable exceptions, e.g., **15d** (Sindelar *et al.*, 1982; Clark *et al.*, 1982), **16j** (Rusterholz *et al.*, 1979), and most of the miscellaneous class of DA receptor agonists, the *meta*-hydroxyphenethylamine unit for most practical purposes can be envisioned as the dopaminergic pharmacophore, with the nitrogen interacting with the receptor in an ammonium form. Clearly, too, N-substitution profoundly influences the mode of interaction of the pharmacophore with the receptor (Seiler and Markstein, 1982).

Conformation is quite significant for interaction of DA with its receptor(s). Studies with rigid analogues suggest that the trans (fully extended, antiperiplanar) conformation is most likely involved; however, the benzazepines, e.g., **12b**, represent an exception (Kaiser *et al.*, 1982). The rotameric conformation of the catecholic ring may not be as significant as originally thought. Thus, either the α or β rotamer may be active, depending on various other factors such as the testing system (Costall *et al.*, 1982) or substitution of the nitrogen (Kohli *et al.*, 1982; Seiler and Markstein, 1982). Near coplanarity of the catechol ring, or a simulating aromatic system, with the nitrogen seems quite important. In general, the variation from coplanarity is about 0.6 Å (Seeman, 1980). The distance between the hydroxyl and amino groups seems of little consequence; it may vary from one as short as 5.5 Å (Hacksell *et al.*, 1981a) to the maximum that DA can attain, i.e., about 7.4 Å. Clearly, a conformational consideration that has been afforded relatively little attention, i.e., the vectorial direction of the lone pair of electrons in the nitrogen p orbital, may be critically important (Goldberg *et al.*, 1978b; Nichols, 1983) for DA-like activity. Lipophilicity often has a potency-enhancing effect; however, overall activity is so dependent on other factors that the precise contribution of lipophilicity is difficult to evaluate. Enantioselectivity, as in the case of other receptor modulators, is uniformly noted among DA receptor agonists (and antagonists).

Lastly, it should be emphasized that structural requirements for the D-1 or DA_1 receptor are generally much more demanding than for the D-2 or DA_2 subpopulations. As a rule, a catecholic system is required for the D-1 or DA_1 systems, and these receptors are usually less tolerant of nitrogen substitution. Until recently it was generally considered that the β rotameric form was more important for D-1 or DA_1 receptor interaction; however, clear exceptions have been identified (Kohli *et al.*, 1982).

5. Conceptual Models of Dopamine Receptor(s)

A number of conceptual models of the DA receptor have been derived from consideration of SAR data from various classes of agonists (Sheppard and Burghardt, 1974; Grol and Rollema, 1977; Goldberg *et al.*, 1978b; Cannon, 1978; McDermed *et al.*, 1979; Erhardt, 1980; 1983a,b; Neumeyer *et al.*, 1981b, 1983; Seeman, 1980; Seiler and Markstein, 1982; Nichols, 1983; Dandridge *et al.*, 1984) and antagonists (Humber *et al.*, 1975, 1979; Clement-Cormier *et al.*, 1972; Philipp *et al.*, 1979; Olson *et al.*, 1981; Smythies, 1981). In derivation of these models, it is essential that not only the structural requirements for DA receptor agonist activity (see Section 4) be recognized but, equally importantly, that some compounds bearing a dopaminergic pharmacophore but lacking activity, e.g., 1-benzylpiperidines, 1-benzyltetrahydroisoquinolines (Cheng *et al.*, 1976), other apomorphine segments (Ginos *et al.*, 1975; Miller, 1978), benzo[*g*]quinolines (e.g., 5) (Cannon *et al.*, 1980a), benz[*h*]isoquinolines (e.g., 6) (Cannon *et al.*, 1980b), be rationalized. Many of the models (e.g., Sheppard and Burghardt, 1974; Grol and Rollema, 1977; Goldberg *et al.*, 1978b; McDermed *et al.*, 1979; Erhardt, 1980; 1983a,b; Neumeyer *et al.*, 1981b, 1983; Seeman, 1980; Nichols, 1983) accomplish this by suggesting specific modes of binding and steric parameters.

Examination of enantioselectivity has played a pivotal role in development of these conceptual models of the DA receptor. As enantiomers

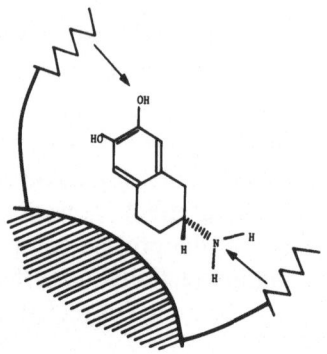

Figure 6. Hypothetical binding of ADTN **(16b)** to a postulated DA receptor (McDermed *et al.*, 1979).

have identical physical properties, they are extraordinarily useful as receptor probes. Unless they are metabolized differently, their effects may reasonably be attributed to events at the receptor. Information derived from examination of the enantioselectivity of aporphines and a number of hydroxyl-substituted 2-amino-1,2,3,4-tetrahydronaphthalene derivatives was employed by McDermed *et al.*, (1979) for derivation of an appealingly simple conceptual model of the DA receptor. This model requires receptor interaction with the hydroxyl group meta to the ethylamine side chain of the dopaminergic pharmacophore, a properly spatially oriented nitrogen, and a region of bulk intolerance, as indicated in Fig. 6 for ADTN **(16b)**. The site of bulk occlusion, depicted by the striped area, was supported by study of the 5- and 8-propyl derivatives; as predicted, the 8- but not the 5-isomer was an effective DA receptor agonist (Freeman and McDermed, 1982). The model clearly rationalizes the inactivity of isoapomorphine (McDermed *et al.*, 1979).

The utility of this model is exemplified in Figs. 7 and 8, which consider the mode of interaction of SK&F 82526 (Weinstock *et al.*, 1980, 1983;

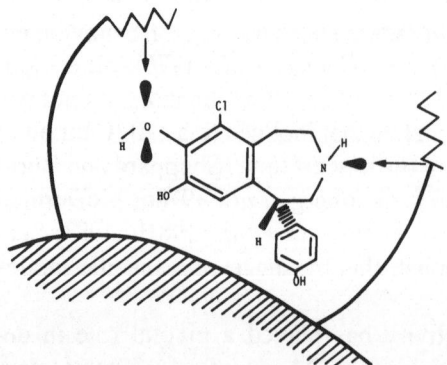

Figure 7. Possible mode of binding of SK&F 82526 to a postulated DA receptor (Kaiser *et al.*, 1983).

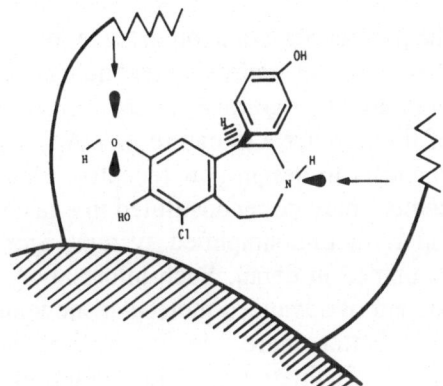

Figure 8. Alternative possible mode of binding of SK&F 82526 to a postulated DA receptor (Kaiser *et al.*, 1983).

Hahn *et al.*, 1982; Ackerman *et al.*, 1983; Kaiser *et al.*, 1983; Dandridge *et al.*, 1984). Some difficulty is encountered in incorporating this molecule into the model. First both of the catecholic hydroxyls are meta to an ethylamine side chain, and both are required for activity (Wilson, 1978; Kaiser *et al.*, 1982). Secondly, either the 6-Cl or 1-(*p*-hydroxyphenyl) group must be directed toward the postulated site of steric occlusion. Figures 7 and 8 (Kaiser *et al.*, 1983) offer two plausible interpretations of the enantioselective interaction of the dopaminergic *R* enantiomer of SK&F 82526 with the model (Kaiser, 1983). As indicated in Fig. 7, the *p*-hydroxyphenyl group might be accommodated as a consequence of its α orientation, which avoids the site of bulk intolerance while the 6-Cl is directed away from this site. Alternatively, as indicated in Fig. 8, perhaps the receptor can accept the relatively small 6-Cl substituent while the 1-(p-hydroxyphenyl) group is directed away from the striped area of steric hindrance. At present, either interpretation might be accepted. Current studies in our laboratories are being directed toward this question (Dandridge *et al.*, 1984).

6. Prospectives for Rational Derivation of New Dopamine Receptor Agonists

The rapidly developing technologies involving protein isolation have made possible the purification of β-adrenergic receptors (cf. Shorr *et al.*, 1981, 1982a,b), with the reasonable assumption that these proteins, or glycoproteins, will be sequenced, and determination of their secondary and tertiary structures will soon follow. Although the lesser accessibility of quantities of DA receptors promises to complicate the problem, it seems very likely that DA receptor(s) will follow a path similar to that of the β-adrenergic (and other) receptors. Thus, it is reasonable to anticipate that with ever-improving technologies the DA receptor(s) will be isolated, purified, and rigorously characterized. In addition to providing final proof of the number and nature of DA receptors, this will position medicinal chemists to design new receptor-selective DA agonists. The purified receptors may be reconstituted in a fashion imitating their natural environment. In this simplified system, agonist–receptor interactions may be examined in detail. Such information might be useful, particularly with the aid of advanced molecular modeling systems, to direct the design of new, better, more selective, and potent DA receptor agonists.

To facilitate separation, determination of enantiomeric excess, and absolute stereochemistry of optical antipodes, it is anticipated that technological advances in high-performance liquid chromatography, NMR, and circular dichroism spectroscopy will be important. It does seem highly probable that solid-state NMR will play a crucial role in understanding the molecular dynamics of agonist–receptor interaction to provide information of benefit in the rational design of new DA-like compounds.

In the past, the imperative synergy of chemists and biologists for derivation of understanding of receptors and their modulators has depended heavily on fortuitous observation and drug probing of the mysterious receptors; it seems reasonable to anticipate that the future promises much more rational development of superior DA—and other—receptor modulators.

References

Ackerman, D. M., Blumberg, A. L., McCafferty, J. P., Sherman, S. S., Weinstock, J., Kaiser, C., and Berkowitz, B., 1983, Potential usefulness of renal vasodilators in hypertension and renal disease: SK&F 82526, *Fed. Proc.* **42:**186–190.

Andén, N.-E., Golembiowska-Nikitin, K., and Thornström, U., 1982, Selective stimulation of dopamine and noradrenaline autoreceptors by B-HT 920 and B-HT 933, respectively, *Naunyn Schmiedebergs Arch. Pharmacol.* **321:**100–104.

Anderson, K., Kuruvilla, A., Uretsky, N., and Miller, D. D., 1981, Synthesis and pharmacological evaluation of sulfonium analogs of dopamine: Non-classical dopamine agonists, *J. Med. Chem.* **24:**683–687.

Andrews, C. D., Davis, A., Freeman, H. S., McDermed, J. D., Poat, J. A., and Woodruff, G. N., 1978, Effects of (+)- and (−)-enantiomers of 2-amino-6,7-dihydroxy-1,2,3,4-tetrahydronaphthalene on dopamine uptake, *Proc. Br. Pharm. Soc.* **1978:**433P.

Arana, G. W., Baldessarini, R. J., and Neumeyer, J. L., 1983, Structure–activity characteristics for high affinity dopamine-agonist binding at central dopamine receptors, *Acta Pharm. Suec. [Suppl.]* **2:**25–36.

Armstrong, J., and Barlow, R. B., 1976, The ionization of phenolic amines, including apomorphine, dopamine and catecholamines and an assessment of zwitterion constants, *Br. J. Pharmacol.* **57:**501–516.

Arnerić, S. P., Maixner, W., Long, J. P., Mott, J., Barfknecht, C. F., Perez, J. A., and Cannon, J. G., 1982, Structure–activity relationships for 2-aminotetralins and 2-aminoindanes: Inhibitory neuroeffector mechanisms in isolated guinea pig ilea, *Arch. Int. Pharmacodyn. Ther.* **258**:84–99.

Arvidsson, L.-E., Hacksell, U., Nilsson, J. L. G., Hjorth, S., Carlsson, A., Lindberg, P., Sanchez, D., and Wikstrom, H., 1981, 8-Hydroxy-2-(di-*n*-propylamino)tetralin, a new centrally acting 5-hydroxytryptamine receptor agonist, *J. Med. Chem.* **24**:921–923.

Bach, N. J., and Kornfeld, E. C., 1978, 4-(Di-*n*-propyl)amino-1,3,4,5-tetrahydrobenz[*cd*]indole, U.S. Patent 4,110,339, *Chem. Abstr.* **90**:121415f.

Bach, N. J., Kornfeld, E. C., Jones, N. D., Chaney, M. O., Dorman, D. E., Paschal, J. W., Clemens, J A., and Smalstig, E. B., 1980a, Bicyclic and tricyclic ergoline partial structures. Rigid 3-(2-aminoethyl)pyrroles and 3- and 4-(2-aminoethyl)pyrazoles as dopamine agonists, *J. Med. Chem.* **23**:481–491.

Bach, N. J., Kornfeld, E. C., Clemens, J. A., Smalstig, E. B., and Fredrickson, R. C. A., 1980b, Preparation and biological evaluation of 2-azaergolines, *J. Med. Chem.* **23**:492–494.

Bach, N. J., Kornfeld, E. C., Clemens, J. A., and Smalstig, E. B., 1980c, Conversion of ergolines to hexahydro- and octahydrobenzo[*f*]quinolines (depyrroloergolines), *J. Med. Chem.* **23**:812–814.

Baggio, G., and Ferrari, F., 1981, DPI, a supposed selective agonist of inhibitory dopamine receptors, strongly increases rat diuresis through α-adrenergic receptor activation, *Life Sci.* **28**:1449–1456.

Bailey, D. M., 1982, Heterocyclic alkyl naphthols, U.S. Patent 4,327,022, April 27, 1982.

Bailey, E. V., and Stone, T. W. 1975, The mechanism of action of amantadine in parkinsonism: A review, *Arch. Int. Pharmacodyn. Ther.* **216**:246–262.

Bannon, M. J., Grace, A. A., Bunney, B. S., and Roth, R. H., 1980, Evidence for an irreversible interaction of bromocriptine with central dopamine receptors, *Naunyn Schmiedebergs Arch. Pharmacol.* **312**:37–41.

Barger, G., and Dale, H. H., 1910, Chemical structure and sympathomimetic action of amines, *J. Physiol. (Lond.)* **41**:19–59.

Barnett, A., and Fiove, J. W., 1971, Hypotensive effects of apomorphine in anesthetized cats, *Eur. J. Pharmacol.* **14**:206–208.

Bergin, R., and Carlström, D., 1968, Structure of the pyrocatecholamines. II. Crystal structure of dopamine hydrochloride, *Acta Crystallogr.* **24B**:1506–1510.

Berney, D., and Schuh, K., 1982, Structural analogues of apophines. Part 1: Synthesis of apomorphines with the catecholic moiety replaced by 5-membered heterocycles, *Helv. Chim. Acta* **65**(4):1304–1309.

Besson, M. J., Cheramy, A., Feltz, P., and Glowinski, J., 1969, Release of newly synthesized dopamine from dopamine-containing terminals in the striatum of the rat, *Proc. Natl. Acad. Sci. U.S.A.* **62**:741–748.

Bird, P., Bruderlein, F. T., and Humber, L. G., 1976, Crystallographic studies on neuroleptics of the benzocycloheptapyridoisoquinoline series. The crystal structure of butaclamol hydrobromide and the absolute configuration and crystal structure of dexclamol hydrobromide, *Can. J. Chem.* **54**:2715–2722.

Birket-Smith, E., Bøttcher, J., Dupont, E., Holm, P., Jensen, J. P. A., Kristensen, O., Køhler, O., and Mikkelsen, B., 1978, Dopaminergic agonist Ro 8-4650 in Parkinson's disease, *Acta Neurol. Scand.* **58**:74–76.

Blaschko, H., 1939, The specific action of *l*-dopa decarboxylase, *J. Physiol. (Lond.)* **96**:50–51P.

Blaschko, H., 1957, Metabolism and storage of biogenic amines, *Experientia* **13**:9–12.

Bockaert, J., 1978, Coupling of neurotransmitter receptors with adenylate cyclase. A tool for studying their pharmacological properties, distribution and modulation in the central nervous system, *J. Physiol. (Paris)* **74**:527–533.

Borgman, R. J., Erhardt, P. W., Gorczynski, R. J., and Anderson, W. G., 1978, (±)-(*E*)-2-(3,4-Dihydroxyphenyl)cyclopropylamine hydrochloride (ASL-7003): A rigid analog of dopamine, *J. Pharm. Pharmacol.* **30**:193–195.

Broll, M., Eymard, P., Lacolle, J.-Y., and Werbenec, J.-P., 1978, Etude pharmacologique d'un antiparkinsonien potentiel: La diprobutine, *J. Pharmacol. (Paris)* **9**(2):121–131.

Burkman, A. M., 1973, Biological activity of apomorphine fragments: Dissociation of emetic and stereotypical effects, *Neuropharmacology* **12**:83–85.

Burkman, A. M., and Cannon, J. G., 1972, Screening nornuciferine derivatives for apomorphine-like activity, *J. Pharm. Sci.* **61**(5):813–814.

Bustard, T. M., and Egan, R. S., 1971, The conformation of dopamine hydrochloride, *Tetrahedron* **27**:4457–4469.

Calne, D. B., and Larsen, T. A., 1983, Potential therapeutic uses of dopamine receptor agonists and antagonists, in: *Dopamine Receptors, American Chemical Society Symposium Series 224* (C. Kaiser and J. W. Kebabian, eds.), American Chemical Society, Washington, pp. 147–153.

Camerman, N., and Camerman, A., 1981, On the stereochemistry of dopaminergic ergoline derivatives, *Mol. Pharmacol.* **19**:517–519.

Camerman, N., Chan, L. Y. Y., and Camerman, A., 1979, Stereochemical characteristics of dopamine agonists: Molecular structure of bromocriptine and structural comparisons with apomorphine, *Mol. Pharmacol.* **16**:729–736.

Cannon, J. G., 1975, Chemistry of dopaminergic agonists, in: *Advances in Neurology,* Volume 9 (D. B. Calne, T. N. Chase, and A. Barbeau, eds.), Raven Press, New York, pp. 177–183.

Cannon, J. G., 1979, Dopamine congeners derived from the benzo[*f*]quinoline ring, in: *Peripheral Dopaminergic Receptors, Advances in the Biosciences,* Volume 20 (J.-L. Imbs and J. Schwartz, eds.), Pergamon Press, New York, pp. 87–94.

Cannon, J. G., Kim, J. C., Aleem, M. A., and Long, J. P., 1972, Centrally acting emetics. Derivatives of β-naphthylamine and 2-indanamine, *J. Med. Chem.* **15**(4):348–350.

Cannon, J. G., Hatheway, G. J., Long, J. P., and Sharabi, F. M., 1976, Centrally acting emetics. 10. Rigid dopamine congeners derived from octahydrobenzo[*f*]quinoline, *J. Med. Chem.* **19**:987–933.

Cannon, J. G., Lee, T., Goldman, H. D., Costall, B., and Naylor, R. J., 1977, Cerebral dopamine agonist properties of some 2-aminotetralin derivatives after peripheral and intracerebral administration, *J. Med. Chem.* **20**:1111–1116.

Cannon, J. G., Costall, B., Laduron, P. M., Leysen, J. E., and Naylor, R. J., 1978, Effects of some derivatives of 2-aminotetralin on dopamine-sensitive adenylate cyclase and on the binding of [³H]haloperidol to neuroleptic receptors in the rat striatum, *Biochem. Pharmacol.* **27**:1417–1420.

Cannon, J. G., Suarez-Gutierrez, C., Lee, T., Long, J. P., Costall, B., Fortune, D. H., and Naylor, R. J., 1979, Rigid congeners of dopamine based on octahydrobenzo[*f*]quinoline: Peripheral and central effects, *J. Med. Chem.* **22**:341–347.

Cannon, J. G., Lee, T., Goldman, H. D., Long, J. P., Flynn, J. R., Verimer, T., Costall, B., and Naylor, R. J., 1980a, Congeners of the β conformer of dopamine derived from *cis*- and *trans*-octahydrobenzo[*f*]quinoline and *trans*-octahydrobenzo[*g*]quinoline, *J. Med. Chem.* **23**(1):1–5.

Cannon, J. G., Lee, T., Hsu, F.-L., Long, J. P., and Flynn, J. R., 1980b, Congeners of the α conformer of dopamine derived from octahydrobenz[*h*]isoquinoline, *J. Med. Chem.* **23**:502–505.

Cannon, J. G., Demopoulos, B. J., Long, J. P., Flynn, J. R., and Sharabi, F. M., 1981, Proposed dopaminergic pharmacophore of lergotrile, pergolide, and related ergot alkaloid derivatives, *J. Med. Chem.* **24**:238–240.

Cannon, J. G., Perez, J. A., Bhatnagar, R. K., Long, J. P., and Sharabi, F. M., 1982, Conformationally restricted congeners of dopamine derived from 2-aminoindan, *J. Med. Chem.* **25**:1442–1446.

Carlsson, A., 1959, The occurrence, distribution and physiological role of catecholamines in the nervous system, *Pharmacol. Rev.* **11**:490–493.

Carlsson, A., Lindqvist, M., Magnusson, T., and Waldeck, B., 1958, On the presence of 3-hydroxytyramine in brain, *Science* **127**:471.

Carlsson, A., Fuxe, K., Hamberger, B., and Lindqvist, M., 1966, Biochemical and histochemical studies on the effects of imipramine-like drugs and (+)-amphetamine on central and peripheral catecholamine neurons, *Acta Physiol. Scand.* **67**:481–497.

Cavero, I., Massingham, R., and Lefèvre-Borg, F., 1982a, Peripheral dopamine receptors, potential targets for a new class of antihypertensive agents. Part I: Subclassification and functional description, *Life Sci.* **31**:939–948.

Cavero, I., Massingham, R., and Lefèvre-Borg, F., 1982b, Peripheral dopamine receptors, potential targets for a new class of antihypertensive agents. Part II: Sites and mechanisms of action of dopamine receptor agonists, *Life Sci.* **31**:1059–1069.

Cheng, H. C., Long, J. P., Van Orden, L. S. III, Cannon, J. G., and O'Donnell, J. P., 1976, Dopaminergic activity of some apomorphine analogs, *Res. Commun. Chem. Pathol. Pharmacol.* **15**(1):89–106.

Clapham, J. C., and Hamilton, T. C., 1982, Involvement of presynaptic dopamine receptors in the antihypertensive response to 2-N,N-dimethylamino-5,6-dihydroxy-1,2,3,4-tetrahydronaphthalene (M-7), *J. Pharm. Pharmacol.* **34**:644–647.

Clark, B. J., 1979, Cardiovascular effects of ergot alkaloids, *J. Pharmacol. (Paris)* **10**(4):439–453.

Clark, J. T., Smith, E. R., Stefanick, M. L., Arneric, S. P., Long, J. P., and Davidson, J. M., 1982, Effects of a novel dopamine-receptor agonist RDS-127 (2-N,N-di-*n*-propylamino-4,7-dimethoxyindane) on hormone levels and sexual behavior in the male rat, *Physiol. Behav.* **29**(1):1–6.

Clement-Cormier, Y. C., Meyerson, L. R., Phillips, H., and Davis, V. E., 1972, Dopamine receptor topography. Characterization of antagonist requirements of striatal dopamine-sensitive adenylate cyclase using protoberberine alkaloids, *Biochem. Pharmacol.* **28**:3123–3129.

Cools, A. R., and van Rossum, J. M., 1976, Excitation-mediating and inhibition-mediating dopamine receptors: A new concept towards a better understanding of electrophysiological, biochemical, pharmacological, functional and clinical data, *Psychopharmacologia* **45**:243–254.

Corrodi, H., Fuxe, K., and Ungerstedt, U., 1971, Evidence for a new type of dopamine receptor stimulating agent, *J. Pharm. Pharmacol.* **23**:989–991.

Corrodi, H., Farnebo, L.-O., Fuxe, K., Hamberger, B., and Ungerstedt, U., 1972, ET495 and brain catecholamine mechanisms: Evidence for stimulation of dopamine receptors, *Eur. J. Pharmacol.* **20**:195–204.

Corrodi, H., Fuxe, K., Hökfelt, T., Lidbrink, P., and Ungerstedt, U., 1973, Effect of ergot drugs on central catecholamine neurons: Evidence for a stimulation of central dopamine neurons, *J. Pharm. Pharmacol.* **25**:409–412.

Costall, B., and Naylor, R. J., 1978, Studies on the dopamine agonist properties of 8-amino-2-methyl-4-(3,4-dihydroxyphenyl)-1,2,3,4-tetrahydroisoquinoline, a derivative of nomifensine, *J. Pharm. Pharmacol.* **30**:514–516.

Costall, B., Naylor, R. J., and Pinder, R. M., 1974, Design of agents for stimulation of neostriatal dopaminergic mechanisms, *J. Pharm. Pharmacol.* **26**:753–762.

Costall, B., Naylor, R. J., Cannon, J. G., and Lee, T., 1977, Differential activation by some 2-aminotetralin derivatives of the receptor mechanisms in the nucleus accumbens of rat which mediate hyperactivity and stereotyped biting, *Eur. J. Pharmacol.* **41**:307–319.

Costall, B., Lim, S. K., Naylor, R. J., and Cannon, J. G., 1982, On the preferred rotameric conformation for dopamine agoinst action: An illusory quest? *J. Pharm. Pharmacol.* **34**:246–254.

Cotzias, G. C., Düby, S., Ginos, J. Z., Steck, A., and Papavasiliou, P. S., 1970, Dopamine analogs for studies of parkinsonism, *N. Engl. J. Med.* **283**(23):1289.

Creese, I., 1974, Behavioural evidence of dopamine receptor stimulation by piribedil (ET495) and its metabolite S584, *Eur. J. Pharmacol.* **28**:55–58.

Creese, I., 1982, Dopamine receptors explained, *Trends Neuropharmacol. Sci.* **5**(2):40–43.

Creese, I., and Leff, S. E., 1982, Dopamine receptors: A classification, *J. Clin. Psychopharmacol.* **2**(5):329–335.

Creese, I., and Sibley, D. R., 1979, Radioligand binding studies: Evidence for multiple dopamine receptors, *Commun. Psychopharmacol.* **3**:385–395.

Crooks, P. A., and Rosenberg, H. E., 1979, Synthesis of 5-hydroxy- and 5,6-dihydroxy-derivatives of spiro[indane-2,2′-pyrrolidine], rigid analogues of tyramine and dopamine respectively, *J. Chem. Soc. [Perkin I]* **1979**:2719–2726.

Crooks, P. A., Szyndler, R., and Cox, B., 1980, 5,6- and 6,7-Dihydroxyspiro (tetralin-1,3′-pyrrolidine): Conformationally restricted analogs of dopamine, *Pharm. Acta Helv.* **55**(5):134–137.

Dandiya, P. C., Sharma, H. L., Patni, S. K., and Gambhir, R. S., 1975, An evaluation of apomorphine action on dopaminergic receptors, *Experientia* **31**:1441–1443.

Dandridge, P. A., Kaiser, C., Brenner, M., Gaitanopoulus, D., David, L. D., Webb, R. L., Foley, J. J., and Sarau, H. M., 1984, Synthesis, resolution, absolute stereochemistry and enantioselectivity of 3′,4′-dihydroxynomifensine, *J. Med. Chem.* **27**:28–35.

Davis, A., Roberts, P. J., and Woodruff, G. N., 1978, The uptake and release of [^{3}H]-2-amino-6,7-dihydroxy-1,2,3,4-tetrahydronaphthalene (ADTN) by striatal nerve terminals, *Br. J. Pharmacol.* **63**:183–190.

DiChiara, G., and Gessa, G. L., 1978, Pharmacology and neurochemistry of apomorphine, in: *Advances in Pharmacology and Chemotherapy,* Volume 15 (S. Garattini, A. Goldin, F. Hawking, I. J. Kopin, and R. J. Schnitzer, eds.), Academic Press, New York, pp. 87–160.

DiChiara, G., Porceddu, M. L., Vargiu, L., and Gessa, G. L., 1978, Stimulation of 'regulatory' dopamine receptors by bromocriptine (CB-154), *Pharmacology* **16**(Suppl. 1):135–142.

Dryer, S. E., Rusterholz, D. B., and Long, J. P., 1980, Biochemical and behavioral actions of 5,8-dimethoxylated aminotetralins, *Fed. Proc.* **39**(3):845.

Enz, H., 1981, Biphasic influence of a 8α-aminoergoline, CU 32-085 on striatal dopamine synthesis and turnover *in vivo* in the rat, *Life Sci.* **29**:2227–2234.

Erhardt, P. W., 1980. Topographical model of the renal vascular dopamine receptor, *J. Pharm. Sci.* **69**(9):1059–1061.

Erhardt, P. W., 1983a, Renal vascular dopamine receptor topography. (*E*)-2-(3,4-Dihydroxyphenyl)cyclopropylamine and renal vascular dopamine receptor topography. Refinement of a receptor model, *Acta Pharm. Suec. [Suppl.]* **2**:56–64.

Erhardt, P. W., 1983b, Renal vascular dopamine receptor topography: Structure–activity relationships that suggest the presence of a ceiling, in: *Dopamine Receptors, American Chemical Society Symposium Series 224* (C. Kaiser and J. W. Kebabian, eds.), American Chemical Society, Washington, pp. 275–280.

Erhardt, P. W., Gorczynski, R. J., and Anderson, W. G., 1979, Conformational analogues of dopamine. Synthesis and pharmacological activity of (*E*)- and (*Z*)-2-(3,4-dihydroxy-phenyl)cyclopropylamine hydrochlorides, *J. Med. Chem.* **22**:907–911.

Ernst, A. M., 1967, Mode of action of apomorphine and dextroamphetamine in gnawing compulsion in rats, *Psychopharmacologia* **10**:316–323.

Ernst, A. M., and Smelik, P. G., 1966, Site of action of dopamine and apomorphine on compulsive gnawing behavior in rats, *Experientia* **22**:(12):837–838.

Euvrard, C., Ferland, L., DiPaolo, T., Beaulieu, M., Labrie, F., Oberlander, C., Raynaud, J. P., and Boissier, J. R., 1980, Activity of two new potent dopaminergic agonists at the striatal and anterior pituitary levels, *Neuropharmacology* **19**:379–386.

Euvrard, C., Ferland, L., Fortin, M., Oberlander, C., Labrie, F., and Boissier, J. R., 1981, Dopaminergic activity of some simplified ergoline derivatives, *Drug Dev. Res.* **1**:151–161.

Feenstra, M. G. P., Rollema, H., Dijkstra, D., Grol, C. J., Horn, A. S., and Westerink, B. H. C., 1980, Effects of non-catecholic 2-aminotetralin derivatives on dopamine metabolism in rat striatum, *Naunyn Schmiedebergs Arch. Pharmacol.* **313**:213–219.

Flueckiger, E., Briner, U., Doepfner, W., Kovacs, E., Marbach, P., and Wagner, H. R., 1978, Prolactin secretion inhibition by a new 8α-amino-ergoline, CH 29-717, *Experientia* **34**:1330–1332.

Flueckiger, E., Briner, U., Buerki, H. R., Marbach, P., Wagner, H. R., and Doepfner, W., 1979, Two novel prolactin release inhibiting 8α-amino-ergolines, *Experientia* **35**:1677–1678.

Freedman, S. B., Templeton, W. W., Poat, J. A., and Woodruff, G. N., 1981, The effect of ADTN and some of its derivatives on dopamine receptor binding in rat striatum, *Proc. Br. Pharmacol. Soc.* **1981**:759P–760P.

Freeman, H. S., and McDermed, J. D., 1982, Interaction of chiral agonists with dopamine receptors, in: *Chemical Regulation of Biological Mechanisms* (A. M. Creighton and S. Turner, eds.), Royal Society of Chemistry, London, pp. 154–166.

Frey, E. A., Cote, T. E., Grewe, C. W., and Kebabian, J. W., 1982, [^{3}H]Spiroperidol identifies a D-2 dopamine receptor inhibiting adenylate cyclase activity in the intermediate lobe of the rat pituitary gland, *Endocrinology* **110**:1897–1904.

Fujita, N., Saito, K., Yonchara, N., and Yoshida, H., 1978, Lisuride inhibits ^{3}H-spiroperidol binding to membranes isolated from striatum, *Neuropharmacology* **17**:1089–1091.

Fuller, R. W., Clemens, J. A., and Hynes, M. D. III, 1982, Degree of selectivity of pre-synaptic versus postsynaptic dopamine receptors: Implications for prevention or treatment of tardive dyskinesia, *J. Clin. Psychopharmacol.* **2**(6):371–375.

Fuxe, K., Fredholm, B. B., Ögren, S.-O., Agnati, L. F., Hökfelt, T., and Gustafsson, J.-Å., 1978, Ergot drugs and central monoaminergic mechanisms: A histochemical, bio-chemical and behavioral analysis, *Fed. Proc.* **37**:2181–2191.

Geissler, H. E., 1977, 3-[2-(Dipropylamino)ethyl]phenol: A new selective dopaminergic agonist, *Arch. Pharm. (Weinheim)* **310**:749–756.

Gershanik, O., Heikkila, R. E., and Duvoisin, R. C., 1983, Effects of dopamine depletion on rotational behavior to dopamine agonists, *Brain Res.* **261**:358–360.

Gianutsos, G., Morrow, G., Light, S., and Sweeney, M. J., 1982, Dopaminergic properties of nomifensine, *Pharmacol. Biochem. Behav.* **17**:951–954.

Giesecke, J., 1980, Refinement of the structure of dopamine hydrochloride, *Acta Crystallogr.* **36B**:178–181.

Geissner-Prettre, C., and Pullman, B., 1975, Molecular-orbital study of the ortho-benzylic long range proton–proton coupling constants $4J_{HH}$ in biological phenethylamines, *J. Mag. Resonance* **18**:564–568.

Ginos, J. Z., Cotzias, G. C., Tolosa, E., Tang, L. C., and LoMonte, A., 1975, Cholinergic effects of molecular segments of apomorphine and dopaminergic effects of N,N-dialkylated dopamine, *J. Med. Chem.* **18**(12):1194–1200.

Goldberg, L. I., and Kohli, J. D., 1983, Differentiation of dopamine receptors in the periphery, in: *Dopamine Receptors, American Chemical Society Symposium Series 224* (C. Kaiser and J. W. Kebabian, eds.), American Chemical Society, Washington, pp. 101–113.

Goldberg, L. I., Sonneville, P. F., and McNay, J. L., 1968, An investigation of the structural requirements for dopamine-like renal vasodilation: Phenylethylamines and apomorphine, *J. Pharmacol. Exp. Ther.* **163**:188–197.

Goldberg, L. I., Volkman, P. H., Kohli, J. D., and Kotake, A. N., 1977, Similarities and differences of dopamine receptors in the renal vascular bed and elsewhere, in: *Advances in Biochemical Psychopharmacology,* Volume 16 (E. Costa and G. L. Gessa, eds.), Raven Press, New York, pp. 251–256.

Goldberg, L. I., Volkman, P. H., and Kohli, J. D., 1978a, A comparison of the vascular dopamine receptor with other dopamine receptors, *Annu. Rev. Pharmacol. Toxicol.* **18**:57–79.

Goldberg, L. I., Kohli, J. D., Kotake, A. N., and Volkman, P. H., 1978b, Characteristics of the vascular dopamine receptor: Comparison with other receptors, *Fed. Proc.* **37**:2396–2402.

Goldstein, M., Lew, J. Y., Nakamura, S., Battista, A. F., Lieberman, A., and Fuxe, K., 1978, Dopaminephilic properties of ergot alkaloids, *Fed. Proc.* **37**:2202–2206.

Goldstein, M., Lieberman, A., Lew, J. Y., Asano, T., Rosenfeld, M. R., and Makman, M. H., 1980, Interaction of pergolide with central dopaminergic receptors, *Proc. Natl. Acad. Sci. U.S.A.* **77**:3725–3728.

Goodale, D. B., Rusterholz, D. B., Long, J. P., Flynn, J. R., Walsh, B., Cannon, J. G., and Lee, T., 1980, Neurochemical and behavioral evidence for a selective presynaptic dopamine receptor agonist, *Science* **210**:1141–1143.

Goodall, McC., 1950a, Dihydroxyphenylalanine and hydroxytryptamine in mammalian suprarenals, *Chem. Abstr.* **44**:8454f.

Goodall, McC., 1950b, Hydroxytyramine in mammalian heart, *Nature* **166**:738.

Goodall, McC., 1951, Adrenaline and nonadrenaline in mammalian heart and suprarenals, *Acta Physiol. Scand. [Suppl.]* **84**:1–51.

Goodall, McC., and Alton, H., 1968, Metabolism of 3-hydroxytyramine (dopamine) in human subjects, *Biochem. Pharmacol.* **17**:905–914.

Gorczynski, R. J., Anderson, W. G., Erhardt, P. W., and Stout, D. M., 1979, Analysis of the cardiac stimulant properties of (3,4-dihydroxyphenyl)-cyclopropylamine (ASL-7003) and 2-amino-6,7-dihydroxy-1,2,3,4-tetrahydronaphthalene (A-6,7-DTN), *J. Pharmacol. Exp. Ther.* **210**:252–258.

Gower, A. J., and Marriott, A. S., 1982, Pharmacological evidence for the subclassification of central dopamine receptors in the rat, *Br. J. Pharmacol.* **77**:185–194.

Grol, C. J., and Rollema, H., 1977, Conformational analysis of dopamine by the INDO molecular orbital method, *J. Pharm. Pharmacol.* **19**:153–156.

Gund, P., 1982, Molecular geometry as an indicator of drug activity, *Trends Pharmacol. Sci.* **3**(2):56–59.

Hacksell, U., Arvidsson, L.-E., Svensson, U., Nilsson, J. L. G., Wikström, H., Lindberg, P., Sanchez, D., Hjorth, S., Carlsson, A., and Paalzow, L., 1981a, Monophenolic 2-(dipropylamino)indans and related compounds: Central dopamine-receptor stimulating activity, *J. Med. Chem.* **24**:429–434.

Hacksell, U., Arvidsson, L.-E., Svensson, U., Nilsson, J. L. G., Sanchez, D., Wikström, H., Lindberg, P., Hjorth, S., and Carlsson, A., 1981b, 3-Phenylpiperidines. Central dopamine-autoreceptor stimulating activity, *J. Med. Chem.* **24**:1475–1482.

Hahn, R. A., 1981, Inhibitory effects of pergolide on peripheral adrenergic neurotransmission in spontaneously hypertensive rats, *Life Sci.* **29**:2501–2509.

Hahn, R. A., Wardell, J. R., Jr., Sarau, H. M., and Ridley, P. T., 1982, Characterization of the peripheral and central effects of SK&F 82526, a novel dopamine receptor agonist, *J. Pharmacol. Exp. Ther.* **223**(2):305–313.

Henkel, J. G., Hane, J. T., and Gianutsos, G., 1982, Structure–anti-parkinson activity relationships in the aminoadamantanes. Influence of bridgehead substitution, *J. Med. Chem.* **25**:51–56.

Hicks, P. E., and Cannon, J. G., 1979, NN-Dialkyl derivatives of 2-amino-5,6-dihydroxy-1,2,3,4-tetrahydronaphthalene as selective agonists at presynaptic α-adrenoceptors in the rat, *J. Pharm. Pharmacol.* **31**:494–496.

Hill, H. F., and Lafferty, J. J., 1975, β-Naphthylmethyl piperazinyl derivatives, U.S. Patent 3,919,230, November 11, 1975.

Hjorth, S., Carlsson, A., Wikström, H., Lindberg, P., Sanchez, D., Hacksell, U., Arvidsson, L.-E., Svensson, U., and Nilsson, J. L. G., 1981, 3-PPP, a new centrally acting DA-receptor agonist with selectivity for autoreceptors, *Life Sci.* **28**:1225–1238.

Hjorth, S., Carlsson, A., Clark, D., Svensson, K., Wikström, H., Sanchez, D., Lindberg, P., Hacksell, U., Arvidsson, L.-E., Johansson, A., and Nilsson, J. L. G., 1982, Pharmacological manipulation of central dopamine (DA) autoreceptors—biochemical and behavioral consequences, in: Symposium on *Dopamine Receptor Agonists* Swedish Academy of Pharmaceutical Sciences, Stockholm, Sweden, April 20–23, 1982.

Hoffmann, I., Ehrhart, G., and Schmitt, K., 1971, 8-Amino-4-phenyl-1,2,3,4-tetrahydroisochinoline, eine neue Gruppe antidepressiver Psyhchopharmaka, *Arzneim. Forsch.* **21**:1045.

Hoffmann, I. S., Naylor, R. J., and Cubeddu, L. X., 1980, Presynaptic effects of 2-aminotetralins on striatal dopaminergic neurons, *J. Pharmacol. Exp. Ther.* **215**:486–493.

Holtz, P., 1939, Dopa decarboxylase, *Naturwissenschaften* **27**:724.

Holtz, P., 1959, Role of L-DOPA decarboxylase in the biosynthesis of catecholamines in nervous tissue and the adrenal medulla, *Pharmacol. Rev.* **11**:317–329.

Holtz, P., Credner, K., and Koeppe, W., 1942, Die enzymatische Entstehung von Oxytyramin in Organismus und die physiologische Bedeutung der Dopadecarboxylase, *Naunyn Schmiedebergs Arch. Exp. Pathol. Pharmakol.* **200**:356–388.

Horn, A. S., 1974, The conformation of dopamine at its uptake site; further studies with rigid analogs, *J. Pharm. Pharmacol.* **26**:735–737.

Horn, A. S., and Rodgers, J. R., 1980, 2-Amino-6,7-dihydroxytetrahydronaphthalene and the receptor-site preferred conformation of dopamine—a commentary, *J. Pharm. Pharmacol.* **32**:521–524.

Hornykiewicz, O., 1971, Dopamine: Its physiology, pharmacology and pathological neurochemistry, in: *Biogenic Amines and Physiological Membranes in Drug Therapy*, (J. H. Biel and L. G. Abood, eds.) Medicinal Research Series, Vol. 5, Part B, Marcel Dekker, New York, pp. 173–258.

Horowski, R., and Wachtel, H., 1976, Direct dopaminergic action of lisuride hydrogen maleate, an ergot derivative, in mice, *Eur. J. Pharmacol.* **36**:373–383.

Humber, L. G., Bruderlein, F. T., and Voith, K., 1975, Neuroleptic agents of the benzocycloheptapyridoisoquinoline series; a hypothesis on their mode of interaction with the central dopamine receptor, *Mol. Pharmacol.* **11**:833–840.

Humber, L. G., Bruderlein, F. T., Philipp, A. H., Götz, M., and Voith, K., 1979, Mapping the dopamine receptor. 1. Features derived from modifications in ring E of the neuroleptic butaclamol, *J. Med. Chem.* **22**(7):761–767.

Ilhan, M., Long, J. P., and Cannon, J. G., 1976, Structure–activity relationship studies of derivatives of aminotetralins and open chain analogs in relation to β and α-agonist activities, *Arch. Int. Pharmacodyn. Ther.* **223**:215–222.

Jacob, J. N., Nichols, D. E., Kohli, J. D., and Glock, D., 1981, Dopamine agonist properties of N-alkyl-4-(3,4-dihydroxyphenyl)-1,2,3,4-tetrahydroisoquinolines, *J. Med. Chem.* **24**:1013–1015.

Jaton, A. L., Loew, D. M., and Vigouret, J. M., 1978, A comparison of apomorphine, bromocriptine and Sandoz CM 29-712 (6-methyl-8a-cyanomethylergoline-I) in four different turning models in the rat, *Br. J. Pharmacol.* **62**:395P.

Jaunin, A., Petcher, T. J., and Weber, H. P., 1977, Conformations of some semi-rigid neuroleptic drugs, Part 2; crystal structures of racemic and of (+)-(S)-octoclothepin [2-chloro-10,11-dihydro-11-(4-methylpiperazin-l-yl)dibenzo[b,f]thiepin] and the absolute configuration of the latter, *J. Chem. Soc.* [*Perkin II*] **1977**:186–190.

Jenner, P., Taylor, A. R., and Campbell, D. B., 1973, Preliminary investigation of the metabolism of piribedil (ET 495); a new central dopaminergic agonist and potential antiparkinsonism agent, *J. Pharm. Pharmacol.* **25**:749–750.

Jenner, P., Clow, A., Reavill, C., Theodorou, A., and Marsden, C. D., 1980, Stereoselective actions of substituted benzemide drugs on cerebral dopamine mechanisms, *J. Pharm. Pharmacol.* **32**:39–44.

Kaiser, C., 1983, Stereoisomeric probes of the dopamine receptor, in: *Dopamine Receptors, American Chemical Society Symposium Series 224* (C. Kaiser and J. W. Kebabian, eds.), American Chemical Society, Washington, pp. 223–246.

Kaiser, C., and Zirkle, C. L., 1983, Enantioselectivity of tricyclic neuroleptics, unpublished observations.

Kaiser, C., Dandridge, P. A., Garvey, E., Hahn, R. A., Sarau, H. M., Setler, P. E., Bass, L. S., and Clardy, J., 1982, Absolute stereochemistry and dopaminergic activity of enantiomers of 2,3,4,5-tetrahydro-7,8-dihydroxy-1-phenyl-1H-3-benzazepine, *J. Med. Chem.* **25**:697–703.

Kaiser, C., Dandridge, P. A., Weinstock, J., Ackerman, D. M., Sarau, H. M., Setler, P. E., Webb, R. L., Horodniak, J. W., and Matz, E. D., 1983, Stereoselectivity of some new dopamine receptor agonists, *Acta Pharm. Suec.* [*Suppl.*] **2**:132–150.

Kebabian, J. W., 1978, Multiple classes of dopamine receptors in mammalian central nervous system: The involvement of dopamine-sensitive adenylyl cyclase, *Life Sci.* **23**:479–484.

Kebabian, J. W., and Calne, D. B., 1979, Multiple receptors for dopamine, *Nature* **277**:93–96.

Kehr, W., 1977, Effect of lisuride and other ergot derivatives on monoaminergic mechanisms in rat brain, *Eur. J. Pharmacol.* **41**:261–273.

Kohli, J. D., and Goldberg, L. I., 1980, Effects of 3'-4'-dihydroxynomifensine on the dopamine vascular receptor, *J. Pharm. Pharmacol.* **32**:225–226.

Kohli, J. D., Goldberg, L. I., and Nand, N., 1979, l-Aminomethyl isochromans: New vascular dopamine agonists, *Pharmacologist* **21**:202.

Kohli, J. D., Weder, A. B., Goldberg, L. I., and Ginos, J. Z., 1980, Structure activity relationships of N-substituted dopamine derivatives as agonists of the dopamine vascular and other cardiovascular receptors, *J. Pharmacol. Exp. Ther.* **213**:370–374.

Kohli, J. D., Goldberg, L. I., and McDermed, J. D., 1982, Modification of cardiovascular actions of 2-amino-5,6-dihydroxytetralin by N,N-di-n-propyl substitution, *Eur. J. Pharmacol.* **81**:293–299.

Ku, T., Bondinell, W. E., Zirkle, C. L., and Setler, P. E., 1983, Aporphine derivatives with central dopamine receptor antagonist activity, unpublished results.

Lafferty, J. J., Kaiser, C., Zirkle, C. L., Hill, H. F., and Setler, P. E., 1983, Structure–activity relationship studies of the dopaminergic piribedil, unpublished observations.

Lal, S., Sourkes, T. L., Missala, K., and Belendiuk, G., 1972, Effects of apormorphine and emetine alkaloids on central dopaminergic mechanisms in rats, *Eur. J. Pharmacol.* **20**:71–79.

Law, S.-J., Morgan, J. M., Masten, L. W., Borne, R. F., Arana, G. W., Kula, N. S., and Baldessarini, R. J., 1982, Rigid analogues of dopamine: Synthesis and interaction of 6-*exo-* and 6-*endo-*(3′,4′-dihydroxyphenyl)-2-aza-bicyclo[2.2.2]octanes with dopamine uptake sites and receptors, *J. Med Chem.* **25**:213–216.

Lemberger, L., and Crabtree. R. E., 1979, Pharmacologic effects in man of a potent, long acting dopamine receptor agonist, *Science* **205**:1151–1153.

Lew, J. Y., Nakamura, S., Battista, A. F., and Goldstein, M., 1979, Dopamine agonist potencies of ergolines, *Commun. Psychopharmacol.* **3**:179–183.

Lichtensteiger, W., Hefti, F., Felix, D., Huwyler, T., Melamed, E., and Schlumpf, M., 1982, Stimulation of nigrostriatal dopamine neurones by nicotine, *Neuropharmacology* **21**:963–968.

Liebowitz, M., Lieberman, A., Goldstein, M., Neophytides, A., Kupersmith, M., Gopinathan, G., and Mehl. S., 1981, Cardiac effects of pergolide, *Clin. Pharmacol. Ther.* **30**(6):718–723.

Loozen, H. J. J., Brands, F. T. L., and de Winter, M. S., 1982, An approach to the synthesis of [2]benzopyrano[3,4-c]pyrroles; alternative dopaminergic molecules, *Rec. Trav. Chem. Pays Bas* **101**(9):298–310.

Maixner, W., Long, J. P., Wright, C. B., Diana, J. N., Cannon, J. G., and Hake, H. L., 1981, Peripheral vascular effects of a new dopamine analog: 5,6-dihydroxy-2-methylaminotetralin (M-8), *J. Cardiovasc. Pharmacol.* **3**:381–389.

Mannich, C., and Jacobsohn, W., 1910, Uber Oxyphenyl-alkylamine und Dioxyphenyl-alkylamine, *Chem. Ber.* **1**:189–197.

Marek, K. L., and Roth, R. H., 1980, Ergot alkaloids: Interaction with presynaptic dopamine receptors in the neostriatum and olfactory tubercles, *Eur. J. Pharmacol.* **62**:137–146.

Markstein, R., Herrling, P. L., Bürki, H. R., Asper, H., and Ruch, W., 1978, The effect of bromocriptine on rat striatal adenylate cyclase and rat brain monoamine metabolism, *J. Neurochem.* **31**:1163–1172.

Martin, G. E., Williams, M., and Haubrich, D. R., 1982a, A pharmacological comparison of 6,7-dihydroxy-2-dimethylaminotetralin (TL-99) and N-*n*-propyl-3-(3-hydroxyphenyl)piperidine (3-PPP) with selected dopamine agonists, *J. Pharmacol. Exp. Ther.* **223**(2):298–304.

Martin, G. E., Williams, M., Clineschmidt, B. V., Yarbrough, G. G., Jones, J. H., and Haubrich, D. R., 1982b, Potent dopamine agonist activity of a novel ergoline, 6-ethyl-9-oxaergoline (EOE), *Life Sci.* **30**:1847–1856.

McDermed, J. D., and Freeman. H. S., 1982, Interactions of chiral agonists of the 2-aminotetralin series with dopamine receptors, in: *Symposium on Dopamine Receptor Agonists, Swedish Academy of Pharmaceutical Sciences, Stockholm, Sweden, April 20–23, 1982,* Swedish Academy of Pharmaceutical Sciences, Stockholm.

McDermed, J.D., and Miller, R. J., 1979, Antipsychotics and dopamine agonists, *Annu. Rep. Med. Chem.* **14**:12–21.

McDermed, J. D., McKenzie, G. M., and Phillips, A. P., 1975, Synthesis and pharmacology of some 2-aminotetralins. Dopamine receptor agonists, *J. Med Chem.* **18**(4):362–367.

McDermed, J. D., McKenzie, G. M., and Freeman, H. S., 1976, Synthesis and dopaminergic activity of (±)-, (+), and (−)-2-dipropylamino-5-hydroxy-1,2,3,4-tetrahydronaphthalene, J. Med Chem. 19:547–549.

McDermed, J. D., Freeman, H. S., and Ferris, R. M., 1979, Enantioselectivity in the binding of (+)- and (−)-2-amino-6,7-dihydroxy-1,2,3,4-tetrahydronaphthalene and related agonists to dopamine receptors, in: Catecholamines: Basic and Clinical Frontiers (E. Usdin, I. J. Kopin, and J. D. Barchas, eds.), Pergamon Press, New York, pp. 568–570.

McKenzie, G. M., and Szerb, J. C., 1968, The effect of dihydroxyphenylalanine, pheniprazine, and dextroamphetamine on the in vivo release of dopamine nucleus, J. Pharmacol. 162:302–308.

McNay, J. L., and Goldberg, L. I., 1966, Comparison of the effects of dopamine, isoproterenol, norepinephrine and bradykinin on canine renal and femoral blood flow, J. Pharmacol. Exp. Ther. 151:23–31.

Metysova, J., and Protiva, M., 1975, Stereospecificity of neuroleptic effects in the 10-piperazino-10,11-dihydrobenzo[b,f]thiepin series, Act. Nerv. Super. 17:218–219.

Miller, D. D., 1978, Steric aspects of dopaminergic drugs, Fed. Proc. 37:2392–2395.

Miller, R. J., and Iversen, L. L., 1974, Stimulation of dopamine-sensitive adenylate cyclase in homogenates of rat striatum by a metabolite of piribedil (ET 495), Naunyn Schiedebergs Arch. Pharmacol. 282:213–216.

Miller, R., Horn, A., Iversen, L., and Pinder, R., 1974, Effects of dopamine-like drugs on rat striatal adenyl cyclase have implications for CNS dopamine receptor topography, Nature 250:238–241.

Miller, R. J., Kelly, P. H., and Neumeyer, J. L., 1976, Aporphines. 15. Action of aporphine alkaloids on dopaminergic mechanisms in rat brain, Eur. J. Pharmacol. 35:77–83.

Montastruc, J. L., and Montastruc, P., 1981, Antihypertensive action of bromocriptine in neurogenic hypertensive dogs, Arch. Int. Pharmacodyn. Ther. 252:210–218.

Moragues, J., Prieto, J., Spickett, R. G. W., Vega, A., Salazar, W., and Roberts, D. J., 1980, Dopaminergic activity in a series of N-substituted 2-aminopyramidines, Farmaco Ed. Sci. 35:951–964.

Nédélec, L., Dumont, C., Oberlander, C., Frechet, D., Laurent, J., and Boissier, J. R., 1978, Syntheses et etude de l'activite dopaminergique de derives de la di(phenethyl)amine, Eur. J. Med. Chem. 13(6):553–563.

Nédélec, L., Guillaume, J., Oberlander, C., Euvrard, C., Labrie, F., Allais, A., and Boissier, J. R., 1980, Synthesis and stimulant dopaminergic activity of 4-(piperidin-3-yl) and 4-(1,2,5,6-tetrahydro-3-pyridinyl)-1H-indoles, Med. Chem. Symp. Abstr. Spain 1980:P168.

Neumeyer, J. L., McCarthy, M., Battista, S. P., Rosenberg, F. J., and Teiger, D. G., 1973a, Aporphines, 9. Synthesis and pharmacological evaluation of (±)-9,10-dihydroxyaporphine [(±)-isoapomorphine],(+)-,(−)-, and (±)-1,2-dihydroxyaporphine, and (+)-1,2,9,10-tetrahydroxyaporphine, J. Med Chem. 16:1228–1233.

Neumeyer, J. L., Neustadt, B. R., Oh, K. H., Weinhardt, K. K., Boyce, C. B., Rosenberg, F. J., and Teiger, D. G., 1973b, Aporphines. 8. Total synthesis and pharmacological evaluation of (±)-apomorphine, (±)-apocodeine, (±)-N-n-propylnorapomorphine and (±)-N-n-propylnorapocodeine, J. Med. Chem. 16:1223–1228.

Neumeyer, J. L., Granchelli, F. E., Fuxe, K., Ungerstedt, U., and Corrodi, H., 1974, Aporphines. 11. Synthesis and dopaminergic activity of monohydroxyaporphines. Total synthesis of (±)-11-hydroxyaporphine, (±)-11-hydroxynoraporphine, and (±)-11-hydroxy-N-n-propylnoraporphine, J. Med. Chem. 17(10):1090–1095.

Neumeyer, J. L., Lal, S., and Baldessarini, R. J., 1981a, Historical highlights of the chemistry, pharmacology, and early clinical uses of apormorphine, in: Apomorphine and

Other Dopaminomimetics, Volume 1: *Basic Pharmacology* (G. L., Gessa and G. U., Corsini, eds.), Raven Press, New York, pp. 1–17.

Neumeyer, J. L., Law, S. J., and Lamont, J. S., 1981b, Apomorphine and related aporphines as probes of the dopamine receptor, in: *Apomorphine and Other Dopaminomimetics*, Volume 1: *Basic Pharmacology* (G. L. Gessa and G. U. Corsini, eds.), Raven Press, New York, pp. 209–218.

Neumeyer, J. L., Arana, G. W., Law, S.-J., Lamont, J. S., Kula, N. S., and Baldessarini, R. J., 1981c, Aporphines. 36. Dopamine receptor interactions of trihydroxyaporphines. Synthesis, radioreceptor binding, and striatal adenylate cyclase stimulation of 2,10,11-trihydroxyaporphines in comparison with other hydroxylated aporphines, *J. Med. Chem.* **24**:1440–1445.

Neumeyer, J. L., Arana, G. W., Ram, V. J., and Baldessarini, R. J., 1983, Synthesis and structure-activity relationships of aporphines at central dopamine receptors, *Acta Pharm. Suec.* [*Suppl.*] **2**:11–24.

Nichols, D. E., 1976, Structural correlation between apomorphine and LSD: Involvement of dopamine as well as serotonin in the actions of hallucinogens. *J. Theor. Biol.* **59**:167–177.

Nichols, D. E., 1983, The development of novel dopamine agonists, in: *Dopamine Receptors, American Chemical Society Symposium Series 224* (C. Kaiser and J. W. Kebabian, eds.), American Chemical Society, Washington, pp. 201–218.

Nichols, D. E., Toth, J. E., Kohli, J. D., and Kotake, C. K., 1978, Dihydroxy-9-amino-9,10-dihydrophenenthrene, a rigid congener of dopamine and isoapomorphine, *J. Med. Chem.* **21**:395–398.

Nilsson, J. L. G., and Carlsson, A., 1982, Dopamine-receptor agonist with apparent selectivity for autoreceptors: A new principle for antipsychotic action?, *Trends Pharmacol. Sci.* **3**(8):322–325.

O'Donnell, J. P., Azzaro, A. J., and Urquilla, P. R., 1979, 2-(3,4-Dihydroxybenzyl)-2-imidazoline (DBHI): An analogue of dopamine, *Res. Commun. Chem. Pathol. Pharmacol.* **26**(2):243–251.

Offermeier, J., and van Rouyen, J. M., 1982, Is it possible to integrate dopamine receptor terminology?, *Trends Pharmacol. Sci.* **3**(8):326–328.

Olson, G. L., Cheung, H.-C., Morgan, K. D., Blount, J. F., Todaro, L., Berger, L., Davidson, A. B., and Boff, E., 1981, A dopamine receptor model and its application in the design of a new class of rigid pyrrolo[2,3-*g*]isoquinoline antipsychotics, *J. Med. Chem.* **24**:1026–1024.

Parli, C. J., Schmidt, B., and Shaar, C. J., 1978, Metabolism of lergotrile to 13-hydroxy lergotrile, a potent inhibitor of prolactin release *in vitro*, *Biochem. Pharmacol.* **27**:1405–1408.

Pendleton, R. G., Samler, L., Kaiser, C., and Ridley, P. T., 1978, Studies on renal dopamine receptors with a new agonist, *Eur. J. Pharmacol.* **51**:19–28.

Petcher, T. J., Schmutz, J., Weber, H. P., and White, T. G., 1975, Chirality of (+)-octoclothepin, a stereospecific neuroleptic agent, *Experientia* **31**:1389–1390.

Philipp, A. H., Humber, L. G. and Voith, K., 1979, Mapping of the dopamine receptor. 2. Features derived from modifications in the rings A/B region of the neuroleptic butaclamol, *J. Med. Chem.* **22**(7):768–773.

Pinder, R. M., Buxton, D. A., and Green, D. M., 1971, On the dopamine-like action of apomorphine, *J. Pharm. Pharmacol.* **23**:995–996.

Pinder, R. M., Buxton, D. A., and Woodruff, G. N., 1972, On apomorphine and dopamine receptors, *J. Pharm. Pharmacol.* **24**:903–904.

Poat, J. A., Woodruff, G. N., and Watling, K. J., 1978, Direct effect of a nomifensine derivative on dopamine receptors, *J. Pharm. Pharmacol.* **30**:495–497.

Poignant, J. C., Gressier, H., Petitjean, M., Regnier, G., and Canevari, R., 1975, A new central direct dopaminergic stimulant: 1-(Coumaran-5-ylmethyl)-4-(2-thiazolyl)piperazine hydrochloride (S 3608), *Experientia* **31**(19):1204–1205.

Rabey, J. M., Passeltiner, P., Markey, K., Asano, T., and Goldstein, M., 1981, Stimulation of pre- and postsynaptic dopamine receptors by an ergoline and by a partial ergoline, *Brain Res.* **225**:347–356.

Remy, D. C., and Martin, G. E., 1980, Antipsychotic agents and dopamine agonists, *Annu. Rep. Med. Chem.* **15**:12–21.

Riffee, W. H., Wilcox, R. E., Smith, R. V., Davis, P. J., and Brubaker, A., 1982, Inhibition of $R(-)$-apomorphine-induced stereotypic cage-climbing behavior in mice by S-$(+)$-apomorphine, in: Advances in the Biosciences, Volume 37, *Advances in Dopamine Research* (M. Kohsaka, T. Shohmori, T. Tsukada, and G. N. Woodruff, eds.), Pergamon Press, London, pp. 357–362.

Rusterholz, D. B., Long, J. P., Flynn, J. R., Cannon, J. G., Lee, T., Pease, J. P., Clemens, J. A., Wong, D. T., and Bymaster, F. P., 1979, Dopaminergic effects of non-hydroxylated rigid analogs of apomorphine, *Eur. J. Pharmacol.* **55**:73–82.

Saari, W. S., King, S. W., and Lotti, V. J., 1973, Synthesis and biological activity of (6a*S*)-10,11-dihydroxyaporphine, the optical antipode of apomorphine, *J. Med. Chem.* **16**:171–172.

Saari, W. S., King, S. W., Lotti, V. J., and Scriabine, A., 1974, Synthesis and biological activity of some aporphine derivatives related to apomorphine, *J. Med. Chem.* **17**(10):1086–1090.

Scharfenberg, P., and Sauer, J., 1980, Biological response as a function of conformation, chirality and electronic characteristics: A catecholamine study, *Int. J. Quantum Chem.* **18**:1309–1337.

Schechter, M. D., and Concannon, J. T., 1982, Dopaminergic activity of quipazine, *Pharmacol. Biochem. Behav.* **17**:393–397.

Schoenfeld, R. I., Neumeyer, J. L., Defeldecker, W., and Roffler-Tarlov, S., 1975, Comparison of structural and stereoisomers of apomorphine on stereotyped sniffing behavior of the rat, *Eur. J. Pharmacol.* **30**:63–68.

Schorderet, M., McDermed, J., and Magistretti, P., 1978, Dopamine receptors and cyclic AMP in rabbit retina—a pharmacological and stereochemical analysis using semi-rigid analogs of dopamine (aminotetralins) and thioxanthene isomers, *J. Physiol. (Paris)* **74**:509–513.

Schuster, D. I., Katerinopoulos, H. E., Holden, W. L., Narula, A. P. S., Libes, R. B., and Murphy, R. B., 1982, Synthesis and dopamine receptor binding of *exo*- and *endo*-2-amino-6,7-dihydroxybenzonorbornene, rigid analogues of 2-amino-6,7-dihydroxytetrahydronaphthalene, *J. Med. Chem.* **25**:850–854.

Seeman, P., 1980, Brain dopamine receptors, *Pharmacol. Rev.* **32**:229–313.

Seeman, P., 1982, Nomenclature of central and peripheral dopaminergic sites and receptors, *Biochem. Pharmacol.* **31**(16):2563–2568.

Seeman, P., Tedesco, J. L., Lee, T., Chau-Wong, M., Muller, P., Bowles, J., Whitaker, P. M., McManus, C., Titeler, M., Weinreich, P., Friend, W. C., and Brown, G. M., 1978a, Dopamine receptors in the central nervous system, *Fed. Proc.* **37**:130–136.

Seeman, P., Titeler, M., Tedesco, J., Weinreich, P., and Sinclair, D., 1978b, in: *Advances in Biochemical Psychopharmacology*, Volume 19 (P. J. Roberts, G. N. Woodruff, and L. L. Iversen, eds.), Raven Press, New York, pp. 167–176.

Seidlova, V., and Protiva, M., 1967, Neutotrope und psychotrope Substanzen. X. Uber die Synthese von 10-(4-Methylpiperazino)-10,11-dihydro-5H-dibenzo-[*a,d*]cyclohepten und seinen 8-Chlorderivat, *Collect. Czech. Chem. Commun.* **32**:1747–1758.

Seiler, M. P., and Markstein, R., 1982, Further characterization of the structural requirements for agonists at the striatal dopamine D-1 receptor. Studies with a series of monohydroxyaminotetralins on dopamine-sensitive adenylate cyclase and comparison with dopamine receptor binding, *Mol. Pharmacol.* **22**:281–289.

Setler, P. E., Sarau, H. M., Zirkle, C. L., and Saunders, H. L., 1978a, The central effects of a novel dopamine agonist, *Eur. J. Pharmacol.* **50**:419–430.

Setler, P. E., Malesky, M., McDevitt, J., and Turner, K., 1978b, Rotation produced by administration of dopamine and related substances directly into the supersensitive caudate nucleus, *Life Sci.* **23**:1277–1284.

Seyfried, C. A., and Fuxe, K., 1982, Neuropharmacological and neurochemical effects of 3-[4-(4-phenyl-1,2,3,6-tetrahydropyridyl-1)-butyl]indole (EMD 23448) a new, long-acting dopamine agonist, *Arzneim. Forsch.* **32**(II):892–893.

Sharabi, F. M., Long, J. P., Cannon, J. G., and Hatheway, G. J., 1976a, Inhibition of the sympathetic nervous system by a series of heterocyclic congeners of dopamine, *J. Pharmacol. Exp. Ther.* **199**:630–638.

Sharabi, F. M., Long, J. P., and Cannon, J. G., 1976b, Hypotensive effect induced by a cyclic dopamine analog, *trans*-4-methyl-7,8-dihydroxy-1,2,3,4,4a,5,6,10b-octahydrobenzo[*f*]quinoline, *J. Pharm. Sci.* **67**(11):1639–1641.

Sheppard, H., and Burghardt, C. R., 1974, The dopamine-sensitive adenylate cyclase of rat caudate nucleus. Comparison with the isoproterenol-sensitive (beta receptor system) of rat erythrocytes in responses to dopamine derivatives, *Mol. Pharmacol.* **10**:721–726.

Sheppard, H., and Burghardt, C. R., 1978, The dopamine-sensitive adenylate cyclase of the rat caudate nucleus. 3. The effect of aporphines and protoberberines, *Biochem. Pharmacol.* **27**:1113–1116.

Sheppard, H., Burghardt, C. R., and Long, J. P., 1978, The effect of dihydroxy-2-aminotetralins (DATS) on dopamine and *beta* type adenylate cyclases, *Res. Commun. Chem. Pathol. Pharmacol.* **19**(2):213–224.

Shorr, R. G. L., Lefkowitz, R. J., and Caron, M. G., 1981, Purification of the β-adrenergic receptor. Identification of the hormone binding subunit, *J. Biol. Chem.* **256**:5820–5826.

Shorr, R. G. L., Heald, S. L., Jeffs, P. W., Lavin, T. M., Strohsacker, M. W., Lefkowitz, R. J., and Caron, M. G., 1982a, The β-adrenergic receptor: Rapid purification and covalent labeling by photoaffinity crosslinking, *Proc. Natl. Acad. Sci. U.S.A.* **79**(9):2778–2782.

Shorr, R. G. L., Strohsacker, M. W., Lavin, T. N., Lefkowitz, R. J., and Caron, M. G., 1982b, The β₁-adrenergic receptor of the turkey erythrocyte. Molecule heterogeneity revealed by purification and photoaffinity labeling, *J. Biol. Chem.* **257**(20):12341–12350.

Sindelar, R. D., Mott, J., Barfknecht, C. F., Arneric, S. P., Flynn, J. R., Long, J. P., and Bhatnagar, R. K., 1982, 2-Amino-4,7-dimethoxyindan derivatives: Synthesis and assessment of dopaminergic and cardiovascular actions, *J. Med. Chem.* **25**:858–864.

Smythies, J. R., 1981, An hypothesis of the molecular structure of the dopamine receptor, *Med. Hypotheses* **7**:1449–1456.

Sokoloff, P., Martres, M. P., and Schwartz, J. C., 1980a, Three classes of dopamine receptor (D-2, D-3, D-4) identified by binding studies with ³H-apomorphine and ³H-domperidone, *Naunyn Schmiedebergs Arch. Pharmacol.* **315**:89–102.

Sokoloff, P., Martres, M.-P., and Schwartz, J.-C., 1980b, ³H-Apomorphine labels both dopamine postsynaptic receptors and autoreceptors, *Nature* **288**:283–286.

Stoof, J. C., Horn, A. S., and Mulder, A. H., 1980, Simultaneous demonstration of the activation of presynaptic dopamine autoreceptors and postsynaptic dopamine receptors *in vitro* by N,N-dipropyl-5,6-ADTN, *Brain Res.* **196**:276–281.

Struyker-Boudier, H., Teppema, L., Cools, A., and van Rossum, J., 1975, (3,4-Dihydroxy-phenylamino)-2-imidazoline (DPI), a new potent agonist at dopamine receptors mediating neuronal inhibition, *J. Pharm. Pharmacol.* **27**:882–883.

Sweet, C. S., Gaul, S. L., Ludden, C. T., and Britt, P. M., 1982, Cardiovascular effects of 6-ethyl-9-oxaergoline (EOE), a potent dopamine agonist, *Fed. Proc.* **41**(5):1587.

Tedesco, J. L., Seeman, P., and McDermed, J. D., 1979, The conformation of dopamine at its receptor: Binding of monohydroxy-2-aminotetralin enantiomers and positional isomers, *Mol. Pharmacol.* **16**:369–381.

Tolosa, E. S., Cotzias, G. C., Burckhardt, P. G., Tang, L. C., and Dahl, K. E., 1977, The dopaminergic and antidopaminergic effects of some aporphines, *Exp. Neurol.* **55**:56–66.

Tsuruta, K., Frey, E. A., Grewe, C. W., Cote, T. E., Eskay, R. L., and Kebabian, J. W., 1981, Evidence that LY-141865 specifically stimulates the D-2 dopamine receptor, *Nature* **292**:463–465.

van Beek, M. C., and Timmerman, H., 1974, Some benzhydryl derivatives as central dopamine receptor stimulating agents, *J. Pharm. Pharmacol.* **26**:57–58.

van der Zee, P., Koger, H. S., Gootjes, J., and Hespe, W., 1980, Aryl 1,4-dialk(en)ylpiperazines as selective and very potent inhibitors of dopamine uptake, *Eur. J. Med. Chem.* **15**(4):363–370.

Van Oene, J. C., Houwing, H. A., and Horn, A. S., 1982a, The purported dopamine agonist (3,4-dihydroxyphenylimino)-2-imidazoline (DPI) acts as a nonselective α-adrenoceptor agonist in inducing hypertension, hypomotility and hypothermia in the rat, *Eur. J. Pharmacol.* **85**:69–77.

Van Oene, J. C., Houwing, H. A., and Horn, A. S., 1982b, Evidence that the purported dopaminergic agonist (3,4-dihydroxyphenylimino)-2-imidazoline (DPI) may reduce rat striatal dopamine turnover by an α₂-adrenergic mechanism, *Eur. J. Pharmacol.* **81**:75–87.

Verimer, T., Long, J. P., Rusterholz, D. R., Flynn, J. R., Cannon, J. G., and Lee, T., 1980, Dopaminergic activity of *cis–trans* isomers of benzhydro[*f*]quinoline analogs, *Eur. J. Pharmacol.* **64**:271–277.

Volkman, P. H., Kohli, J. D., Goldberg, L. I., Cannon, J. G., and Lee, T., 1977, Conformational requirements for dopamine-induced vasodilation, *Proc. Natl. Acad. Sci. U.S.A.* **74**:3602–3606.

Wardell, J. R., Jr., Hahn, R. A., and Stefankiewicz, J. S., 1979, in: *Peripheral Dopaminergic Receptors* (J. Imbs and J. Schwartz, eds.), Pergamon Press, New York, pp. 389–399.

Watling, K. J., 1982, Dopamine receptors and 3-PPP, a P-ossible P-referential P-resynaptic agonist? *Trends Pharmacol. Sci.* **3**(6):232.

Watling, K. J., and Williams, M., 1982, Interaction of the putative dopamine autoreceptor agonists, 3-PPP and TL-99, with the dopamine-sensitive adenylate cyclase of carp retina, *Eur. J. Pharmacol.* **77**:321–326.

Weinstock, J., Wilson, J. W., Ladd, D. L., Brush, C. K., Pfeiffer, F. R., Kuo, G. Y., Holden, K. G., Yim, N. C. F., Hahn, R. A., Wardell, J. R., Jr., Tobia, A. J., Setler, P. E., Sarau, H. M., and Ridley, P. T., 1980, Separation of potent central and renal dopamine agonist activity of substituted 6-chloro-2,3,4,5-tetrahydro-7,8-dihydroxy-1-phenyl-1*H*-3-benzazepines, *J. Med. Chem.* **23**:973–975.

Weinstock, J., Wilson, J. W., Ladd, D. L., Brenner, M., Ackerman, D. M., Blumberg, A. L., Hahn, R. A., Hieble, J. P., Sarau, H. M., and Wiebelhaus, V. D., 1983, Dopaminergic benzazepines with divergent cardiovascular profiles, in: *Dopamine Receptors, American Chemical Society Symposium Series 224* (C. Kaiser and J. W. Kebabian, eds.), American Chemical Society, Washington, pp. 157–169.

Weir, R. L., Hruska, R. E., and Silbergeld, E. K., 1981, Binding of antiparkinsonian ergot derivatives to the dopamine receptor, *Psychopharmacology* **75**:119–123.

Wikström, H., Sanchez, D., Lindberg, P., Arvidsson, L.-E., Hacksell, U., Johansson, A., Nilsson, J. L. G., Hjorth, S., and Carlsson, A., 1982, Monophenolic octahydrobenzo[f]quinolines: Central dopamine- and serotonin-receptor stimulating activity, *J. Med. Chem.* **25**:925–931.

Wilk, S., Mizoguchi, H., and Orlowski, M., 1978, Gamma-glutamyl dopa: A kidney specific dopamine precursor, *J. Pharmacol. Exp. Ther.* **206**(1):227–232.

Wilson, J. W., 1978, 3-Benzazepine derivatives with peripheral and central dopaminergic properties, in: *Program and Abstracts, 16th National Medicinal Chemical Symposium of the American Chemical Society, Kalamazoo, Michigan, June 18–22, 1978*, American Chemical Society, Washington, p. 155.

Woodman, O. L., Medgett, I. C., Lang, W. J., and Rand, M. J., 1981, Agonist actions of DPI [2-(3,4-dihydroxyphenylimino)-imidazolidine] on α-adrenoceptors and dopamine receptors, *Eur. J. Pharmacol.* **75**:11–19.

Woodruff, G. N., 1971, Dopamine receptors: A review, *Comp. Gen. Pharmacol.* **2**:439–455.

Woodruff, G. N., 1982, ADTN-a potent dopamine receptor agonist, *Trends Pharmacol. Sci.* **3**:59–61.

Woodruff, G. N., Elkhawad, A. O., and Pinder, R. M., 1974, Long lasting stimulation of locomotor activity produced by the intraventricular injection of a cyclic analogue of dopamine into conscious mice, *Eur. J. Pharmacol.* **25**:80–86.

5

Peripheral Dopamine Receptors

*M. G. BOGAERT, W. A. BUYLAERT, R. A. LEFEBVRE, and
J. L. WILLEMS*

1. Introduction

In the last 20 years there has been increasing interest in the effects of
dopamine both in the CNS and in the periphery. Moreover, much work
has been done to elucidate which receptors are involved in these effects.

The first evidence for the existence of a peripheral dopamine receptor
was found in the dog renal artery (McNay *et al.*, 1965). Since then, dopamine receptors have been described in other blood vessels and organs
as well as in orthosympathetic ganglia and on nerve endings. Dopamine
and dopamine agonists and antagonists possess a variety of effects in
different parts of the organism. However, in observing such effects, one
should refrain from claiming too easily that *peripheral* receptors are involved. It is well known that, e.g., in the cardiovascular and gastrointestinal systems, some effects are mediated by interaction with central
receptors, and it is not easy to exclude in *in vivo* experiments a central
site of action of agonists or antagonists.

Moreover, one has to prove with appropriate experiments that the
effects seen cannot be explained by interaction with receptors other than
dopamine receptors. That one should be very cautious is illustrated by
recent findings in the rat vas deferens. The presence of dopamine receptors was suggested for the rat vas deferens in a number of publications
(Ferrini and Miragoli, 1972; Simon and Van Maanen, 1976; Tayo, 1979).
However, in recent pharmacological studies, two groups of authors concluded that the contractile effect of dopamine on the rat vas deferens can

M. G. BOGAERT, W. A. BUYLAERT, R. A. LEFEBVRE, and J. L. WILLEMS • Heymans
Institute of Pharmacology, University of Gent Medical School, B-9000 Gent, Belgium.

be explained satisfactorily by interaction with postsynaptic α receptors (Langeloh and Jurkiewicz, 1982; Leedham and Pennefather, 1982). This illustrates clearly that before one can postulate the presence of a dopamine receptor in an organ, several dopamine agonists and antagonists should be studied, and, moreover, agonists and antagonists for other receptors should also be included in the study. It should be added that in a recent publication Relja *et al.* (1982) found evidence for the presence of dopamine binding sites in the rat vas deferens.

In view of the numerous reviews available (Goldberg, 1972; Goldberg *et al.*, 1978; Buylaert *et al.*, 1981; Schmidt *et al.*, 1981; Brodde, 1982; Lokhandwala and Barrett, 1982), no attempt will be made to discuss all problems concerning peripheral dopamine receptors, and this chapter is limited to some particular aspects.

In the first part, peripheral dopamine receptors in the cardiovascular system are dealt with. There is a wealth of data concerning the cardiovascular system, and these data suggest that there are at least two different types of dopamine receptors; their characteristics and similarities and dissimilarities to central dopamine receptors are discussed.

In the second part, ganglionic dopamine receptors are dealt with. Dopamine inhibits transmission in autonomic sympathetic ganglia: the dopamine receptor that is involved in this effect is compared to the dopamine receptors found in the cardiovascular system.

Finally, there is a discussion about whether or not peripheral dopamine receptors are present in the gastrointestinal system, mediating effects on motility and on secretion.

2. Dopamine Receptors in the Cardiovascular System

The first description of a peripheral dopamine receptor was in the renal artery of the dog, located on the smooth muscle cell and mediating vasodilatation (McNay *et al.*, 1965); since then, postsynaptic receptors have been described on smooth muscle of many other blood vessels.

Later, dopamine receptors were also found on the sympathetic nerve endings leading to the cat heart (Long *et al.*, 1975), to the canine femoral arteries (Buylaert *et al.*, 1977, 1978), and to a number of other organs (see reviews cited above). Stimulation of these presynaptic receptors leads to inhibition of transmitter release from the sympathetic nerve endings.

2.1. Differences between Pre- and Postsynaptic Receptors

There is much interest in the possibility that several classes of dopamine receptors are present in the central nervous system (for discussion, see Kebabian and Calne, 1979; Seeman, 1980, 1982; Creese and Sibley, 1982). The question about multiple dopamine receptors has also been raised for the peripheral dopamine receptors in the cardiovascular system. Indeed, soon after the discovery of presynaptic dopamine receptors on orthosympathetic nerve endings leading to the heart and to the femoral vasculature, it was suggested that the dopamine receptors located at pre- and postsynaptic sites were different (Willems *et al.*, 1979): phenoxybenzamine antagonizes the effects mediated by presynaptic receptors, whereas the postsynaptic receptor, e.g., in the renal artery, is typically studied in the presence of phenoxybenzamine. Other differences emerged, and this led to the nomenclature of DA_1 for postsynaptic and DA_2 for presynaptic dopamine receptors (Goldberg and Kohli, 1979; Langer, 1981).

The evidence for the existence of at least two classes of peripheral dopamine receptors in the cardiovascular system comes mainly from *in vivo* studies of the pharmacological effects of agonists and antagonists. It should be stressed that in such *in vivo* studies, the requirements for a valid receptor characterization, e.g., presence of steady-state concentrations of the agonists and antagonists and involvement of only one receptor type in the response seen, are not fulfilled (Furchgott, 1972). Therefore, a very careful experimental approach and cautious interpretation of the results are mandatory. What are the results of these studies with agonists and antagonists?

2.1.1. Studies with Agonists

Structural requirements for the postsynaptic receptor are very restrictive, and only few compounds are active at these receptors, whereas a large number of compounds are agonists at the presynaptic receptors.

For example, dimethyldopamine, several ergot derivatives, and piribedil are active on presynaptic receptors but not on postsynaptic receptors. For some compounds, conflicting results have been reported in the literature. For example, Volkman and Goldberg (1976) found no vasodilatation with bolus injections of bromocriptine in the renal artery of the dog; however, others reported a postsynaptic effect of the substance (Imbs *et al.*, 1979; Schmidt *et al.*, 1982), and Brodde *et al.* (1981) confirmed the postsynaptic effect of bromocriptine on isolated rabbit mesenteric strips. Differences in species used and in experimental protocol and problems of solubility of bromocriptine could be responsible for these discrepancies.

Other agonists, although active on both pre- and postsynaptic receptors, are much more potent on the presynaptic receptor. Apomor-

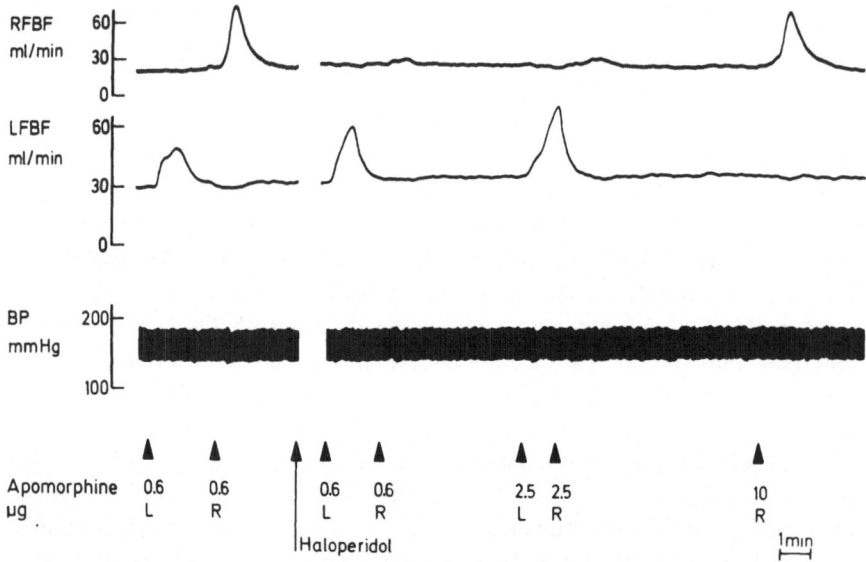

Figure 1. The effect of apomorphine (▲) injected into the right (R) and left (L) femoral artery of the dog. RFBF, right femoral blood flow; LFBF, left femoral blood flow; BP, systemic blood pressure. ↑ indicates the injection of 30 μg of haloperidol into the right femoral artery; right tracing starts 5 min after haloperidol administration. The doses of apomorphine are shown below the figure. (From Buylaert *et al.*, 1977, with permission of *The Journal of Pharmacology and Experimental Therapeutics.*)

phine, for instance, is only a partial agonist on the renal artery postsynaptic receptor but has a marked activity on presynaptic dopamine receptors (Fig. 1), and this at a much lower dose range.

There has been recently much interest in substances such as SK&F 38393 and SK&F 82526. SK&F 38393 is an agonist at postsynaptic dopamine receptors (Pendleton *et al.*, 1978) but lacks presynaptic activity (Roby and Orzechowski, 1979). For SK&F 82526, which is a full dopamine agonist at the postsynaptic level, absence of a peripheral presynaptic effect has been suggested but not been shown until recently (Hahn *et al.*, 1982).

There is also a difference between the pre- and postsynaptic activity of aminotetralins. 2-Amino-6,7-dihydroxy-1,2,3,4-tetrahydronaphtalene is active at both pre- and postsynaptic dopamine receptors, whereas 2-amino-5,6-dihydroxy-1,2,3,4-tetrahydronaphtalene is only active at the presynaptic dopamine receptor (Goldberg and Kohli, 1979). However, it is hazardous to draw firm conclusions from such observations regarding the characteristics of the receptors and the receptor-preferred dopamine conformation, as shown by the fact that the same group recently reported that dipropyl substitution in the nitrogen position of the 5,6-analogue leads to a high agonist potency on postsynaptic receptors (Kohli *et al.*, 1982).

2.1.2. Studies with Antagonists

Differences between peripheral pre- and postsynaptic dopamine receptors in the cardiovascular system have also been seen in studies with antagonists.

As already described, phenoxybenzamine antagonizes effects mediated by presynaptic dopamine receptors, whereas the postsynaptic receptor is classically studied in the presence of phenoxybenzamine (Willems *et al.*, 1979).

Haloperidol has a very narrow range of specificity against dopamine at postsynaptic sites. This is in marked contrast with the ease with which the specific antagonism by haloperidol can be shown at presynaptic sites, as illustrated in our work on presynaptic receptors on the orthosympathetic nerve endings leading to the canine femoral vasculature (Buylaert *et al.*, 1977) and shown in Fig. 1; this is also true for a number of other butyrophenones and for phenothiazines.

For some substances that are highly active at presynaptic receptors, postsynaptic activity cannot even be shown. A good example is domperidone, which blocks the apomorphine-induced femoral vasodilatation (Willems *et al.*, 1981) but does not antagonize the dopamine-induced renal vasodilatation (Glock *et al.*, 1982).

Bulbocapnine and sulpiride were reported to be highly selective antagonists at postsynaptic sites (Goldberg and Kohli, 1981). Moreover, the study of the enantiomers of sulpiride showed that (*S*)-sulpiride is more active than (*R*)-sulpiride on presynaptic dopamine receptors of the canine femoral artery (Goldberg and Kohli, 1979), of the rabbit ear artery (Brown and O'Connor, 1981), and of the perfused cat spleen (Dubocovich and Langer, 1980). In contrast, (*R*)-sulpiride is more active than (*S*)-sulpiride on the postsynaptic renal artery dopamine receptor (Goldberg and Kohli, 1979) or at least as active on the postsynaptic receptor in the superior mesenteric artery of the dog (Shepperson *et al.*, 1982).

Shepperson *et al.* (1982) studied several dopamine antagonists at presynaptic (heart and nictitating membrane) and postsynaptic (superior mesenteric artery) dopamine receptors in the dog. They confirmed the differences in relative potency of these antagonists at pre- and postsynaptic dopamine receptors but could not confirm the finding by Goldberg and Kohli (1981) that sulpiride is more potent as a postsynaptic antagonist than either haloperidol or bulbocapnine. Although this discrepancy could result from differences in experimental design, this finding is not without importance for the comparison of peripheral and central dopamine receptors.

Although studies *in vivo* should be used cautiously for characterization of receptors, the studies with agonists and antagonists discussed above point to the existence of at least two different types of dopamine receptors in the cardiovascular system.

It is possible that even more subtypes of dopamine receptors will be identified. Steinsland and Hieble (1979) suggested the presence of different type of prejunctional dopamine receptors in the rabbit ear artery. Lang and Woodman (1982) reported that the postsynaptic dopamine agonist SK&F 38393 increases renal blood flow in the dog but is without dilator activity in the coronary vasculature; dopamine itself dilated both vascular beds, and these authors conclude that there is a difference between the dopamine receptors present in renal and coronary vasculature.

2.2. Comparison of Peripheral with Central Dopamine Receptors

In view of the finding that cardiovascular receptors belong to at least two distinct types, it is tempting to compare the peripheral receptors to the central dopamine receptors. Such attempts are hazardous. Indeed, there is no agreement on the exact classification of central dopamine receptors (Kebabian and Calne, 1979; Seeman, 1980, 1982; Creese and Sibley, 1982). Moreover, characterization of central dopamine receptors is mainly based on *in vitro* data, e.g., ligand binding and adenylate cyclase stimulation, whereas for the peripheral receptor characterization, pharmacological effects obtained mainly *in vivo* are considered. There are data suggesting that dopamine-sensitive adenylate cyclase exists in the canine renal artery (see Murphy *et al.*, 1976), but there is no proof of a correlation of renal vasodilatation with adenylate cyclase activity.

Comparison of the activity of agonists and antagonists on the CNS and in the periphery suggests a similarity between peripheral presynaptic receptors (DA_2) and the D_2 receptor of Kebabian and Calne (1979). It is not clear how far DA_1 and D_1 receptors are comparable. Thus, sulpiride, for example, which does not inhibit dopamine stimulation of central adenylate cyclase, a D_1 phenomenon, was found to be mainly a DA_1 antagonist (Goldberg and Kohli, 1981); in a recent study, Shepperson *et al.*, (1982) could, however, not confirm this. SK&F 82526, a full agonist on DA_1 receptors, has no inhibitory effect on prolactin release, a D_2-receptor-mediated phenomenon, although it stimulates striatal adenylate cyclase, a D_1 phenomenon (Hahn *et al.*, 1982).

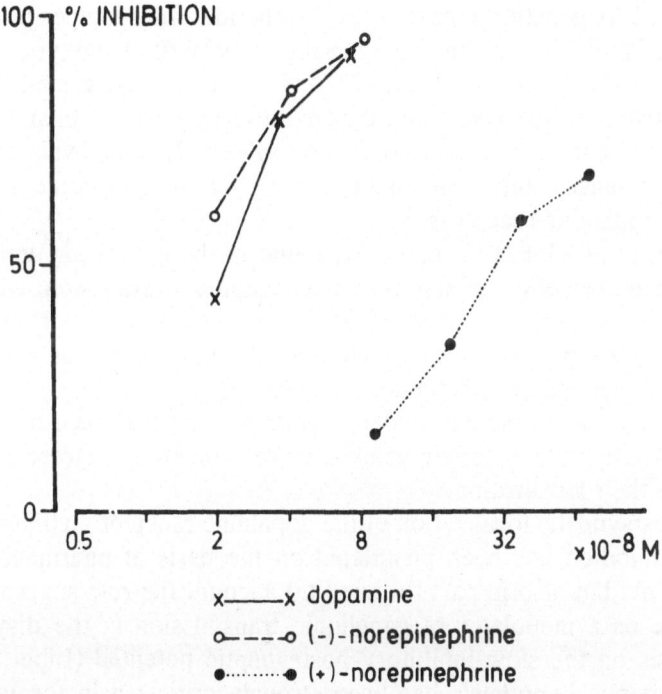

Figure 2. Dose–response curves for the inhibitory effect of dopamine, (−)-norepinephrine, and (+)-norepinephrine on the postganglionic action potential evoked by preganglionic electrical stimulation on the dog lumbar paravertebral ganglion.

3. Dopamine Receptors Mediating Ganglionic Inhibition

Dopamine, as do other catecholamines, inhibits ganglionic transmission. It is not well accepted that, at least for some ganglia and some species, this occurs through interaction with dopamine receptors. For the lumbar paravertebral ganglion of the dog, for example, the possibility that dopamine inhibits ganglionic transmission via a receptor different from the α receptor was first suggested on the basis of the observation that dopamine is equipotent with (−)-norepinephrine and much more potent than (+)-norepinephrine, as shown in Fig. 2 (Willems, 1973). Studies with dopamine agonists and antagonists confirmed that the inhibition of transmission is mediated through a specific dopamine receptor (Willems, 1973; Willems *et al.*, 1979).

How does the dopamine receptor involved in this ganglionic inhibition compare to the dopamine receptors found in the cardiovascular system? On the basis of the equipotence of apomorphine with dopamine, the potent and long-lasting blockade by haloperidol and domperidone, the activity of piribedil, and the antagonistic activity of phenoxybenzamine (Willems, 1973; Willems *et al.*, 1979, 1981), it can be suggested that the characteristics of the ganglionic dopamine receptor are similar to those of the DA_2 receptor in the cardiovascular system. Lokhandwala and Barrett (1982) suggest the term "neurotropic" for the ganglionic and presynaptic dopamine receptors.

Horn *et al.* (1982a,b), however, found in the guinea pig and in the dog a facilitatory effect of sulpiride on ganglionic transmission, with (*R*)-sulpiride being more potent in this regard than (*S*)-sulpiride; (*R*)-sulpiride was also more potent than (*S*)-sulpiride in antagonizing the inhibitory effect of dopamine on ganglionic transmission.

Although experimental evidence points to the existence of specific dopamine receptors in certain ganglia, there is much less agreement with regard to their localization.

A postsynpatic localization of the dopamine receptor mediating ganglionic inhibition has been postulated on the basis of pharmacological experiments but also in part to take into account the role suggested for dopamine as a modulator of ganglionic transmission in the disynaptic hypothesis on the slow inhibitory postsynaptic potential (Libet, 1970). The disynaptic hypothesis has been strongly criticized in the last few years; moreover, there is no direct pharmacological evidence for a postsynaptic localization of a dopamine receptor, and Brown and Caulfield (1979) concluded that the postsynaptic hyperpolarization by dopamine is mediated by an α_2 receptor.

There are a number of arguments in favor of a presynaptic role for dopamine (and other catecholamines), with inhibition of the release of the neurotransmitter acetylcholine from presynaptic nerve endings. In one study attempts were made to characterize the presynaptic receptor, but there was no evidence that this is a specific dopamine receptor (Nakamura, 1978).

4. *Peripheral Dopamine Receptors in the Gastrointestinal System*

The question of whether peripheral dopamine receptors are present in the gastrointestinal system is at this moment unanswered. As already presented, conclusions about the presence or the absence of a particular receptor, such as a dopamine receptor, should be based on extensive studies with agonists and antagonists. Moreover, many substances that affect the gastrointestinal system act on the central nervous system, for example, on the chemoreceptor trigger zone. It is often difficult to exclude *in vivo* an effect on these central structures, even for substances that do not cross the blood–brain barrier such as dopamine and domperidone; indeed, the chemoreceptor trigger zone is not protected by the blood–brain barrier. Therefore, studies *in vivo* will often not allow conclusions about the existence of peripheral dopamine receptors mediating effects on gastrointestinal motility and gastrointestinal secretion, and the evidence should come from studies *in vitro* or studies *in vivo* with appropriate experimental design.

4.1. Gastrointestinal Secretion

There are a number of studies on peripheral dopamine receptors and secretion in organs such as stomach, pancreas, and salivary glands.

Involvement of dopamine receptors has been postulated for the inhibitory effect of dopamine on gastric acid secretion in dog and man (Valenzuela and Grossman, 1976; Valenzuela *et al.*, 1979). However, these suggestions are based on very limited experimental evidence, and in these studies only one or no antagonist was used. Others have found that the inhibitory action of dopamine on acid secretion in the dog can be satisfactorily explained by an interaction with β_1 receptors (Hovendal *et al.*, 1982). Suggestions that dopamine receptors are involved in the pathogenesis of duodenal ulceration (Szabo, 1979) are not substantiated.

There has been much interest in a stimulatory effect of dopamine on pancreatic secretion and in the possibility that this effect is mediated by a dopamine receptor. There is good evidence from studies with antagonists and agonists that such a receptor does in fact exist in the dog (Hashimoto *et al.*, 1971; Bastie *et al.*, 1977; Satoh *et al.*, 1980). No such evidence is, however, present in other species such as rat (Furuta *et al.*, 1978) and man (Lankisch and Koop, 1978).

Involvement of a dopamine receptor was also suggested for the stimulatory effect of dopamine on amylase secretion in the guinea pig submandibular gland (Carlsöo *et al.*, 1974; Bloom *et al.*, 1975). The stimulatory effect of dopamine on parotid and submandibular protein secretion in the rat is thought to involve activation of α, β, and dopamine receptors (Abe and Dawes, 1982).

4.2. Gastrointestinal Motility

Interest in the possibility that dopamine receptors are involved in the effect of some substances on gastrointestinal motility, and even that dopamine receptors are involved physiologically in the regulation of gas-

trointestinal motility, stems mostly from the observation of the therapeutic effects of substances such as metoclopramide and domperidone in
gastroesophageal reflux, nausea, and vomiting.

Metoclopramide (Baumann *et al.*, 1979) and domperidone (Weihrauch *et al.*, 1979) increase lower esophageal sphincter pressure, and L-
dopa decreases this pressure, a phenomenon antagonized by metoclopramide (Baumann *et al.*, 1979). Such findings do not prove the presence
of peripheral dopamine receptors in the gastrointestinal tract; for example, gastric relaxation by apomorphine in the conscious dog is mainly
of central origin, as can be shown by comparison of intravenous and
intracerebroventricular administrations (Blancquaert *et al.*, 1982).

Some experimental observations suggest the presence of peripheral
dopamine receptors mediating changes in gastrointestinal motility. Studies *in vitro* and *in vivo* provide rather strong evidence for the presence of
dopamine receptors in the opossum lower esophageal sphincter (De Carle
and Christensen, 1976; Rattan and Goyal, 1976; Mukhopadhyay and Weisbrodt, 1977). This is, however, not true in other species. The effects of
dopamine on the lower esophageal spincter in the guinea pig for instance
can be satisfactorily explained by interaction with α and β receptors (Cox
and Ennis, 1980; Sahyoun *et al.*, 1982b). The observations in man do not
permit any conclusions to be drawn.

Van Nueten and collaborators (Van Nueten and Janssen, 1978; Van
Nueten *et al.*, 1978: Schuurkes and Van Nueten, 1981) have done extensive studies on a guinea pig whole stomach preparation under different
conditions; on the basis of experiments with agonists and antagonists they
inferred the existence of dopamine receptors. From the evidence available
it is not clear where these receptors are localized and how their existence
can be integrated into the regulation of gastric motility. Furthermore,
evidence for the presence of dopamine receptors was not found in studies
on strips of guinea pig stomach (Costall *et al.*, 1982; Sahyoun *et al.*, 1982a).

On the basis of limited experimental evidence, the presence of dopamine receptors was also suggested for the human stomach (Lanfranchi
et al., 1978b) and for the human sigmoid colon (Lanfranchi *et al.*, 1978a).
Dopamine receptors were also suggested to be present on the intramural
cholinergic neurons of the guinea pig ileum (Ennis *et al.*, 1979), but other
authors were not able to confirm this (Görich *et al.*, 1982; Zar *et al.*,
1982).

In view of the ongoing discussion about the presence of peripheral
dopamine receptors in the gastrointestinal system, we have studied this
problem in rat stomach fundus strips. In these strips, dopamine inhibits
contractions elicited by transmural electrical stimulation more than contractions of similar amplitude induced by mecholyl. The postsynaptic ef-

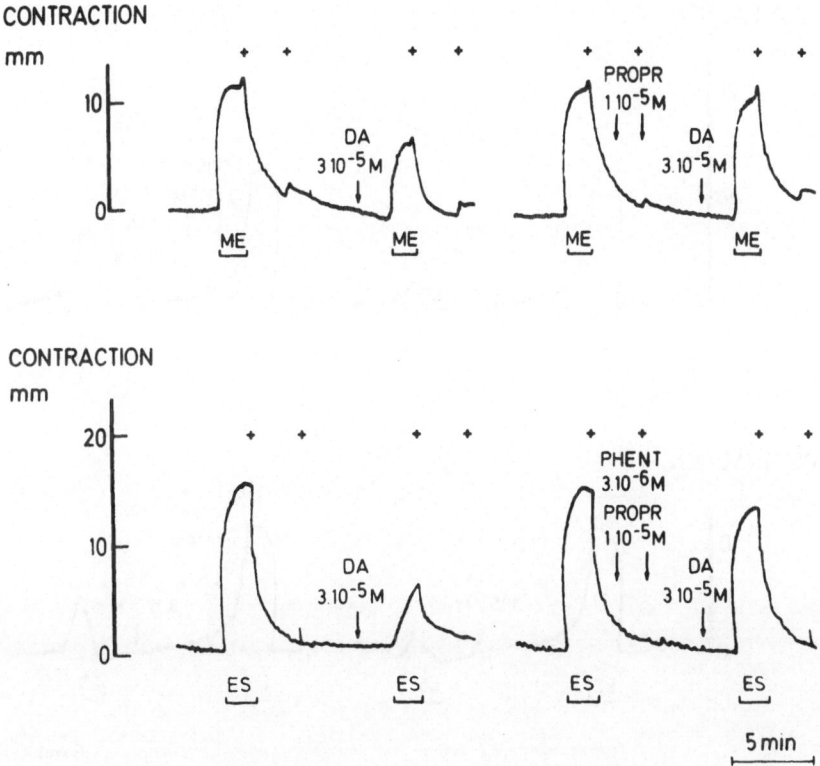

Figure 3. Inhibitory influence of dopamine (DA) on contractions induced by mecholyl (ME, $1 \cdot 10^{-7}$ M, 2 min, upper panel) and by transmural electrical stimulation (ES, 1 Hz, 2 min, lower panel) in rat fundus strips. The right tracings show the influence of propranolol (PROPR) and of phentolamine (PHENT) with propranolol (PROPR) on the inhibition by dopamine. + denotes rinsing.

fect of dopamine, as studied on mecholyl-induced contractions, can be blocked by propranolol. Phentolamine has hardly any effect on the inhibition of the mecholyl contraction, but the inhibitory effect of dopamine on electrically induced contractions is partially blocked by phentolamine, and in the presence of both phentolamine and propranolol, this inhibitory effect of dopamine is no longer seen (Fig. 3). It can be concluded from these experiments that in rat fundus strips the inhibitory effect of dopamine at the postsynaptic site is mediated by β receptors, the effect at the presynaptic site by α receptors. The presynaptic α receptors involved were further studied by use of α_1 and α_2 receptor agonists and antagonists. It was not possible, however, to conclude the existence of pure α_1 or pure α_2 characteristics, and the presence of both α_1 and α_2 receptors or of an

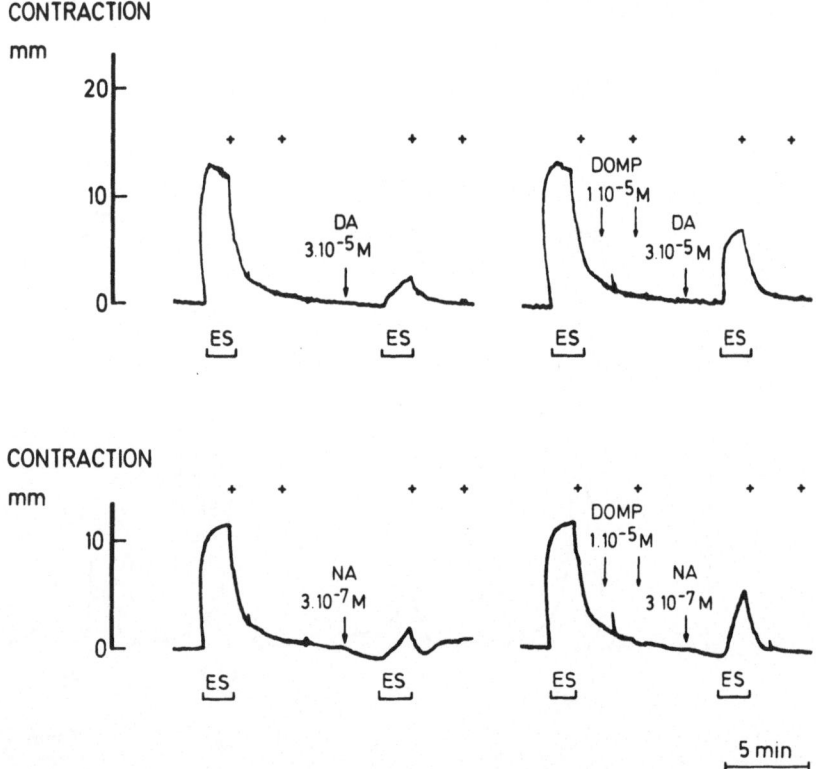

Figure 4. Inhibitory influence of dopamine (DA, upper panel) and norepinephrine (NA, lower panel) on contractions induced by transmural electrical stimulation (ES, 1 Hz, 2 min) in rat fundus strips. The right tracings show the influence of domperidone (DOMP) on the inhibition by dopamine or norepinephrine. + denotes rinsing.

α receptor combining α_1 and α_2 characteristics was postulated (Lefebvre *et al.*, 1983). Experiments in reserpinized animals and experiments with cocaine show that the effect of dopamine on electrically induced contractions in the rat fundus strips is largely indirect, occurring by release of norepinephrine from sympathetic nerve endings. Several dopamine antagonists [haloperidol, domperidone, *(RS)*-sulpiride, *cis*-flupenthixol, metoclopramide] were also studied. When at a given concentration these antagonists diminished the inhibitory effect of dopamine, the same diminution was also seen for the effect of norepinephrine on these strips (Fig. 4).

Experiments on strips of dog fundus likewise did not provide evidence that dopamine receptors were present.

5. Conclusion

There is now good evidence for the presence of peripheral dopamine receptors in the cardiovascular system, in orthosympathetic ganglia, and in a number of other systems; however, in some organs dopamine receptors do not exist, or earlier suggestions about their presence could not be confirmed when extensive studies involving agonists and antagonists were performed. In the gastrointestinal tract, for example, only for the opossum lower esophageal spincter and the dog pancreas is there good experimental evidence for the presence of peripheral dopamine receptors; in other parts of the gastrointestinal system, dopamine receptors were not found or the evidence was not satisfactory, e.g., because an effect on central structures such as the chemoreceptor trigger zone could not be excluded.

In the cardiovascular system, there are at least two types of dopamine receptors present, and although one should be aware of the limitations of the *in vivo* approach used, one can say that postsynaptic dopamine receptors (DA_1 receptors) are different from presynaptic dopamine receptors (DA_2 receptors). The question of how these receptors in the cardiovascular system compare to the receptors found in the central nervous system is not yet answered, but there seems to be some similarity between DA_2 receptors and central D_2 receptors, and perhaps also between DA_1 receptors and central D_1 receptors.

The dopamine receptor mediating ganglionic inhibition in orthosympathetic ganglia shows some similarities to the DA_2 receptor in the cardiovascular system, but its localization (presynaptic or postsynaptic) is not clear.

ACKNOWLEDGMENT. This research was supported by grants 3.0026.78 and 3.0019.82 from the Belgian Fund for Medical Research (F.G.W.O.).

References

Abe, K., and Dawes, C., 1982, Dopamine-induced secretion of protein and of some electrolytes by rat submandibular and parotid glands *Arch. Oral Biol.* **27**:635–643.

Bastie, M. J., Vaysse, N., Brenac, B., Pascal, J. P., and Ribet, A., 1977, Effects of catecholamines and their inhibitors on the isolated canine pancreas. II. Dopamine, *Gastroenterology* **72**:719–723.

Baumann, H. W., Sturdevant, R. A. L., and McCallum, R. W., 1979, L-Dopa inhibits metoclopramide stimulation of the lower esophageal sphincter in man, *Dig. Dis. Sci.* **24**:289–295.

Blancquaert, J. P., Lefebvre, R. A., and Willems, J. L., 1982, Gastric relaxation by intravenous and intracerebroventricular administration of apomorphine, morphine and fentanyl in the conscious dog. *Arch. Int. Pharmacodyn* **256**:153–154.

Bloom, G. D., Carlsöö, B., and Danielsson, Å., 1975, Dopamine-induced amylase secretion from guinea-pig submandibular gland, *Br. J. Pharmacol.* **54**:523–528.

Brodde, O.-E., 1982, Vascular dopamine receptors: Demonstration and characterization by *in vitro* studies. *Life Sci.* **31**:289–306.

Brodde, O. E., Meyer, F. J., Schemuth, W., and Freistühler, J., 1981, Demonstration of specific vascular dopamine receptors mediating vasodilatation in the isolated rabbit mesenteric artery, *Naunyn Schmiedebergs Arch. Pharmacol.* **316**:24–30.

Brown, D. A., and Caulfield, M. P., 1979, Hyperpolarizing α_2-adrenoceptors in rat sympathetic ganglia, *Br. J. Pharmacol.* **65**:435–445.

Brown, R. A., and O'Connor, S. E., 1981, Stereoselective antagonism of prejunctional dopamine receptors in the rabbit ear artery by sulpiride, *Br. J. Pharmacol.* **73**:189P–190P.

Buylaert, W. A., Willems, J. L., and Bogaert, M. G., 1977, Vasodilatation produced by apomorphine in the hindleg of the dog, *J. Pharmacol. Exp. Ther.* **201**:738–746.

Buylaert, W. A., Willems, J. L., and Bogaert, M. G., 1978, The receptor mediating the apomorphine vasodilatation in the hindleg of the dog, *J. Pharm. Pharmacol.* **30**:113–115.

Buylaert, W. A., Willems, J. L., and Bogaert, M. G., 1981, Peripheral prejunctional dopamine receptors, in: *Vasodilatation* (P. M. Vanhoutte and I. Leusen, eds.), Raven Press, New York, pp. 125–130.

Carlsöö, B., Danielsson, Å., Marklund, S., and Stigbrand, T., 1974, Effects of alpha- and beta-receptor blocking agents on catecholamine and 5-hydroxytryptamine induced peroxidase and amylase secretion from guinea pig submandibular gland, *Acta Physiol. Scand.* **92**:263–271.

Costall, B., Gunning, S. J., and Naylor, R. J., 1982, Apomorphine contracts and relaxes circular smooth muscle of guinea-pig stomach via action on adrenoceptor mechanisms, *Naunyn Schmiedebergs Arch. Pharmacol.* **319**:226–230.

Cox, B., and Ennis, C., 1980, Mechanism of action of dopamine on the guinea-pig gastroesophageal junction *in vitro*, *Br. J. Pharmacol.* **71**:177–184.

Creese, I., and Sibley, D. R., 1982, Comments on the commentary by Dr. Seeman, *Biochem. Pharmacol.* **31**:2568–2569.

De Carle, D. J., and Christensen, J., 1976, A dopamine receptor in esophageal smooth muscle of the opossum, *Gastroenterology* **70**:216–219.

Dubocovich, M. L., and Langer, S. Z., 1980, Dopamine and alpha adrenoceptor agonists inhibit neurotransmission in the cat spleen through different presynaptic receptors, *J. Pharmacol. Exp. Ther.* **212**:144–152.

Ennis, C., Janssen, P. A. J., Schnieden, H., and Cox, B., 1979, Characterization of receptors on postganglionic cholinergic neurons in the guinea-pig isolated ileum, *J. Pharm. Pharmacol.* **31**:217–221.

Ferrini, R., and Miragoli, G., 1972, Selective antagonism of dopamine by apomorphine, *Pharmacol. Res. Commun.* **4**:347–352.

Furchgott, R. F., 1972, The classification of adrenoceptors. An evaluation from the standpoint of receptor theory, in: *Catecholamines, Handbuch der Experimentellen Pharmakologie*, Volume 33 (H. Blaschko and E. Muscholl, eds.), Springer-Verlag Berlin, pp. 283–335.

Furuta, Y., Hashimoto, K., and Washizaki, M., 1978, β-Adrenoceptor stimulation of exocrine secretion from the rat pancreas, *Br. J. Pharmacol.* **62**:25–29.

Glock, D., Kohli, J. D., and Goldberg, L. I., 1982, Domperidone: A potent and highly selective DA$_2$, peripheral dopamine receptor, antagonist, *Fed. Proc.* **41**:1651.

Goldberg, L. I., 1972, Cardiovascular and renal actions of dopamine: Potential clinical applications, *Pharmacol. Rev.* **24**:1–29.

Goldberg, L. I., and Kohli, J. D., 1979, Peripheral pre- and post-synaptic dopamine receptors: Are they different from dopamine receptors in the central nervous system? *Commun. Psychopharmacol.* **3**:447–456.

Goldberg, L. I., and Kohli, J. D., 1981, Agonists and antagonists of peripheral pre- and post-synaptic dopamine receptors: Clinical implications, in: *Apomorphine and other dopaminomimetics: Basic Pharmacology*, Volume 1 (G. L. Gessa and G. U. Corsini, eds.), Raven Press, New York, pp. 273–284.

Goldberg, L. I., Volkman, P. H., and Kohli, J. D., 1978, A comparison of the vascular dopamine receptor with other dopamine receptors, *Annu. Rev. Pharmacol. Toxicol.* **18**:57–79.

Görich, R., Weihrauch, T. R., and Kilbinger, H., 1982, The inhibition by dopamine of cholinergic transmission in the isolated guinea-pig ileum, *Naunyn Schmiedebergs Arch. Pharmacol.* **318**:308–312.

Hahn, R. A., Wardell, J. R., Sarau, H. M., and Ridley, P. T., 1982, Characterization of the peripheral and central effects of SK&F 82526, a novel dopamine receptor agonist, *J. Pharmacol. Exp. Ther.* **223**:305–313.

Hashimoto, K., Satho, S., and Takeuchi, O., 1971, Effect of dopamine on pancreatic secretion in the dog, *Br. J. Pharmacol.* **43**:739–746.

Horn, P. T., Kohli, J. D., and Goldberg, L. I., 1982a, Facilitation of ganglionic transmission by sulpiride: Evidence for an inhibitory role of dopamine in the canine sympathetic ganglion, *J. Pharmacol. Exp. Ther.* **223**:462–468.

Horn, P. T., Kohli, J. D., and Goldberg, L. I., 1982b, Effects of dopamine, N-N-di-*n*-propyl dopamine, and (*R*)- and (*S*)-sulpiride on guinea pig blood pressure, *J. Cardiovasc. Pharmacol.* **4**:668–675.

Hovendal, C. P., Bech, K., Gottrup, F., and Andersen, D., 1982, Effect of dopamine on pentagastrin-stimulated gastric acid secretion and mucosal blood flow in dogs with gastric fistula, *Scand. J. Gastroenterol.* **17**:97–102.

Imbs, J. L., Schmidt, M., Ehrhardt, J. D., and Schwartz, J., 1979, Renal dopaminergic mechanisms, in: *Advances in the Biosciences: Peripheral Dopaminergic Receptors*, Volume 20 (J. L. Imbs and J. Schwartz, eds.), Pergamon Press, Oxford, New York, pp. 331–343.

Kebabian, J. W., and Calne, D. B., 1979, Multiple receptors for dopamine, *Nature* **277**:93–96.

Kohli, J. D., Goldberg, L. I., and McDermed, J. D., 1982, Modification of cardiovascular actions of 2-amino-5,6-dihydroxytetralin by N,N-di-*n*-propyl substitution, *Eur. J. Pharmacol.* **81**:293–299.

Lanfranchi, G. A., Marzio, L., Cortini, C., and Osset, E. M., 1978a, Motor effect of dopamine on human sigmoid colon. Evidence for specific receptors, *Am. J. Dig. Dis.* **23**:257–263.

Lanfranchi, G. A., Marzio, L., Cortini, C., Trento, L., and Labó, G., 1978b, Effect of dopamine on gastric motility in man: Evidence for specific receptors, in: *Gastrointestinal Motility in Health and Disease, Proceedings of the 6th International Symposium on Gastrointestinal Motility* (H. L. Duthie, ed.), MTP Press, Lancaster, pp. 161–172.

Lang, W. J., and Woodman, O. L., 1982, Comparison of the vasodilator action of dopamine and dopamine agonists in the renal and coronary beds of the dog, *Br. J. Pharmacol.* **77**:23–28.

Langeloh, A., and Jurkiewicz, A., 1982, Analysis of the effects of dopamine and noradrenaline in relation to the proposed postsynaptic dopamine receptor in rat vas deferens, *Naunyn Schmiedebergs Arch. Pharmacol.* **318:**202–209.

Langer, S. Z., 1980, Presynaptic regulation of the release of catecholamines, *Pharmacol. Rev.* **32:**337–362.

Lankisch, P. G., and Koop, H., 1978, Dopamine-Wirkung auf die basale Pankreas-sekretion des Menschen, *Dtsch. Med. Wochenschr.* **103:**391–392.

Leedham, J. A., and Pennefather, J. N., 1982, Dopamine acts at the same receptors as noradrenaline in the rat isolated vas deferens, *Br. J. Pharmacol.* **77:**293–299.

Lefebvre, R. A., Blancquaert, J. P., Willems, J. L., and Bogaert, M. G., 1983, *In vitro* study of the inhibitory effects of dopamine on the rat gastric fundus, *Naunyn Schmiedebergs Arch. Pharmacol.* **322:**228–236.

Libet, B., 1970, Generation of slow inhibitory and excitatory postsynaptic potentials, *Fed. Proc.* **29:**1945–1956.

Lokhandwala, M. F., and Barrett, R. J., 1982, Cardiovascular dopamine receptors: Physiological, pharmacological and therapeutic implications, *J. Autonom. Pharmacol.* **3:**189–215.

Long, J. P., Heintz, S., Cannon, J. G., and Kim, J., 1975, Inhibition of the sympathetic nervous system by 5,6-dihydroxy-2-dimethylamino tetralin (M-7), apomorphine and dopamine, *J. Pharmacol. Exp. Ther.* **192:**336–342.

McNay, J. L., McDonald, R. H., and Goldberg, L. I., 1965, Direct renal vasodilatation produced by dopamine in the dog, *Circ. Res.* **16:**510–517.

Mukhopadhyay, A. K., and Weisbrodt, N., 1977, Effect of dopamine on esophageal motor function, *Am. J. Physiol.* **232:**E19–E24.

Murphy, V. V., Gilbert, J. C., Goldberg, L. I., and Kuo, J. F., 1976, Dopamine-sensitive adenylate cyclase in canine renal artery, *J. Pharm. Pharmacol.* **28:**567–571.

Nakamura, J., 1978, The effect of neuroleptics on the dopaminergic and cholinergic systems in sympathetic ganglia, *Kurume Med. J.* **25:**241–253.

Pendleton, R. G., Samler, L., Kaiser, C., and Ridley, P. T., 1978, Studies on renal dopamine receptors with a new agonist, *Eur. J. Pharmacol.* **51:**19–28.

Rattan, S., and Goyal, R. K., 1976, Effect of dopamine on the esophageal smooth muscle *in vivo*, *Gastroenterology* **70:**377–381.

Relja, M., Lacković, Z., and Neff, N. H., 1982, Evidence for the presence of dopaminergic receptors in vas deferens, *Life Sci.* **31:**2571–2575.

Roby, A., and Orzechowski, R. F., 1979, Selective postsynaptic dopamine receptor stimulation by SK&F 38393 in canine mesenteric vasculature, *Pharmacologist* **21:**239.

Sahyoun, H. A., Costall, B., and Naylor, R. J., 1982a, On the ability of domperidone to selectively inhibit catecholamine-induced relaxation of circular smooth muscle of guinea-pig stomach, *J. Pharm. Pharmacol.* **34:**27–33.

Sahyoun, H. A., Costall, B., and Naylor, R. J., 1982b, Catecholamine-induced relaxation and contraction of the lower oesophageal and pyloric sphincters of guinea-pig stomach: Modification by domperidone, *J. Pharm. Pharmacol.* **34:**318–324.

Satoh, Y., Satoh, H., and Honda, F., 1980, Dopamine receptor blocking activity of sulpiride in the canine exocrine pancreas, *Jpn. J. Pharmacol.* **30:**689–699.

Schmidt, M., Imbs, J. L., and Schwartz, J., 1981, The vascular dopamine receptor: A review, *J. Pharmacol. (Paris)* **12:**355–382.

Schmidt, M., Imbs, J. L., Giesen, E. M., and Schwartz, J., 1982, Vasodilator effects of dopaminomimetics in the perfused rat kidney, *Eur. J. Pharmacol.* **84:**61–70.

Schuurkes, J. A. J., and Van Nueten, J. M., 1981, Effects of dopamine and its antagonist domperidone cannot be explained by an effect on α_1-adrenergic receptors, *Arch. Int. Pharmacodyn.* **250:**324–327.

Seeman, P., 1980, Brain dopamine receptors, *Pharmacol. Rev.* **32**:229–313.

Seeman, P., 1982, Nomenclature of central and peripheral dopaminergic sites and receptors, *Biochem. Pharmacol.* **31**:2563–2568.

Shepperson, N. B., Duval, N., Massingham, R., and Langer, S. Z., 1982, Differential blocking effects of several dopamine receptor antagonists for peripheral pre- and postsynaptic dopamine receptors in the anesthetized dog, *J. Pharmacol. Exp. Ther.* **221**:753–761.

Simon, A., and Van Maanen, E. F., 1976, Dopamine receptors and dopaminergic nerves in the vas deferens of the rat, *Arch. Int. Pharmacodyn.* **222**:4–15.

Steinsland, O. S., and Hieble, J. P., 1979 Activities of structural analogues of dopamine on prejunctional dopaminergic and alpha adrenergic receptors, in: *Advances in the Biosciences: Presynaptic receptors,* Volume 18 (S. Z. Langer, K. Starke, and M. L. Dubocovich, eds.), Pergamon Press, Oxford, New York, pp. 93–98.

Szabo, S., 1979, Dopamine disorder in duodenal ulceration, *Lancet* **2**:880–882.

Tayo, F. M., 1979, Occurrence of excitatory dopaminoceptors in the rat and guinea-pig vas deferens, *Clin. Exp. Pharmacol. Physiol.* **6**:275–279.

Valenzuela, J. E., and Grossman, M. I., 1976, Dopamine stimulates pancreatic secretion and inhibits gastric secretion in dogs, *Clin. Res.* **24**:292A.

Valenzuela, J. E., Defilippi, C., Diaz, G., Navia, E., and Merino, Y., 1979, Effect of dopamine on human gastric and pancreatic secretion, *Gastroenterology* **76**:323–326.

Van Nueten, J. M., and Janssen, P. A. J., 1978, Is dopamine an endogenous inhibitor of gastric emptying? in: *Gastrointestinal Motility in Health and Disease, Proceedings of the 6th International Symposium on Gastrointestinal Motility* (H. L. Duthie, ed.), MTP Press, Lancaster, pp. 173–180.

Van Nueten, J. M., Ennis, C., Helsen, L., Laduron, P. M., and Janssen, P. A. J., 1978, Inhibition of dopamine receptors in the stomach: An explanation of the gastrokinetic properties of domperidone, *Life Sci.* **23**:453–457.

Volkman, P. H., and Goldberg, L. I., 1976, Lack of correlation between inhibition of prolactin release and stimulation of dopaminergic renal vasodilatation, *Pharmacologist* **18**:130.

Weihrauch, T. R., Förster, Ch.F., and Krieglstein, J., 1979, Evaluation of the effect of domperidone on human esophageal and gastroduodenal motility by intraluminal manometry, *Postgrad. Med. J.* **55**(1):7–10.

Willems, J. L., 1973, Dopamine-induced inhibition of synaptic transmission in lumbar paravertebral ganglia of the dog, *Naunyn Schmiedebergs Arch. Pharmacol.* **279**:115–126.

Willems, J. L., Buylaert, W. A., and Bogaert, M. G., 1979, Evidence that dopamine receptors mediate the neurogenic vasodilatation by dopaminergic agents, in: *Advances in the Biosciences: Peripheral Dopaminergic Receptors,* Volume 20 (J. L. Imbs and J. Schwartz, eds.), Pergamon Press, Oxford, New York, pp. 299–307.

Willems, J. L., Bogaert, M. G., and Buylaert, W., 1981, Preliminary observations on the interaction of domperidone with peripheral dopamine receptors, *J. Pharmacol.* **31**:131–133.

Zar, M. A., Ebong, O. O., and Bateman, D. N., 1982, Effect of metoclopramide in guinea-pig ileum longitudinal muscle: Evidence against dopamine mediation, *Gut* **23**:66–70.

6

Pharmacological Significance of Pre- and Postsynaptic Dopamine Receptors

SALOMON Z. LANGER AND SONIA ARBILLA

1. Introduction

Stimulation of dopamine receptors of the D-2 subtype reduces the release of various neurotransmitters in the peripheral and central nervous systems (for reviews, see Langer, 1980; Langer and Lehmann, 1984).

In the peripheral nervous system, dopamine receptor agonists inhibit the stimulation-evoked release of norepinephrine as well as the postsynaptic responses elicited by sympathetic nerve stimulation under *in vitro* as well as *in vivo* experimental conditions (Langer, 1973; Enero and Langer, 1975; Dubocovich and Langer, 1980; Massingham *et al.*, 1980; Shepperson *et al.*, 1982b). The presynaptic inhibition of peripheral noradrenergic neurotransmission is mediated by the D-2 dopamine receptor subtype. At the postsynaptic level, dopamine produces vasodilatation of certain vascular beds through the stimulation of dopamine receptors of the D-1 subtype located in vascular smooth muscle.

In the central nervous system, a number of presynaptic, release-modulating dopamine receptors have been reported. The calcium-dependent, electrically evoked release of [^{3}H]-dopamine in the striatum of several species is modulated by presynaptic inhibitory dopamine autoreceptors with the pharmacological characteristics of the D-2 subtype (for reviews see Langer, 1980; Langer and Lehmann, 1984; Lehmann and Langer, 1983). The dopamine autoreceptors that regulate the release of dopamine in the striatum appear to play a physiological role in dopaminergic neurotransmission (Langer *et al.*, 1980a; Kamal *et al.*, 1981; Arbilla

SALOMON Z. LANGER and SONIA ARBILLA • Department of Biology, Laboratoires d'Etudes et de Recherches Synthélabo, 75013 Paris, France.

and Langer, 1981). On the other hand, there is no evidence in support of a physiological role for the presynaptic dopamine receptors that mediate inhibition of peripheral noradrenergic neurotransmission (Langer and Dubocovich, 1979) or of central noradrenergic neurotransmission (Galzin *et al.*, 1982).

The electrically evoked release of [^{3}H]-acetylcholine from the cholinergic interneuron of the striatum of various species is inhibited by dopamine receptor agonists (Hertting *et al.*, 1980; Scatton, 1982; Lehmann *et al.*, 1983a; Langer *et al.*, 1983a). This inhibitory dopamine receptor is also of the D-2 subtype and appears to be localized on the terminals rather than on the dendrites of the cholinergic interneuron (Lehmann and Langer, 1983).

Presynaptic release-modulating receptors are generally believed to act on voltage-dependent calcium channels to inhibit the depolarization-evoked release of the transmitter (Pellmar, 1981). On the other hand, postsynaptic neurotransmitter receptors activate a specific ion channel, resulting in either excitatory or inhibitory postsynaptic potentials. Differences appear to exist between the pharmacological properties of the dopamine receptor that modulates the release of dopamine or acetylcholine in the striatum and the postynaptic dopamine receptors that modulate the electrical activity of striatal neurons and mediate locomotor activation and stereotyped behavior induced by dopamine receptor agonists (Lehmann and Langer, 1983).

The aim of the present chapter is to review the pharmacological properties of the presynaptic release-modulating dopamine receptors in the peripheral and central nervous systems and to compare them with the postsynaptic dopamine receptors.

2. Dopamine Receptors Mediating the Inhibition of Peripheral Noradrenergic Neurotransmission

The inhibition of norepinephrine release by dopamine and other dopamine receptor agonists was first reported in the isolated nictitating membrane and perfused spleen of the cat (Langer, 1973; Enero and Langer, 1975). These presynaptic inhibitory dopamine receptors differ from the α_2 adrenoceptors that mediate the autoinhibition of noradrenergic neurotransmission (Dubocovich and Langer, 1980).

The presynaptic dopamine receptor that inhibits peripheral noradrenergic neurotransmission can be characterized as a D-2 receptor, and it is blocked stereoselectively by the D-2 dopamine receptor antagonist sulpiride both under *in vitro* and under *in vivo* conditions (Langer and Dubocovich, 1980; Massingham *et al.*, 1980; Shepperson *et al.*, 1982b).

Within the concentration range of (*S*)-sulpiride in which there is complete antagonism of the inhibitory effects of dopamine receptor agonists on norepinephrine release, there is no increase in the release of the noradrenergic transmitter during nerve stimulation (Langer and Dubocovich, 1980; Massingham *et al.*, 1980; Shepperson *et al.*, 1982b). These results are compatible with the view that the presynaptic dopamine receptors that mediate the inhibition of peripheral noradrenergic neurotransmission do not play a physiological role in the regulation of norepinephrine release (Langer and Dubocovich, 1979; Langer, 1980).

Although blockade of dopamine receptors with sulpiride or pimozide fails to enhance norepinephrine release, it is well established that blockade of presynaptic inhibitory α_2 adrenoceptors with antagonists such as phentolamine, yohimbine, or RX 781094 increases the release of the noradrenergic transmitter elicited by postganglionic sympathetic stimulation (for review see Langer, 1981). It can therefore be concluded that in contrast with the presynaptic α_2 adrenoceptors, the presynaptic inhibitory dopamine receptors do not play a physiological role in the modulation of peripheral noradrenergic neurotransmission. Nevertheless, the presynaptic inhibitory dopamine receptors on peripheral noradrenergic neurons are attractive targets for selective agonists that produce hypotensive and bradycardic actions through the reduction of norepinephrine output in the peripheral sympathetic system (Langer *et al.*, 1980b).

In addition to dopamine, which stimulates D-1 and D-2 receptors (Table I), a number of preferential D-2 receptor agonists can activate the presynaptic inhibitory dopamine receptors on peripheral noradrenergic nerve terminals. These drugs include apomorphine and N,N-di-*n*-propyldopamine (DPDA) (Langer and Dubocovich, 1981; Massingham *et al.*, 1980; Shepperson *et al.*, 1982b). In addition, pergolide, another preferential D-2 receptor agonist (Table I), is also a potent inhibitor of noradrenergic neurotransmission in the perfused cat spleen (Fig. 1). The inhibition by pergolide of [^{3}H]-norepinephrine release in the perfused cat spleen is still present when the presynaptic α_2 adrenoceptors are blocked with phentolamine (Fig. 2). Sulpiride, a selective D-2 receptor antagonist (Table I), completely blocks the inhibition by pergolide of noradrenergic neurotransmission (Figs. 1 and 2) but does not by itself significantly enhance the release of [^{3}H]-norepinephrine elicited by nerve stimulation. In the perfused cat spleen, blockade of presynaptic α_2 adrenoceptors increases the overflow of norepinephrine during sympathetic nerve stimulation (Dubocovich and Langer, 1974, 1976).

Table I. Relative Order of Selectivities of Agonists and Antagonists for Dopamine
Receptor Subtypes in the Periphery[a]

Relative order of selectivity of agonists	
SK&F 38393	D-1
Dopamine	D-1 = D-2
Apomorphine < pergolide < DPDA < LY 141865	D-2
Relative order of selectivity of antagonists	
Bulbocapnine	D-1
(+)-Butaclamol	D-1 = D-2
Haloperidol < domperidone < S-sulpiride	D-2

[a] The results are derived from data obtained under *in vitro* and *in vivo* conditions at peripheral noradrenergic neuroeffector junctions in several species. D-1 corresponds to the postsynaptic dopamine
receptor mediating vasodilatation in vascular smooth muscle (renal, mesenteric, and coronary vascular
beds). D-2 corresponds to the presynaptic dopamine receptor, which mediates the inhibition of norepinephrine release elicited by postganglionic sympathetic stimulation. SK&F 38393, 2,3,4,5-tetrahy-
dro-7,8-dihydroxy-1-phenyl-1H-3-benzazepine; LY 141865: *trans*(±)-4,4a,5,6,7,8a,9-octahydro-5-pro-
pyl-2H-pyrazolo[3,4-g]quinoline; DPDA, N,N-di-(n-propyl)dopamine.

In support of the view that the presynaptic dopamine receptor that
inhibits peripheral noradrenergic transmission corresponds to the D-2 subtype is the fact that (S)-sulpiride and (+)-butaclamol, but not bulbocapnine, block the inhibitory effects of DPDA on norepinephrine release in
the anesthetized dog (Shepperson et al., 1982b). As shown in Table I,
bulbocapnine is a preferential D-1 receptor antagonist, and, as expected,
it does not block the presynaptic effects of DPDA on noradrenergic neurotransmission in the anesthetized dog (Shepperson et al., 1982b). The
presynaptic inhibitory effects of DPDA on noradrenergic transmission in
the anesthetized dog are also blocked by haloperidol and (+)-butaclamol
(Shepperson et al., 1982b). Both dopamine receptor antagonists, haloperidol and (+)-butaclamol, have either nonselective or preferential affinity for the D-2 subtype of peripheral dopamine receptor (Table I).

As indicated in Table I, LY 141865 is considered to be the most
selective D-2 receptor agonist available at present. Nevertheless, it was
recently reported that LY 141865 in addition to stimulating D-2 receptors
is a potent histamine H-2 receptor agonist (Armstrong et al., 1983). The
stimulating effects of LY 141865 on histamine receptors has been demonstrated in the coronary circulation of the dog (Armstrong et al., 1984)
and in isolated guinea pig atria. These recent observations are of considerable interest because until recently LY 141865 was considered to be a
pure D-2 receptor agonist without affinity or intrinsic activity for other
receptors.

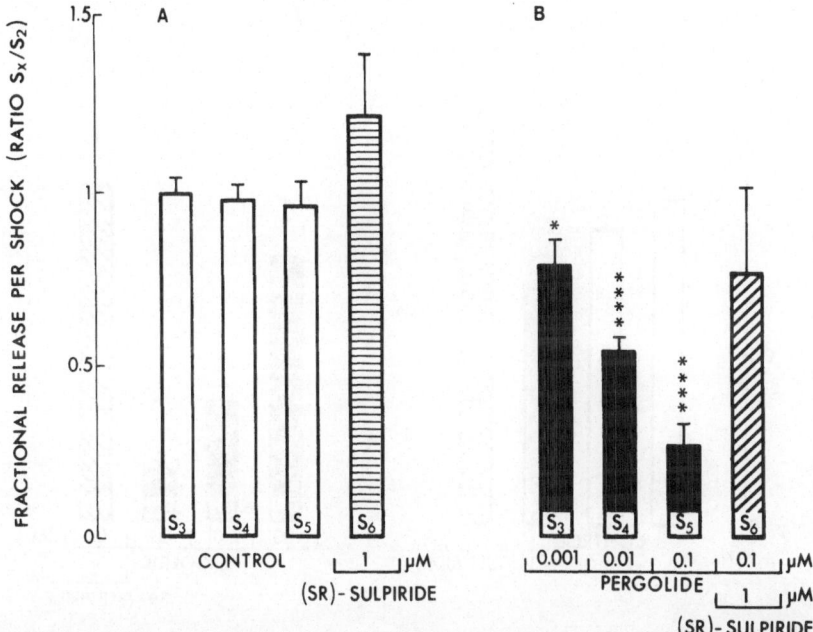

Figure 1. Inhibition by pergolide of the stimulation-evoked overflow of [^{3}H]-norepinephrine in the perfused cat spleen. Ordinate: fractional release per shock expressed as the ratio obtained between different periods of stimulation (S_3, S_4, S_5, and S_6) and the corresponding control (S_2) within the same experiment. For details of the experimental set-up see Dubocovich and Langer (1980). The splenic nerves were stimulated at 1 Hz for 5 min (0.5 msec, supramaximal voltage). Cocaine 29 μM was present in the perfusion medium from 60 min before the first period of stimulation and kept throughout the experiment. (S,R)-Sulpiride, 1 μM in A and B, was present in the perfusion medium 23 min before and during the sixth period of stimulation (S_6). Pergolide, 0.001, 0.01, and 0.1 μM in B, was present, respectively, 23 min before and during the stimulation periods S_3, S_4, and S_5. □, controls; ▤, (S,R)-sulpiride; ■, pergolide; and ▨, pergolide in the presence of (S,R)-sulpiride. Note that (S,R)-sulpiride, 1 μM, completely antagonized the inhibitory effects of the highest concentration of pergolide (0.1 μM) but failed on its own to increase the overflow of [^{3}H]-norepinephrine elicited by sympathetic nerve stimulation. Shown are mean values ± S.E.M. of at least four experiments per group. *$P < 0.05$ and ****$P < 0.001$ when compared with the corresponding control group.

3. Postsynaptic Dopamine Receptors in Vascular Smooth Muscle

Dopamine produces vasodilatation in the renal and mesenteric vascular beds through the stimulation of postsynaptic D-1 receptors in vascular smooth muscle (Goldberg, 1979; Shepperson *et al.*, 1982a; Goldberg

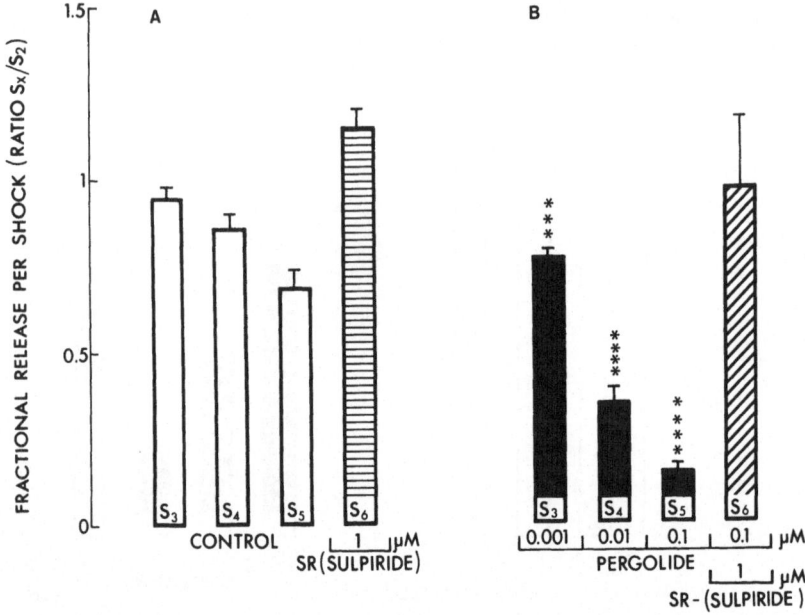

Figure 2. Blockade of presynaptic α_2 adrenoceptors does not influence the inhibition by pergolide of the stimulation evoked overflow of [^{3}H]-norepinephrine in the perfused cat spleen. Ordinate: fractional release per shock expressed as the ratio obtained between different periods of stimulation (S_3, S_4, S_5, and S_6) and the corresponding control (S_2) within the same experiment. For details of the experimental set-up see Dubocovich and Langer (1980). The nerves were stimulated at 1 Hz for 5 min (0.5 msec, supramaximal voltage). Cocaine, 29 μM, and phentolamine, 1 μM, were present in the perfusion medium from 60 min before the first period of stimulation and kept throughout the experiment. (S,R)-Sulpiride, 1 μM in A and B, was present in the perfusion medium 23 min before and during the sixth period of stimulation (S_6). Pergolide, 0.001, 0.01, and 0.1 μM in B, was present, respectively, 23 min before and during the stimulation periods S_3, S_4, and S_5. □, Controls; ▤, (S,R)-sulpiride; ■, pergolide; and ▨, pergolide in the presence of (S,R)-sulpiride. Note that (S,R)-sulpiride, 1 μM, antagonized completely the inhibitory effects of the highest concentration of pergolide (0.1 μM) but did not increase on its own the overflow of [^{3}H]-norepinephrine elicited by sympathetic nerve stimulation. Shown are mean values ± S.E.M. of at least four experiments per group. ***$P < 0.005$ and ****$P < 0.001$ when compared with the corresponding control group.

and Kohli, 1983). In support of the view that the dopamine-induced vasodilatation involves the D-1 subtype of receptor, it was recently reported that the vasodilatation produced by dopamine in the mesenteric bed of the dog is antagonized by bulbocapnine, whereas it is resistant to blockade by (S)-sulpiride (Shepperson *et al.*, 1982b). Butaclamol, which blocks both D-1 and D-2 receptors (Table I), was also effective in antagonizing the increase in mesenteric blood flow produced by dopamine in the anesthetized dog (Shepperson *et al.*, 1982b).

It is of interest to note that in order to study the D-1-mediated dilatation by dopamine in the mesenteric vascular bed, it is necessary to block β-adrenoceptors with propranolol and α-adrenoceptors with phenoxybenzamine (Shepperson *et al.*, 1982b). When the effects of dopamine are tested on mesenteric blood flow in the anesthetized dog in the absence of α-adrenoceptor blockade, then an α_2-adrenoceptor-mediated decrease in blood flow can be demonstrated for dopamine injected intraarterially (Shepperson *et al.*, 1982b). The fact that dopamine, in the absence of α-adrenoceptor blockade, can stimulate α_2 adrenoceptors in vascular smooth muscle is of considerable interest (Langer and Shepperson, 1982). Additional experiments are necessary to establish if dopamine can stimulate α_2 adrenoceptors in the smooth muscle of other vascular beds.

The D-1 receptors in the mesenteric vascular smooth muscle of the dog are blocked by low doses of the preferential D-1 antagonist bulbocapnine (Shepperson *et al.*, 1982b). These D-1 receptors mediating dilatation are also blocked stereoselectively by the nonselective dopamine receptor antagonist butaclamol (Table I; Shepperson *et al.*, 1982b).

Dopamine receptors of the D-1 subtype mediate dilatation in the rabbit splenic artery (Massingham *et al.*, 1980) and in the coronary vessels of the anesthetized dog (Armstrong *et al.*, 1982)- Dopamine injected intraarterially increases coronary blood flow in a dose-dependent manner, and these effects are attributable to stimulation of D-1 receptors because they are blocked by bulbocapnine or butaclamol but not by the D-2 receptor antagonist (*S*)-sulpiride (Armstrong *et al.*, 1982). It was therefore surprising to see that the selective D-2 receptor agonist LY 141865 (Table I) was equipotent with dopamine in increasing the coronary flow in the anesthetized dog (Fig. 3). It is of interest that in this preparation, the preferential D-2 receptor agonist pergolide was approximately five times less potent than LY 141865 (Fig. 3), whereas on D-2 receptors pergolide is usually ten times more potent than LY 141865 (Lehmann *et al.*, 1983b). The dilatation of the coronary vascular bed induced by LY 141865 or pergolide is insensitive to blockade by bulbocapnine, (+)-butaclamol or (*S*)-sulpiride and does not involve the activation of dopamine receptors (Armstrong *et al.*, 1982). Recent experiments indicate that LY 141865 stimulates histamine H_2 receptors to produce this increase in coronary flow, and these effects are completely blocked with cimetidine (Armstrong *et al.*, 1983a).

Further support for the view that LY 141865 stimulates histamine H_2 receptors was obtained in isolated, spontaneously beating guinea pig atria. In this tissue, cimetidine blocks the positive chronotropic effects induced

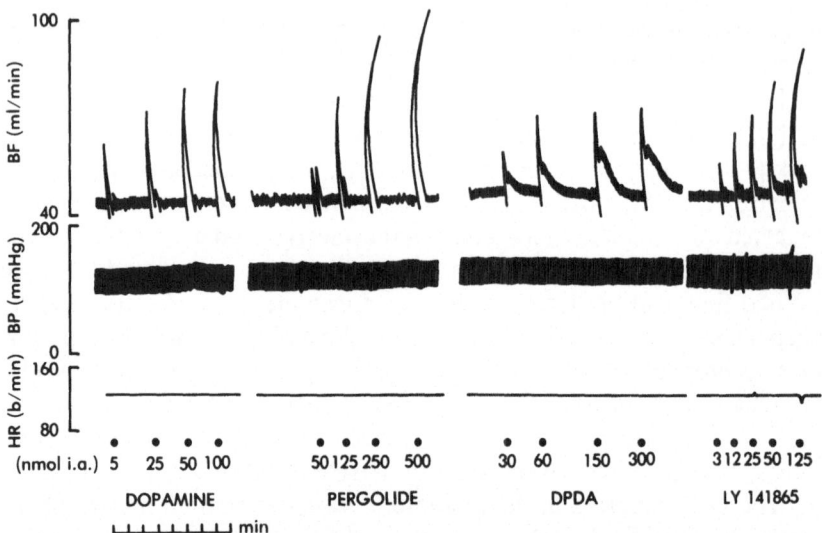

Figure 3. Coronary blood flow in the anaesthetized dog: responses to intraarterial doses of dopamine agonists. The figure reproduces a representative recording of mean circumflex coronary arterial blood flow (BF), pulsatile aortic blood pressure (BP, mm Hg), and heart rate (HR) (beats per min) in a dog anesthetized with pentobarbital. The corresponding scales are indicated by the vertical bars. Intracoronary arterial injections of dopamine and other dopamine receptor agonists produced increases in blood flow without affecting systemic arterial pressure or heart rate. Drugs were injected intraarterially in volumes of 0.05–0.2 ml containing the drugs in the nanomolar quantities indicated below the points. The intervals (min) between the injections of the agonists are given by the scale at the bottom of the figure.

by both histamine and LY 141865 (Armstrong *et al.*, 1984). Attention should therefore be drawn to the fact that LY 141865, which is considered to be the most selective D-2 receptor agonist available (Tsuruta *et al.*, 1981; see Table I), is also a potent agonist at histamine H_2 receptors. The recent finding about the H_2 agonist effects of LY 141865 (Armstrong *et al.*, 1983, 1984) indicates that the results obtained with this dopamine receptor agonist should be interpreted with caution, particularly when the tissue under study possesses histamine H_2 receptors.

4. Inhibition of Central Noradrenergic Neurotransmission by Dopamine Receptor Agonists

Dopamine receptor agonists such as apomorphine and pergolide inhibit the calcium-dependent, electrically evoked release of [³H]-norepinephrine from slices of the hypothalamus and cerebral cortex of the rabbit

(Galzin *et al.*, 1982). These inhibitory effects of dopamine receptor agonists on central noradrenergic neurotransmission are more clearly seen when the presynaptic α_2 adrenoceptors are blocked by either phentolamine or yohimbine (Galzin *et al.*, 1982). The inhibitory effects of dopamine receptor agonists on the electrically evoked release of [^{3}H]-norepinephrine are blocked stereoselectively by sulpiride or butaclamol in a range of concentrations (below 1 μM) that do not by themselves enhance the release of [^{3}H]-norepinephrine elicited by electrical stimulation (Galzin *et al.*, 1982). These results indicate that the dopamine D-2 receptors involved in the inhibition of central noradrenergic neurotransmission do not play a physiological role in the modulation of norepinephrine release.

Exposure to concentrations of sulpiride higher than those required to block the dopamine receptors (3 to 30 μM) induces an increase in the overflow of [^{3}H]-norepinephrine without changes in the basal outflow of radioactivity (Galzin *et al.*, 1982). The facilitation of central noradrenergic neurotransmission by high concentrations of sulpiride does not occur through inhibition of neuronal uptake of norepinephrine or blockade of presynaptic α_2 adrenoceptors by this drug (Langer *et al.*, 1983b). The facilitation by sulpiride of the electrically evoked release of [^{3}H]-norepinephrine is not stereoselective, because both the *S* and *R* isomers of sulpiride produced this effect in the same range of concentrations (Langer *et al.*, 1983b).

Additional studies are needed to establish the significance of the inhibition of central noradrenergic neurotransmission by dopamine receptor agonists observed in brain slices (Galzin *et al.*, 1982; Langer *et al.*, 1983b). There is, as yet, no evidence that these effects can be observed under *in vivo* experimental conditions when dopamine receptor agonists that readily cross the blood–brain barrier are administered.

5. Presynaptic Dopamine Autoreceptors and the Modulation of the Release of Dopamine in the Central Nervous System

Three basic functions are modulated by dopamine autoreceptors localized to dopaminergic neurons: (1) inhibition of the calcium-dependent, depolarization-evoked release of the neurotransmitter; (2) inhibition of the synthesis of dopamine, and (3) inhibition of the firing of the dopaminergic neuron.

In perfused slices of the striatum of several species, the electrically evoked release of [^{3}H]-dopamine is inhibited by low concentrations of dopamine receptor agonists such as apomorphine and pergolide and enhanced stereoselectively by the dopamine receptor antagonists sulpiride and butaclamol (Starke *et al.*, 1978; Langer *et al.*, 1981a; Kamal *et al.*, 1981; Lehmann *et al.*, 1981; Arbilla and Langer, 1981). The calcium-independent release of [^{3}H]-dopamine elicited by tyramine or amphetamine is not affected by dopamine receptor agonists or antagonists (Kamal *et al.*, 1981).

A large number of dopamine receptor agonists inhibit the electrically evoked release of [^{3}H]-dopamine from the striatum of various species (Lehmann *et al.*, 1983b). However, 3-(3-hydroxyphenyl)-N-(*n*-propyl)piperidine (3-PPP), which has been suggested to be a selective dopamine autoreceptor agonist (Nilsson and Carlsson, 1982), fails to stimulate the dopamine autoreceptor in the *in vitro* model of perfused striatal slices (Langer *et al.*, 1983a; Arbilla and Langer, 1983). Neither racemic 3-PPP nor its active (−) isomer was able to inhibit the electrically evoked release of [^{3}H]-dopamine in slices of the rat or rabbit striatum (Langer *et al.*, 1983a; Arbilla and Langer, 1983). In fact, the (—) isomer of 3-PPP increased both the spontaneous outflow of radioactivity and the electrically evoked release of [^{3}H]-dopamine when tested at concentrations of 1 and 10 μM, suggesting that (−)-3-PPP may block rather than stimulate the dopamine autoreceptor that modulates dopaminergic neurotransmission (Arbilla and Langer, 1983).

In contrast to the results obtained on central and peripheral noradrenergic neurotransmission, low concentrations of (*S*)-sulpiride or (+)-butaclamol enhance the electrically evoked release of [^{3}H]-dopamine (Arbilla and Langer, 1981). Since blockade of the presynaptic dopamine autoreceptors increases transmitter release evoked by electrical stimulation, it can be concluded that the dopamine autoreceptors play a physiological role in the modulation of dopaminergic neurotransmission in the striatum (Langer *et al.*, 1980a).

6. *Dopamine Receptors Modulating the Release of Acetylcholine from the Striatum*

It is by now well established that dopamine receptor agonists inhibit the depolarization-evoked release of [^{3}H]-acetylcholine from the striatum of different species (Hertting *et al.*, 1980; Scatton, 1982; Lehmann *et al.*, 1983a,c; Langer *et al.*, 1983a). This effect is mediated through the activation of the D-2 subtype of dopamine receptor and is antagonized by (*S*)-sulpiride or haloperidol. In contrast to the results obtained with the dopamine autoreceptor that modulates dopaminergic neurotransmission, exposure to (*S*)-sulpiride or to other dopamine receptor antagonists does not by itself increase the overflow of [^{3}H]-acetylcholine elicited by electrical stimulation in striatal slices of the cat (Lehmann *et al.*, 1983a) or the rabbit (Langer *et al.*, 1983b). Yet, in slices of the rabbit striatum, a small but significant increase of [³H]-acetylcholine overflow can be observed in the presence of haloperidol (Hertting *et al.*, 1980).

It is possible that the effect of endogenously released dopamine on [³H]-acetylcholine release in the striatum is very small or absent, because the dopamine terminal does not form a synapse with cholinergic elements and must diffuse a relatively long distance to interact with dopamine receptors on cholinergic nerve terminals. In support of this view, it has been reported that inhibition of neuronal uptake of dopamine with nomifensine, cocaine, or benzotropine, by increasing the extracellular concentration of released dopamine, can inhibit the electrically evoked release of [³H]-acetylcholine (Hertting *et al.*, 1980; S. Arbilla and S. Z. Langer, unpublished observations). However, it is likely that the experimental conditions (inhibition of neuronal uptake of dopamine) under which released dopamine can be shown to exert an important modulatory effect on cholinergic neurons may not necessarily represent the physiological situation.

7. Inhibition by d-Amphetamine of the Electrically Evoked Release of [³H]-Acetylcholine from the Rat Striatum

It is generally well established that neither amphetamine nor tyramine directly stimulate dopamine receptors but that each produces its effect indirectly through the release of the catecholamine. In rabbit striatal slices, amphetamine and tyramine are practically equipotent in releasing recently taken up [³H]-dopamine (Kamal *et al.*, 1981). Amphetamine has been shown to be a full agonist at inhibiting the electrically evoked release of [³H]-acetylcholine in slices of rabbit and rat striatum with an IC$_{50}$ of approximately 1 μM (Langer *et al.*, 1983b). On the other hand, tyramine produces only a 25% inhibition of [³H]-acetylcholine release at 10 μM, and it is inactive at lower concentrations (Langer *et al.*, 1983b). This small but significant inhibition in the release of [³H]-acetylcholine elicited by 10 μM tyramine is entirely abolished by pretreatment with reserpine (Langer *et al.*, 1983b). In sharp contrast to the results obtained with tyramine, pretreatment with reserpine failed to modify the inhibition by amphetamine of the electrically evoked release of [³H]-acetylcholine (Langer *et al.*, 1983b; Cantrill *et al.*, 1983a).

These results indicate that amphetamine, in contrast to tyramine, can inhibit the electrically evoked release of [³H]-acetylcholine through the release of dopamine from a special pool that is resistant to pretreatment with reserpine. It appears that the reserpine-resistant pool of dopamine that can be released by amphetamine corresponds to a pool of recently synthetized transmitter, which originates in dopaminergic nerve terminals. In support of this view, it has been reported that (1) after pretreatment with reserpine, the inhibition by amphetamine of [^{3}H]-acetylcholine release can be completely antagonized in the presence of the inhibitor of tyrosine hydroxylase, α-methyl-*para*-tyrosine (Cantrill *et al.*, 1983b), and (2) chemical denervation with 6-hydroxydopamine reduces the inhibitory effects of amphetamine on the release of [^{3}H]-acetylcholine in the rat striatum without affecting the inhibitory action of the directly acting dopamine receptor agonist apomorphine (Cantrill *et al.*, 1983b).

As shown in Table II, the inhibition of [^{3}H]-acetylcholine release by apomorphine and *d*-amphetamine is mediated through the activation of dopamine receptors, since they are blocked by low concentrations of (*S*)-sulpiride, which on its own does not enhance the release of [^{3}H]-acetylcholine elicited by electrical stimulation.

It is of interest that (−)-3-PPP at 1 μM does not stimulate the dopamine receptors that modulate [^{3}H]-acetylcholine release but effectively blocks the inhibition by amphetamine of the electrically evoked release of [^{3}H]-acetylcholine (Table II).

Further support for the involvement of dopamine in the inhibition by amphetamine of the release of [^{3}H]-acetylcholine in rats pretreated with reserpine is provided by the effects of inhibition of monoamine oxidase with pargyline. As shown in Table II, exposure to 10 μM pargyline did not by itself modify the electrically evoked release of [^{3}H]-acetylcholine but significantly potentiated the inhibition by amphetamine of [^{3}H]-acetylcholine release.

Several authors have postulated direct effects of amphetamine on dopamine receptors in the striatum (Feltz and De Champlain, 1973) and on amphetamine recognition sites in the hypothalamus (Paul *et al.*, 1982). Our results do not support the view that amphetamine could directly stimulate a dopamine receptor subtype. In our experimental model of [^{3}H]-acetylcholine release from the striatum, it appears that amphetamine releases newly synthesized dopamine from a reserpine-resistant pool and can thus stimulate the inhibitory dopamine receptors present on the cholinergic interneuron. The fact that amphetamine is also able to inhibit neuronal uptake of dopamine should be taken into consideration in the analysis of its inhibitory effects on [^{3}H]-acetylcholine release. Inhibition of neuronal uptake of dopamine with nomifensine, benzotropine, or cocaine reduces the electrically evoked release of [^{3}H]-acetylcholine (S. Arbilla and S. Z. Langer, unpublished observations), probably by allowing higher

Table II. Antagonism by S-Sulpiride and $(-)$-3-PPP of the Inhibition by d-Amphetamine of the Electrically Evoked Release of [³H]-ACh in Striatal Slices from Rats Pretreated with Reserpine[a]

		Concn. (µM)	n	S_1[b]	S_2/S_1[b]
Control			13	2.95 ± 0.24	0.79 ± 0.02
(S)-Sulpiride	(S_2)	0.01	1	2.55 ± 0.11	0.70 ± 0.04
(S)-Sulpiride	(S_2)	0.1	5	2.75 ± 0.27	0.75 ± 0.02
($-$)-3-PPP	(S_2)	1	4	2.97 ± 0.39	0.78 ± 0.02
Apomorphine	(S_2)	0.03	4	2.12 ± 0.17	0.28 ± 0.01[c]
d-Amphetamine	(S_2)	1	6	2.22 ± 0.28	0.37 ± 0.02[c]
(S)-Sulpiride + apomorphine	($S_1 + S_2$)	0.01			
	(S_2)	0.03	4	2.71 ± 0.33	0.58 ± 0.05[d]
(S)-Sulpiride + d-amphetamine	($S_1 + S_2$)	0.1			
	(S_2)	1	5	2.76 ± 0.35	0.97 ± 0.03[d]
($-$)-3-PPP + d-amphetamine	($S_1 + S_2$)	1			
	(S_2)	1	3	2.73 ± 0.29	0.80 ± 0.01[d]
Pargyline	($S_1 + S_2$)	10	4	3.92 ± 1.20	0.85 ± 0.05
Pargyline + d-amphetamine	($S_1 + S_2$)	10			
	(S_2)	1	4	3.78 ± 1.36	0.16 ± 0.04[e,f]

[a] Rats received reserpine (5 mg/kg, i.p.) 24 hr before the experiment. Slices of the corpus striatum were labeled with [³H]-methylcholine and perfused with Krebs medium. For additional details of the methods, see Lehmann et al. (1983a).

[b] S_1 corresponds to the percent of total tissue radioactivity released by the first period of electrical stimulation (1 Hz, 2 msec, 2 min), and S_2 to the second one obtained 44 min later. Drugs were added 20 min before the second period of stimulation (S_2) or when indicated, they were added 20 min before the first period of stimulation and kept throughout the experiment ($S_1 + S_2$). Values are mean ± S.E.M. of n experiments per group.

[c] $P < 0.001$ when compared with the control group.

[d] $P < 0.001$ when compared with the effect of the agonist alone.

[e] $P < 0.001$ when compared with the effect of pargyline alone.

[f] $P < 0.001$ when compared with amphetamine, 1 µM, in the absence of pargyline.

concentrations of released dopamine to accumulate and reach the dopamine receptors on the cholinergic nerve endings of the striatum.

The ability of amphetamine to stimulate dopamine receptors in the cholinergic neuron even after pretreatment with reserpine is of particular interest because it is well established that amphetamine can produce schizophrenic symptoms in man (Angrist and Gershon, 1970) that are antagonized by α-methyltyrosine (Jönsson et al., 1971). It is possible that further studies on the mechanism involved in the inhibitory effects of amphetamine on [³H]-acetylcholine release and on the role of this reserpine-resistant pool of dopamine may help to clarify the mechanism whereby amphetamine, in preference to other directly acting dopamine receptor agonists, can produce schizophrenic symptoms in man.

8. Dopamine Receptors Involved in the Inhibition of the Release of Other Neurotransmitters

The possibility that presynaptic dopamine receptors located on the GABAergic nerve endings of the substantia nigra facilitate the release of GABA was suggested by Reubi *et al.* (1977). However, a subsequent study by Arbilla *et al.* (1981) concluded that apomorphine inhibited the potassium-evoked release of [^{3}H]-GABA without affecting the spontaneous outflow of radioactivity and that these inhibitory effects of apomorphine were antagonized by haloperidol. In addition, under these experimental conditions, exogenous dopamine did not affect the spontaneous or the potassium-evoked release of [^{3}H]-GABA from the rat substantia nigra (Arbilla *et al.*, 1981). It therefore appears unlikely that in the rat substantia nigra, the dendritic release of dopamine could modulate the spontaneous or stimulation-evoked release of GABA (Arbilla *et al.*, 1981). Additional studies are necessary to further clarify the possible influence of dopamine receptor agonists on GABAergic neurotransmission.

The situation appears to be clearer concerning the inhibition by dopamine receptor agonists of the potassium-evoked release of [^{3}H]-glutamate in the striatum. This effect appears to result from the activation of the D-2 subtype of dopamine receptor (Mitchell and Doggett, 1980). These dopamine receptors, which inhibit [^{3}H]-glutamate release, appear to be localized on corticostriatal afferent terminals. It is possible that [^{3}H]-sulpiride may label dopamine receptors modulating the release of [^{3}H]-gultamate, because there is a 37% loss of [^{3}H]-sulpiride binding sites in the striatum following decortication (Jenner and Marsden, 1981).

9. Dopamine Receptor Subtypes: Pharmacological Characterization of Presynaptic and Postsynaptic Dopamine Receptors

As shown in Table I, a clear relative order of selectivities exists for the characterization of D-1 and D-2 receptor subtypes in the periphery when agonists as well as antagonists are taken into consideration. This situation results from the clear advantage of measuring responses at the level of D-2 receptors (inhibition of norepinephrine release) and at the level of the D-1 receptor (vasodilatation in certain vascular beds). Figure 4 shows a schematic representation of the presynaptic and postsynaptic receptors for catecholamines in a peripheral neuroeffector junction in vascular smooth muscle.

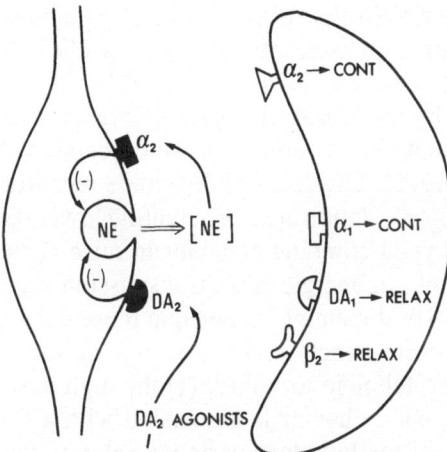

Figure 4. Schematic representation of a peripheral neuroeffector junction in vascular smooth muscle. Norepinephrine (NE) released from the noradrenergic varicosity activates presynaptic α_2 adrenoceptors to inhibit its own release. Activation of presynaptic inhibitory dopamine receptors of the D-2 subtype can also reduce the release of NE. At the level of the vascular smooth muscle, both α_1 and α_2 adrenoceptors mediate contraction. Relaxation of vascular smooth muscle is mediated by β_2-adrenoceptors and, in some vascular beds (renal, mesenteric, coronary, and cerebral), by postsynaptic dopamine receptors of the D-1 subtype.

Another useful scheme for subclassification of dopamine receptors is based on the observation that the D-1 dopamine receptor subtype is linked to adenylate cyclase whereas the D-2 subtype is not (Garau *et al.*, 1978; Kababian and Calne, 1979). In the central nervous system, the D-1 receptor is localized to neurons of striatal origin (McGeer *et al.*, 1976), whereas the D-2 receptor subtype is localized to corticostriatal afferents, neurons of striatal origin, and possibly glial elements in the striatum (for review, see Seeman, 1981). The dopamine receptor modulating the release of norepinephrine, acetylcholine, dopamine, and glutamate corresponds to the D-2 subtype.

Although the pharmacological properties of the dopamine autoreceptor and the dopamine receptor modulating acetylcholine release appear to be very similar, there are differences between the dopamine autoreceptor and the postsynaptic dopamine receptors that control the electrical activity of striatal neurons and mediate locomotor activation and stereotyped behavior induced by dopamine receptor agonists. Consequently, it appears that the dopamine receptor modulating acetylcholine release is unlikely to be an adequate model for the postsynaptic dopamine receptor mediating these behavioral effects and modulating the electrical activity of striatal neurons.

It is well established that postsynaptic dopamine receptors mediate locomotor stimulation and stereotyped behavior elicited by dopamine receptor agonists (Strömbom, 1976; Voith, 1980). On the other hand, locomotor sedation by low doses of dopamine receptor agonists is thought to result from stimulation of dopamine autoreceptors (Di Chiara *et al.*, 1976; Strömbom, 1976). The doses of dopamine receptor agonists needed to produce locomotor sedation are about tenfold lower than those required to produce stereotyped climbing behavior in mice (Costall *et al.*, 1981). If the modulation of cholinergic neurotransmission represents the direct postsynaptic action of dopamine involved in these behavioral effects, one should expect opposite effects of low and high doses of apomorphine to be reflected in acetylcholine turnover: (1) the high dose of apomorphine producing stereotyped behavior is associated with a decrease in acetylcholine turnover; (2) the low dose of apomorphine producing locomotor sedation should be expected to elicit an increase in acetylcholine turnover. However, there is not such biphasic curve on acetylcholine turnover (Choi and Roth, 1978). In fact, the decrease in acetylcholine levels by apomorphine is obtained at doses considerably lower than those required to induce sterotypy (Choi and Roth, 1978; Costall *et al.*, 1981).

It is therefore clear that in order to characterize *in vitro* the pharmacological properties of the dopamine receptors mediating the postsynaptic effects of dopamine at the behavioral and electrophysiological level, we require new experimental models, and the modulation by dopamine of acetylcholine release is not an adequate model for these postsynaptic effects of dopamine.

10. Conclusions

The dopamine receptors involved in the modulation of the release of various neurotransmitters in the peripheral as well as in the central nervous system appear to be of the D-2 subtype. In the periphery, D-1 receptors in vascular smooth muscle produce vasodilatation in certain vascular beds. The physiological role of the D-1 receptor (which is coupled to adenylate cyclase) in the central nervous system remains to be elucidated.

The presence of presynaptic release-modulating dopamine receptors can be demonstrated through the inhibitory effects of dopamine receptor agonists on transmitter release and the selective blockade of these actions by specific D-2 dopamine receptor antagonists.

Only at the level of the dopamine autoreceptors can it be clearly demonstrated that the dopamine receptor-blocking agent has on its own a facilitating effect on transmitter release. The latter indicates that the dopamine autoreceptors are likely to play a physiological role in the regulation of the release of dopamine. The dopamine receptors that inhibit the release of other transmitters (norepinephrine, acetylcholine, glutamate) are potential targets for the effects of agonist drugs that will reduce the release of the corresponding neurotransmitter.

Amphetamine does not directly stimulate dopamine receptors, but it can release dopamine from a strategic pool of newly synthetized transmitter that is resistant to pretreatment with reserpine. Amphetamine may act by promoting a latent dopaminergic transmission, which may play an important role under physiological or pathological conditions. The latter may be of particular interest because of the well-established ability of amphetamine in high doses to produce schizophrenic symptoms in man.

The stimulation of peripheral presynaptic D-2 receptors on noradrenergic nerve terminals produces a hypotensive and bradycardic action, which has a promising therapeutic potential in hypertension. In addition, stimulation by D-1 dopamine receptor agonists, by producing vasodilatation in certain vascular beds, may be of potential interest in the therapy of hypertension and other cardiovascular diseases.

Dopamine receptor agonists that selectively stimulate the dopamine autoreceptor in the CNS and have a low or negligible affinity for the postsynaptic dopamine receptor may represent a novel therapeutic approach to the treatment of schizophrenia by reducing presynaptically the release of dopamine.

Additional studies on the facilitation by amphetamine of the latent dopaminergic neurotransmission and the postsynaptic dopamine receptor subtypes involved in this process may provide a new insight in the pathophysiology of certain psychiatric diseases such as schizophrenia.

References

Angrist, B. M., and Gershon, S., 1970, The phenomenology of experimentally induced amphetamine psychosis. Preliminary observations, *Biol. Psychiatry* **2**:95–107.

Arbilla, S., and Langer, S. Z., 1981, Stereoselectivity of presynaptic autoreceptors modulating dopamine release, *Eur. J. Pharmacol.* **76**:345–351.

Arbilla, S., and Langer, S. Z., 1983, Blockade by (−)3PPP of the dopamine receptors that modulate the release of ^{3}H-acetylcholine in rat striatal slices, *Br. J. Pharmacol.* **79**:193.

Arbilla, S., Kamal, L., and Langer, S. Z., 1981, Inhibition by apomorphine of the potassium-evoked release of ^{3}H-γ-aminobutyric acid from the rat substantia nigra *in vitro*, *Br. J. Pharmacol.* **74**:389–397.

Armstrong, J. M., Duval, N., and Langer, S. Z., 1982, Possible heterogeneity of dopamine receptors in coronary vascular smooth muscle of the anaesthetised dog, *Br. J. Pharmacol.* **77**:471P.

Armstrong, J. M., Duval, N. and Langer, S. Z., 1983, LY 141865 stimulates histamine-2 (H_2) receptors and dopamine-2 (DA_2) receptors in the anaesthetised dog, *Eur. J. Pharmacol.* **87**:165–166.

Armstrong, J. M., Duval, N., and Langer, S. Z., 1984, Characterization of the postsynaptic receptors mediating dilatation of the coronary vascular bed produced by dopamine-like agents in anesthetized dogs, *Naunyn Schmiedebergs Arch. Pharmacol.* (in press).

Cantrill, R., Arbilla, S., and Langer, S. Z., 1983a, Inhibition by *d*-amphetamine of the electrically-evoked release of ^{3}H-acetylcholine from slices of the rat striatum: Involvement of dopamine receptors, *Eur. J. Pharmacol.* **87**:167–168.

Cantrill, R., Arbilla, S., Zivkovic, B., and Langer, S. Z., 1983b, Amphetamine enhances latent dopaminergic neurotransmission in the rat striatum: effects on ^{3}H-acetylcholine release, *Naunyn Schmiedebergs Arch. Pharmacol.* **322**:322–324.

Choi, R. L., and Roth, R. H., 1978, Development of supersensitivity of apomorphine induced increases in acetylcholine levels and stereotypy after chronic fluphenazine treatment, *Neuropharmacology* **17**:59–64.

Costall, B., Lim, S. K., and Naylor, R. J., 1981, Characterisation of the mechanisms by which purported dopamine agonists reduce spontaneous locomotor activity of mice, *Eur. J. Pharmacol.* **73**:175–188.

DiChiara, G., Porceddu, M. L., Vargin, L., Stefanini, E., and Gessa, G. L., 1976, Evidence for dopamine receptors mediating sedation in the mouse brain, *Nature* **264**:564–567.

Dubocovich, M. L., and Langer, S. Z., 1974, Negative feed-back regulation of noradrenaline release by nerve stimulation in the perfused cat's spleen: Differences in potency of phenoxybenzamine in blocking the pre- and post-synaptic adrenergic receptors, *J. Physiol. (Lond.)* **237**:505–519.

Dubocovich, M. L., and Langer, S. Z., 1976, Influence of the frequency of nerve stimulation on the metabolism of ^{3}H-norepinephrine released from the perfused cat spleen: Differences observed during and after the period of stimulation, *J. Pharmacol. Exp. Ther.* **198**:83–101.

Dubocovich, M. L., and Langer, S. Z., 1980, Dopamine and *alpha*-adrenoceptor agonists inhibit neurotransmission in the cat spleen through different presynaptic receptors, *J. Pharmacol. Exp. Ther.* **212**:144–152.

Enero, M. A., and Langer, S. Z., 1975, Inhibition by dopamine of ^{3}H-noradrenaline release elicited by nerve stimulation in the isolated cat's nictitating membrane, *Naunyn Schmiedebergs Arch. Pharmacol.* **289**:179–203.

Feltz, P., and De Champlain, J., 1973, The postsynaptic effects of amphetamine on striatal dopamine-sensitive neurons, in: *Frontiers in Catecholamine Research*, Pergamon Press, Oxford, pp. 951–956.

Galzin, A. M., Dubocovich, M. L., and Langer, S. Z., 1982, Presynaptic inhibition by dopamine receptor agonists of noradrenergic neurotransmission in the rabbit hypothalamus, *J. Pharmacol. Exp. Ther.* **221**:461–471.

Garau, L., Govoni, S., Stefanini, E., and Spano, P. F., 1978, Dopamine receptors: Pharmacological and anatomical evidences indicate that two distinct dopamine receptor populations are present in rat striatum, *Life Sci.* **23**:1745–1750.

Goldberg, L. I., 1979, The dopamine vascular receptor: Agonists and antagonists. *Advances in Biosciences: Peripheral Dopaminergic Receptors*, Volume 20 (J. L. Imbs and J. Schwartz, eds.), Pergamon Press, Oxford, pp. 1–12.

Goldberg, L. I., and Kohli, J. D., 1983, Peripheral dopamine receptors: A classification based on potency series and specific antagonism, *Trends Pharmacol. Sci.* **4**:64–66.

Hertting, G., Zumstein, A., Jackisch, R., Hoffmann, I., and Starke, K., 1980, Modulation by endogenous dopamine of the release of acetylcholine in the caudate nucleus of the rabbit, *Naunyn Schmiedebergs Arch. Pharmacol.* **315**:111–117.

Jenner, P., and Marsden, C. D., 1981, Substitute benzamide drugs as selective neuroleptic agents, *Neuropharmacology* **20:**1285–1293.

Jönsson, L. E., Ånggard, E., and Gunne, L. M., 1971, Blockade of intravenous amphetamine euphoria in man, *Clin. Pharmacol. Ther.* **12:**889–896.

Kamal, L., Arbilla, S., and Langer, S. Z., 1981, Presynaptic modulation of the release of dopamine from the rabbit caudate nucleus: Differences between electrical stimulation, amphetamine and tyramine, *J. Pharmacol. Exp. Ther.* **216:**592–598.

Kebabian, J. W., and Calne, D. B., 1979, Multiple receptors for dopamine, *Nature* **277:**93–96.

Langer, S. Z., 1973, The regulation of transmitter release elicited by nerve stimulation through a presynaptic feed-back mechanism, in: *Frontiers in Catecholamine Research* (E. Usdin and S. Snyder, eds.), Pergamon Press, Oxford, New York, pp. 543–549.

Langer, S. Z., 1981, Presynaptic regulation of the release of catecholamines, *Pharmacol. Rev.* **32:**337–362.

Langer, S. Z., and Dubocovich, M. L., 1979, Physiological and pharmacological role of the regulation of noradrenaline release by presynaptic dopamine receptors, in: *Peripheral Dopamine Receptors* (J. L. Imbs and J. Schwartz, eds.), Pergamon Press, Oxford, New York, pp. 233–245.

Langer, S. Z., and Dubocovich, M. L., 1981, Cocaine and amphetamine antagonize the decrease of noradrenergic transmission elicited by oxymetazoline but potentiate the inhibition by α-methylnorepinephrine in the perfused cat spleen, *J. Pharmacol. Exp. Ther.* **216:**162–171.

Langer, S. Z., and Lehmann, J., 1984, Presynaptic receptors on catecholamine neurons, in: *Catecholamine II* (U. Trendelenburg and N. Weiner, eds.), Springer-Verlag, Berlin, Heidelberg, New York (in press).

Langer, S. Z., and Shepperson, N. B., 1982, Recent developments in vascular smooth muscle pharmacology: The postsynaptic α_2-adrenoceptor, *Trends Pharmacol. Sci.* **3:**440–444.

Langer, S. Z., Arbilla, S., and Kamal, L., 1980a, Autoregulation of noradrenaline and dopamine release through presynaptic receptors, in: *Neurotransmitters and Their Receptors* (U. Z. Littauer, Y. Dudai, I. Silman, V. I. Teichberg, and Z. Vogel, eds.), John Wiley & Sons, New York, pp. 7–21.

Langer, S. Z., Cavero, I., and Massingham, R., 1980b, Recent developments in noradrenergic neurotransmission and its relevance to the mechanism of action of certain antihypertensive agents, *Hypertension* **2:**372–382.

Langer, S. Z., Arbilla, S., Kamal, L., and Cantrill, R., 1983a, Peripheral and central dopamine receptors modulating the release of neurotransmitters. *Acta Pharm. Suec.* Suppl. 1 (A. Carlsson and J. L. G. Nilsson, eds), Swedish Pharmaceutical Press, Stockholm, pp. 108–117.

Langer, S. Z., Arbilla, S., Galzin, A. M., and Cantrill, R., 1983b, Stereoselective blockade by sulpiride or the effects of dopamine agonists on the release of dopamine, noradrenaline and acetylcholine, in: *Special Aspects of Psychopharmacology* (M. Ackenheil and N. Matrssek, eds.), Expansion Scientifique Française, Paris, pp. 103–111.

Lehmann, J., and Langer, S. Z., 1983, Dopamine receptors modulating striatal cholinergic function: A valid model for the postsynaptic actions of dopamine? *Neuroscience*, **10:** 1105–1120.

Lehmann, J., Arbilla, S., and Langer, S. Z., 1981, Dopamine receptor mediated inhibition by pergolide of electrically-evoked ^{3}H-dopamine release from striatal slices of cat and rat: slight effect of ascorbate, *Naunyn Schmiedebergs Arch. Pharmacol.* **317:**31–35.

Lehmann, J., Smith, R. V., and Langer, S. Z., 1983a, Stereoisomers of apomorphine differ in affinity and intrinsic activity at presynaptic dopamine receptors modulating (^{3}H)-

dopamine and (^{3}H)-acetylcholine release in slices of cat caudate, *Eur. J. Pharmacol.*, **88**:81–88.

Lehmann, J., Briley, M., and Langer, S. Z., 1983b, Characterization of classical and novel dopamine receptor agonists at dopamine autoreceptor and ^{3}H-spiperone binding sites *in vitro*, *Eur. J. Pharmacol*, **88**:11–26.

Lehmann, J., Lee, C., and Langer, S. Z., 1983c, Dopamine receptors modulating ^{3}H-acetylcholine release in slices of the cat caudate: effects of (–)-N-(2-chloroethyl)-norapomorphine, *Eur. J. Pharmacol.*, **90**:393–400.

Massingham, R., Dubocovich, M. L., and Langer, S. Z., 1980, The role of presynaptic receptors in the cardiovascular action of N,N-di-*n*-propyldopamine in the cat and dog, *Naunyn Schmiedebergs Arch. Pharmacol.* **314**:17–28.

McGeer, E. G., Innanen, V. T., and McGeer, P. L., 1976, Evidence on the cellular localization of adenylcyclase in the neostriatum, *Brain Res.* **118**:356–358.

Mitchell, P. R., and Doggett, N. S., 1980, Modulation of striatal [^{3}H]-glutamic acid release by dopaminergic drugs, *Life Sci.* **26**:2073–2081.

Nilsson, L. J. G., and Carlsson, A., 1982, Dopamine-receptor agonist with apparent selectivity for autoreceptors: A new principle for antipsychotic action? *Trends Pharmacol. Sci.* **3**:322–325.

Paul, S. M., Hulihan-Giblin, B., and Skolnick, P., 1982, (+)Amphetamine binding to rat hypothalamus: Relation to anorexic potency of phenyl ethylamines, *Science* **218**:487–490.

Pellmar, T. C., 1981, Transmitter control of voltage-dependent currents, *Life Sci.* **28**:2199–2205.

Reubi, J. C., Iversen, L. L., and Jessell, T. M., 1977, Dopamine selectively increases ^{3}H-GABA release from slices of rat substantia nigra *in vitro*, *Nature* **268**:652–654.

Scatton, B., 1982, Effect of dopamine agonists and neurologic agents on striatal acetylcholine transmission in the rat: Evidence against dopamine receptor multiplicity, *J. Pharmacol. Exp. Ther.* **220**:197–202.

Seeman, P., 1980, Brain dopamine receptors, *Pharmacol. Rev.* **32**:229–313.

Shepperson, N. B., Duval, N., and Langer, S. Z., 1982a, Dopamine decreases mesenteric blood flow in the anaesthetized dog through the stimulation of postsynaptic α_2-adrenoceptors, *Eur. J. Pharmacol.* **81**:627–635.

Shepperson, N. B., Duval, N., Massingham, R., and Langer, S. Z., 1982b, Differential blocking effects of several dopamine receptor antagonists for peripheral pre- and postsynaptic dopamine receptors in the anaesthetized dog, *J. Pharmacol. Exp. Ther.* **221**:753–761.

Starke, K., Reimann, W., Zumstein, A., and Hertting, G., 1978, Effect of dopamine receptor agonists and antagonists on the release of dopamine in the rabbit caudate nucleus *in vitro*, *Naunyn Schmiedebergs Arch. Pharmacol.* **305**:27–36.

Strömbom, U., 1976, Catecholamine receptor agonists: Effects on motor activity and rate of tyrosine hydroxylation in mouse brain, *Naunyn Schmiedebergs Arch. Pharmacol.* **292**:167–176.

Tsuruta, K., Frey, E. A., Grewe, C. W., Cote, T. E., Eskay, R. L., and Kebabian, J. W., 1981, Evidence that LY-141865 specifically stimulates the D-2 dopamine receptor, *Nature* **292**:463–466.

Voith, K., 1980, Supersensitivity to apomorphine in experimentally induced hypokinesia and drug-induced modifications of the apomorphine response, *Psychopharmacology* **79**:247–254.

DOPAMINE AGONIST FUNCTION AND PHARMACOLOGY

Dopamine
An Endogenous Peripheral Neurotransmitter

N. H. NEFF, M. HADJICONSTANTINOU, and Z. LACKOVIC

1. Introduction

There is now considerable evidence for the presence of dopamine receptors in peripheral tissues, as is documented throughout this volume. There has been, however, a reluctance to accept the possibility of a peripheral dopaminergic neuronal system to innervate these receptors for several reasons. Traditionally, students are taught that the autonomic nervous system is composed of only two types of neurons, cholinergic and noradrenergic. It is difficult to break with tradition. Dopamine is present in autonomic nerves, and it represents about 5–10% of the norepinephrine content. Therefore, it is assumed to be solely a precursor for norepinephrine synthesis and not a neurotransmitter. We should recall that dopamine in the spinal cord represents about 5–10% of the norepinephrine, and, until recently, it was considered to be only a precursor for norepinephrine. There is now a vast literature on the presence of dopaminergic neurons in the cord together with speculation about their possible physiological role (Commissiong *et al.*, 1978; Gentleman *et al.*, 1981; Commissiong and Neff, 1979). What percentage of dopamine should be found in a nerve or tissue to raise suspicion that dopaminergic neurons are present within a structure? Is the percentage of dopamine present meaningful if it is concentrated in a few neurons and nerve endings? Moreover,

N. H. NEFF and M. HADJICONSTANTINOU • Laboratory of Preclinical Pharmacology, National Institute of Mental Health, Saint Elizabeths Hospital, Washington, D. C. 20032. *Z. LACKOVIC* • Department of Pharmacology, Medical Faculty University of Zagreb, Zagreb, Yugoslavia.

the quantity of amine stored in a nerve ending may not be as important as its rate of formation and release onto receptors.

Based on pharmacological studies, two populations of peripheral dopamine receptors have been identified (for recent reviews, see Goldberg *et al.*, 1978; Lokhandwala, 1979; Cavero *et al.*, 1982a,b; Brodde, 1982). Type DA_1 dopamine receptors are found postjunctionally, primarily on renal and mesenteric vascular beds, and their activation leads to direct myorelaxation. These receptors are activated by dopamine, SK&F 38393, and SK&F 82526 and are preferentially blocked by bulbocapnine. Type DA_2 dopamine receptors are found prejunctionally on noradrenergic axonal varicosities and on some sympathetic ganglion cell bodies, and their activation leads to reduced release of norepinephrine. The consequences of stimulating these receptors is diminished release of norepinephrine, resulting in decreased heart rate and passive vasodilation, which would be most evident when there is significant sympathetic drive. These receptors are activated by dopamine or N,N-di-*n*-propyldopamine (DPDA) and are blocked by haloperidol but are resistant to bulbocapnine. DA_1 and DA_2 receptors are associated primarily with the cardiovascular system and therefore have received a great deal of investigation because of their potential importance in controlling blood pressure. It now appears, however, that dopamine receptors are associated with a wide variety of physiological responses in addition to cardiovascular responses. It is our contention that these receptors were not put there for the pharmacologist to activate them with drugs. Indeed, there is now a body of evidence supporting the hypothesis that there is a widely distributed peripheral dopaminergic neuronal system to innervate peripheral dopamine receptors. Our objective in this chapter is to present evidence from a variety of experimental approaches suggesting that there are, indeed, peripheral dopaminergic neurons.

2. Peripheral Nerves where Dopamine is Postulated to Function as a Neurotransmitter

Dopaminergic neurons have been identified in mammals by a variety of techniques. In some cases, a physiological role for these neurons has been proposed.

2.1. Sympathetic Ganglion Small Intensely Fluorescent Cells

In 1963, Eränkö and Härkönen reported the presence of small cells in the rat superior cervical ganglion that fluoresce intensely when exposed to formaldehyde vapor. These cells are intensely fluorescent because they contain a high content of catecholamine. In the rat, the predominate catecholamine is dopamine (Bjorklund *et al.*, 1970). In some species the small intensely fluorescent (SIF) cell system may contain norepinephrine (Wamsley *et al.*, 1978) or epinephrine (Koslow *et al.*, 1975). Recently, Verhofstad *et al.* (1981) identified a separate SIF cell system in the rat that contains serotonin (Hadjiconstantinou *et al.*, 1982). The SIF cells have been divided into two types based on their location and morphology (Williams *et al.*, 1976). Type I SIF cells are solitary and situated by the principal ganglionic neurons and appear to be interneurons. Type II SIF cells are found in clusters in proximity to blood vessels and therefore may have a neuroendocrine or chemoreceptive function (Matthews, 1980). There is a considerable difference in the percentage of type I and II SIF cells in sympathetic ganglia of different species (Williams *et al.*, 1976).

The physiological role of the dopamine-containing SIF cells is most likely to modulate ganglionic transmission, probably by altering the sensitivity of the principal neurons to acetylcholine released from preganglionic neurons (Libet and Tosaka, 1970). Within the ganglion, dopamine released from SIF cells is apparently responsible for an initial S-IPSP followed by a S-EPSP of the principal neurons to a direct muscarinic action of acetylcholine (Libet and Owman, 1974; Libet, 1977). The first response to dopamine is associated with suppression of ganglionic transmission, whereas the second response to dopamine may be associated with enhanced ganglionic transmission, although this remains to be demonstrated. Release of dopamine from the SIF cells, especially in the celiac ganglion, following preganglionic cholinergic nerve activity could modulate postganglionic sympathetic activity to the kidneys and visceral arteries and thus affect blood pressure. The dopamine receptors on the sympathetic neuron cell bodies appear to be of the DA_2 type (Cavero *et al.*, 1982a,b), whereas the dopamine-containing SIF cells may be the neurons that innervate these receptors. Because of the importance of sympathetic ganglia for blood pressure regulation, it is necessary that we understand the factors that control SIF cell dopamine metabolism.

The major metabolite of dopamine in the rat sympathetic ganglion is 3,4-dihydroxyphenylacetic acid (DOPAC), although small quantities of homovanillic acid (HVA) are present (Karoum *et al.*, 1977). The acidic metabolites do not freely diffuse into the circulation, as treatment with probenecid to block acid transport results in the accumulation of HVA and DOPAC within the ganglia. Decentralization of the ganglion does not change dopamine content but results in a significant fall of DOPAC, suggesting that preganglionic neurons are responsible, in part, for maintaining the metabolism of dopamine. This hypothesis is supported by the finding that the administration of carbachol increases the content of DOPAC in the ganglion whereas atropine pretreatment blocks the increase of DOPAC after carbachol (Lutold *et al.*, 1979). Indeed, there is a direct correlation between the content of DOPAC in the ganglion and the rate of formation of dopamine. Of the three ganglia we have studied in the rat (superior cervical ganglion, middle–inferior cervical ganglia, and celiac ganglion), the celiac ganglion is the most responsive to stimulation by muscarinic agonists (Lutold *et al.*, 1979). In the normal rat, the rate of dopamine formation is severalfold more rapid than the formation of dopamine in the striatum (Karoum *et al.*, 1977). The rapid rate of dopamine formation supports the notion that dopamine plays a role in ganglionic transmission.

The SIF cells respond to pharmacological agents similarly to striatal dopaminergic neurons. Treatment of rats with dopamine receptor antagonists such as haloperidol results in increased activity of striatal dopaminergic neurons, and, as a result, dopamine metabolites increase, presumably via activation of a neuronal feedback loop system (Carlsson and Lindquist, 1963). A similar control system appears likely for rat sympathetic ganglia. Haloperidol treatment results in increased DOPAC formation in ganglia, suggesting the presence of a local neuronal feedback loop system (Karoum *et al.*, 1980).

Sympathetic ganglion dopamine-containing SIF cells are apparently modulated by α-adrenergic receptors also (Karoum *et al.*, 1980). Phenylephrine treatment results in a fall of DOPAC content, which can be blocked by treatment with phenoxybenzamine. This observation suggests a model for future studies. Perhaps norepinephrine released from the cell bodies or dendrites of sympathetic neurons onto SIF cells inhibits dopamine release and metabolism by acting at α-adrenergic receptors. Thus, SIF cell activity would be modulated by preganglionic cholinergic neurons via muscarinic receptors and also by information they receive from the principal neurons via α-adrenergic receptors. Such a reciprocal system could serve to modulate information transfer between SIF cells and sympathetic neurons.

Dopamine-containing SIF cells are not exclusive to sympathetic ganglia. Rabbit nodose (Kojima *et al.*, 1981) and petrosal (Katz *et al.*, 1982) ganglia contain both dopamine- and norepinephrine-containing SIF cells. Interestingly, the dopamine content is higher than the norepinephrine content in rabbit nodose ganglia, although the opposite is true for superior cervical ganglia. The high dopamine content in nodose ganglion is consistent with the observation that human vagus nerve contains about equal quantities of norepinephrine and dopamine (Lackovic *et al.*, 1981) (Table I). Moreover, the metabolites HVA and DOPAC are also found within

Table I. Content of Catecholamines and Metabolites in Human Peripheral Nerves

	Content (nmole/g)			
	NE	DA	HVA	DOPAC
Superior cervical ganglion	2.6 ± 0.53	0.28 ± 0.12 (11)[a]	2.9 ± 0.27	0.23 ± 0.13
Splanchnic N.	1.0 ± 0.03	0.23 ± 0.05 (23)	4.0 ± 1.1	1.43 ± 0.68
Genitofemoral N.	0.39 ± 0.34	0.19 ± 0.03 (49)	2.3 ± 0.14	0.59 ± 0.30
Vagus N.	0.21 ± 0.08	0.25 ± 0.02 (119)	0.55	0.36
Intercostal N.	0.27	0.14 ± 0.03 (52)	0.93	0.22
Phrenic N.	0.28	0.007 (2.5)	0.87	0.44
Ilioinguinal N.	0.79	0.22 (28)	0.32	0.13

[a] Values in parentheses represent percentage of dopamine.

the vagus. The presence of dopamine in the vagus may indicate that do-pamine-containing SIF cells or other cell types within the nodose ganglion send axons to peripheral structures via the vagus nerve. It is now universally accepted that SIF cells of many species contain dopamine as a neurotransmitter.

Recently, Bell and Muller (1982) suggested that there are autonomic neurons in the dog that contain dopamine as a neurotransmitter and not norepinephrine. These neurons were identified by the absence of dopamine-β-hydroxylase-like immunoreactivity and the presence of catecholamine histofluorescence. The apparent dopamine-containing cells were localized mainly in L6–S2 and T8–L1 paravertebral ganglia. The L6–S2 ganglia correspond to the origins of the vasodilator nerves supplying the dog hind paw, which are thought to be dopaminergic (Beck *et al.*, 1966; Rolewicz and Zimmerman, 1972).

2.2. *Dopamine-Containing Peripheral Nerves*

Spinal nerve roots are a principal source of peripheral nerves. The majority of the nerves leaving the spinal cord (somatic and preganglionic autonomic nerves) via the ventral roots are cholinergic, whereas the neurotransmitter associated with neurons entering the spinal cord via the dorsal roots is unclear. Substance P and somatostatin may be neurotransmitters for some of these neurons (Hokfelt *et al.*, 1975; Nagy and Hunt, 1982). Dahlstrom and Fuxe (1965) reported that catecholamine histofluorescence was present in the ventral nerve roots of the rat spinal cord. Subsequently, adrenergic nerve fibers were observed in spinal ganglia (Owman and Santini, 1966). There are now several reports that ventral roots in animals and man contain relatively large quantities of dopamine compared to norepinephrine (Lackovic *et al.*, 1981; Lackovic and Neff, 1980). For human ventral nerve roots from thoracic regions of the cord, the contents of norepinephrine and dopamine were much higher than in the roots from lumbar regions of the cord. In general, the pattern of distribution and concentrations of dopamine and norepinephrine were similar (Lackovic *et al.*, 1981).

Recently, Price and Mudge (1983) found evidence for dopamine-containing neurons in a subpopulation of rat dorsal root ganglia. They used antisera against tyrosine hydroxylase and dopamine-β-hydroxylase as well as catecholamine histofluorescence to identify these neurons. The neurons were positive for tyrosine hydroxylase and negative for dopamine-β-hydroxylase. Positive-staining cells were small (diameter about 20 μm), distributed throughout a ganglion, and represented about 1% of the sensory neurons of the L5 ganglia. The cells were not uniformly distributed among the ganglia, and no positive cells were observed in ganglia T13 to L4 or in any of the cervical ganglia. Price and Mudge (1983) postulate that the dopamine-containing neurons are sensory and, because of their small diameter, probably play a role in either temperature or pain pathways.

2.3. Measurement of Dopamine and Its Metabolite in Peripheral Nerves

Some investigators contend that dopamine-containing nerves are best identified by their ratio of dopamine to norepinephrine. An arbitrary value of greater than 10% dopamine is often used as evidence for the presence of dopaminergic neurons. Indeed, if this criterion is used, almost all of the peripheral human nerves that have been surveyed (Table I) would qualify as containing dopaminergic neurons (Lackovic *et al.*, 1981). Interestingly, the superior cervical ganglion contains SIF cells yet only contains about 11% dopamine, whereas the vagus nerve, considered to be cholinergic, contains about 119% dopamine. The high dopamine content is consistent with the observation that dopamine SIF cells are present in the nodose ganglion (Kojima *et al.*, 1981). The possible presence of dopamine neurons in the vagus might explain the evidence presented for dopaminergic innervation of the lower esophageal sphincter and the gastrointestinal tract (Mukhopadhyay and Weisbrodt, 1977).

Norepinephrine is metabolized in nerve endings and in cell somata (Costa and Neff, 1966). Metabolism in the soma is faster than in nerve endings. Therefore, it would be expected that dopaminergic nerves would show evidence of dopamine metabolism, and indeed human peripheral nerves do. Both HVA and DOPAC have been found in all human peripheral nerves in which dopamine is present (Table I). Furthermore, the metabolites are present in higher concentration than dopamine, suggesting that dopamine metabolism is rather rapid (Lackovic *et al.*, 1981).

Two arguments have often been raised in the past against the possibility that dopamine might be a neurotransmitter in peripheral nerves: (1) it is found in low concentration in comparison with norepinephrine; and (2) it is not metabolized in peripheral nerves. Clearly, these arguments are not valid for man. The presence of dopamine and its metabolites in most of the nerves surveyed suggests that there is a widespread system of dopaminergic neurons in man.

3. Peripheral Tissues and Organs where There is Evidence for Dopaminergic Innervation

In the previous sections we have documented the presence of dopamine and its metabolites in the major neuronal systems as they proceed from the CNS to peripheral structures. We now present evidence favoring the view that dopaminergic neurons are present and functional in peripheral structures.

3.1. The Gastrointestinal Tract

The administration of dopamine produces a dose-dependent decrease in lower esophageal sphincter pressure and a dose-dependent increase in contractile activity in the body of the esophagus (Mukhopadhyay and Weisbrodt, 1977). Haloperidol and bulbocapnine antagonize the effect of dopamine. The amplitude of esophageal contraction and esophageal distention in response to pharyngeal stimulation was increased after haloperidol treatment. Mukhopadhyay and Weisbrodt (1977) speculate that dopamine receptors in the body of the esophagus may have a physiological role in controlling the amplitude of esophageal contraction during swallowing and in response to esophageal distention. These observations are consistent with the finding that dopamine is present in the gastrointestinal tract of several species (Heilman and Lum, 1971).

Dopamine administration induces relaxation of the stomach, which is specifically blocked by pimozide and metoclopramide (Valenzuela, 1976). The administration of dopamine antagonists alone increases intragastric pressure. Thus, it has been suggested that dopamine might be a neurotransmitter mediating gastric relaxation.

Collins and West (1968) prelabeled the rabbit ileum with radioactive dopamine and found a rather large increase in dopamine release following stimulation of sympathetic nerves. They concluded that the dopamine appeared to be released from sites that had many of the characteristics of other sympathetically innervated structures. We suggest that the release of dopamine may have been from endogenous dopaminergic neurons in the ileum.

3.2. The Reproductive System

In 1976, Simon and Van Maanen proposed that vas deferens is innervated by dopaminergic neurons. Indeed, most of the structures of the urogenital system contain substantial quantities of dopamine and metabolites (Lackovic et al., 1981). Boadle-Biber and Roth (1975) found that large quantities of dopamine were formed from radioactive precursors and released by depolarization of the rat vas deferens. Metabolism of dopamine takes place within neurons, as the administration of the neurotoxin 6-hydroxydopamine diminished endogenous dopamine and metabolites in rat seminal vesicles (Lackovic et al., 1982). Not only is there physiological evidence for the presence of dopamine receptors in vas deferens (Tayo, 1979, 1981; Badia et al., 1982), but dopamine receptor binding sites have been identified with radioactive haloperidol (Relja et al., 1982).

Dopamine-activated adenylate cyclase has been described in rat prostate gland (Shima et al., 1980). Cyclase activation was exclusively inhibited by dopamine antagonists.

The available evidence supports the hypothesis that a dopaminergic neuronal system is present in the reproductive system. If a dopaminergic neuronal system is present in the reproductive system, it would imply that administered dopaminergic drugs would act at these receptors as well as in the CNS. Perhaps some of the action of dopaminergic drugs on sexual function might be mediated by a direct action of these drugs on dopaminergic receptors in the reproductive system and not only via a central action, as is generally thought.

3.3. The Endocrine and Exocrine Glands

The administration of metoclopramide, a potent dopamine receptor antagonist, induces a doubling of plasma aldosterone content in man (Norbiato et al., 1977; Carey et al., 1979; Noth et al., 1980). Infusion of dopamine blocks the rise of plasma aldosterone induced by antagonists, suggesting that there is tonic inhibition of aldosterone release by endogenous dopamine. Dopamine has also been shown to suppress the aldosterone secretory response to angiotensin II in suspensions of isolated bovine adrenal glomerulosa cells (McKenna *et al.*, 1979). Aldosterone is produced almost entirely in the zona glomerulosa of the adrenal gland, and recently Dunn and Bosmann (1981) identified specific dopaminergic receptor binding sites there. The receptors appeared to be of the D_2 subclass as defined by Kebabian and Calne (1979).

There is evidence that dopaminergic receptors are present on parathyroid cells. Activation of these receptors by dopamine agonists results in activation of adenylate cyclase and the release of parathyroid hormone (Brown *et al.*, 1977, 1980; Attie *et al.*, 1980). Specific dopaminergic antagonists block the response to dopamine or to dopamine agonists.

George and Rayfield (1974) reported that the administration of L-DOPA induced the release of pancreatic glucagon. Based on the rapid response to administered L-DOPA, they postulated that dopaminergic receptors may be associated with the pancreatic α cells.

Furuta *et al.* (1973) found that L-DOPA or dopamine increased the secretion of pancreatic juice in the perfused canine pancreas. The response to L-DOPA could be blocked with a decarboxylase inhibitor and enhanced with a monoamine oxidase inhibitor. Haloperidol attenuated the dopamine-induced secretion. The authors concluded that the dog pancreas might contain specific receptors for dopamine. Several amino-acid-conjugated derivatives of dopamine were evaluated in the same model system and were found to have a longer duration of action than dopamine (Iwatsuki and Chiba, 1980).

Pancreatic polypeptide (PP) secretion in man may be regulated by dopamine receptors (Spitz *et al.*, 1979; Sowers *et al.*, 1982). Administration of domperidone or metoclopramide induces a rise of PP, whereas bromocriptine can reverse the postural and exercise-induced increase of PP. The finding that dopamine antagonists induce a rise of PP suggests that their secretion is normally tonically inhibited by endogenous dopamine.

3.4. The Kidney and Renal Vessels

The presence of a peripheral dopaminergic system in kidney was originally proposed based on its high content of dopamine (Bell, 1982a; Bell *et al.*, 1978a,b). In the dog renal cortex, dopamine represents about 10% of the catecholamine present, as compared with other kidney structures, where it represents about 3% or less of the catecholamine. Indeed, the kidney contains one of the only visualized dopaminergic neuronal elements in a peripheral organ (Dinerstein *et al.*, 1979). Dopaminergic elements are located at the glomerular vascular poles. Because of this location, they might be involved with regulation of renal blood flow and renin release.

Injection of dopamine into the canine renal artery produces a biphasic response of vasoconstriction followed by vasodilation. The vasoconstriction response is blocked by α-adrenergic antagonists, whereas the vasodilation is blocked by the specific dopamine antagonist sulpiride. From numerous studies, the kidney receptor has been characterized as a postsynaptic DA_1 receptor (for reviews see Goldberg, 1972; Goldberg et al., 1978).

The innervated kidney releases both norepinephrine and dopamine (Stephenson et al., 1982; Morgunov and Baines, 1981). Renal artery (Murthy et al., 1976) and a kidney particulate preparation (Nakajima et al., 1977) contain specific noradrenergic and dopaminergic coupled adenylate cyclase systems. The cyclase systems are similar to those found in brain. There is evidence that dopamine is a physiologically significant natriuretic factor and norepinephrine a significant antinatriuretic factor (Alexander et al., 1974; Ball et al., 1978; Morgunov and Baines, 1981).

There is no doubt that a dopaminergic neuronal system is present in the kidney. All of the criteria proposed by Bell (1982a) for identifying postganglionic autonomic dopaminergic nerves are satisfied in the kidney, including its presence in defined structures, release by activation of renal nerves, and the presence of receptors that modulate specific physiological functions.

3.5. The Cardiovascular System

There is now universal agreement that dopamine receptors are present in the cardiovascular system. For major reviews see Goldberg (1972). Goldberg et al. (1978). Lokhandwala (1979), Cavero et al., 1982a,b), Brodde (1982), Bell (1982), and other chapters in this volume. Blood vessels contain postjunctional DA_1 receptors, and their activation results in direct smooth muscle relaxation. Heart and sympathetic ganglia contain DA_2 receptors, and their activation results in a reduction of norepinephrine release from sympathetic nerves. Thus, the administration of a dopamine agonist would result in a fall of blood pressure because of a fall in peripheral resistance.

Receptors are present in cardiovascular tissue, but are dopaminergic nerves present? As we have documented in previous sections, there are substantial quantities of dopamine in the major nerves that innervate peripheral structures. These nerves also contain HVA and DOPAC; thus, dopamine is not solely a precursor for norepinephrine synthesis.

Long *et al.* (1975) were the first to report that activation of presynaptic dopamine receptors by agonists resulted in the inhibition of the responses to stimulation of the right postganglionic cardioaccelerator nerves. The inhibitory effect could be blocked by treatment with dopamine antagonists. There have been many reports confirming this observation (see Lokhandwala, 1979). The implication is that dopaminergic neurons are present in the cardioaccelerator nerve and, thus, dopamine can be released by nerve stimulation. The response to antagonist, therefore, might not be apparent unless there were sufficient sympathetic drive to the heart.

For most vessels, dopamine represents 3–8% of the catecholamine present (Head and Berkowitz, 1979; Bell and Gillespie, 1981). In the renal cortex, it represents about 10% of norepinephrine (Bell, 1982a), and there are identified dopaminergic neuronal elements present (Dinerstein *et al.*, 1979). There are other vessels in which the dopamine content is high also. There is a surprisingly high dopamine content, about 50% of norepinephrine, in cerebral microvessels (Head *et al.*, 1980). Sympathetic innervation of the cerebral vessels arises from the superior cervical ganglia, as ganglionectomy depletes specific catecholamine histofluorescence (Nielson and Owman, 1967). Recently, Suzuki *et al.* (1983) reported that the loss of dopamine from cerebral vessels after ganglionectomy was substantially different from the loss of norepinephrine. They suggested that dopamine may play a role other than that of a precursor for norepinephrine. In addition to the presence of a high dopamine content and a different distribution and origin compared with norepinephrine, there are specific dopamine receptors in cerebral vessels that induce vasodilation (Edvinsson *et al.*, 1978; Altura *et al.*, 1980). Thus, there is support for the presence of dopaminergic innervation of cerebral vessels.

Bell (1982a) has put together a convincing body of evidence favoring the presence of postganglionic dopaminergic autonomic nerves in the paw pad of the dog. This evidence includes identification of sympathetic ganglion cell bodies that appear to contain only dopamine and should project to the hindlimbs (Bell and Muller, 1982), the presence of relatively large quantities of dopamine in the paw pad (Bell *et al.*, 1978a), the presence of catecholamine nerve endings supplying the arteriovenous anastomoses of the paw pad that by pharmacological criteria appear to be dopaminergic (Bell *et al.*, 1978b), increased femoral blood flow following stimulation of the cut tibial nerve that is blocked by dopamine antagonists (Bell and Lang, 1979), and increased response to nerve stimulation by the presence of dopamine uptake-blocking drugs (Bell, 1982b).

Presently, there is substantial evidence that some blood vessels are innervated by dopaminergic neurons. These vessels include the kidney glomerular vascular poles, some cerebral vessels, and the arteriovenous anastomoses of the canine paw pad. Are these exceptions, or do they contain the most easily identified dopaminergic vascular nerves? In our view, these vascular elements are not exceptions; they are part of a vast dopaminergic system that innervates many peripheral structures.

4. Conclusions

The following arguments were often cited in the past to support the notion that dopamine is only a precursor for norepinephrine synthesis in peripheral tissues: (1) there are no specific dopamine receptors, and its pharmacology is related to its weak sympathetic amine activity; (2) the concentration is low in peripheral tissue, as might be expected for a precursor; and (3) the dopamine in peripheral tissue is converted to norepinephrine and is not metabolized. We have documented in this chapter that these arguments are not valid. There is one unifying concept that would explain all of the data: there is a widely distributed peripheral dopaminergic neuronal system.

References

Alexander, R. W., Gill, T. R., Jr., Yamabe, H., Lovenberg, W., and Keiser, H. R., 1974, Effects of dietary sodium and acute saline infusion on the interrelationship between dopamine excretion and adrenergic activity in man, *J. Clin. Invest.* **54**:194–200.

Altura, B. M., Gebrewold, A., and Lassoff, S., 1980, Biphasic responsiveness of rat pial arterioles to dopamine: Direct observations on the microcirculation, *Br. J. Pharmacol.* **69**:543–544.

Attie, M. F., Brown, E. M., Gardner, D. G., Spiegel, A. M., and Aurbach, G. D., 1980, Characterization of the dopamine-responsive adenylate cyclase of bovine parathyroid cells and its relationship to parathyroid hormone secretion, *Endocrinology* **107**:1776–1781.

Badia, A., Bermejo, P., and Jane, F., 1982, Pre- and postsynaptic effects of sulpiride in the rat isolated vas deferens, *J. Pharm. Pharmacol.* **34**:266–268.

Ball, S. G., Oats, N. S., and Lee, M. R., 1978, Urinary dopamine in man and rat: Effects of inorganic salts on dopamine excretion, *Clin. Sci. Mol. Med.* **55**:167–173.

Beck, L., Pollard, A. A., Kayaalp, S. O., and Weiner, L. M., 1966, Sustained dilatation elicited by sympathetic nerve stimulation, *Fed. Proc.* **25**:1596–1606.

Bell, C., 1982a, Dopamine as a postganglionic autonomic neurotransmitter, *Neuroscience* **7**:1–8.

Bell, C., 1982b, Benztropine-induced prolongation of responses to vasodilator nerve stimulation in the canine paw pad, *Br. J. Pharmacol.* **76**:231–233.

Bell, C., and Gillespie, J. S., 1981, Dopamine and noradrenaline levels in peripheral tissues of several mammalian species, *J. Neurochem.* **36**:703–706.

Bell, C., and Lang, W. J., 1979, Evidence for dopaminergic vasodilator innervation of the canine paw pad, *Br. J. Pharmacol.* **67**:337–343.

Bell, C., and Muller, B. D., 1982, Absence of dopamine-β-hydroxylase in some catecholamine-containing sympathetic ganglion cells of the dog: Evidence for dopaminergic autonomic neurones, *Neurosci. Lett.* **31**:31–35.

Bell, C., Lang, W. J., and Laska, F., 1978a, Dopamine-containing vasomotor nerves in the dog kidney, *J. Neurochem.* **31**:77–83.

Bell, C., Lang, W. J., and Laska, F., 1978b, Dopamine-containing axons supplying the arterio-venous anastomoses of the canine paw pad, *J. Neurochem.* **31**:1329–1333.

Bjorklund, A., Cegrell, L., Falck, B., Ritzin, M., and Rosengren, E., 1970, Dopamine-containing cells in sympathetic ganglia, *Acta Physiol. Scand.* **78**:334–338.

Boadle-Biber, M. C., and Roth, R. H., 1975, Formation of dopamine and noradrenaline in rat vas deferens: Comparison with guinea pig vas deferens, *Br. J. Pharmacol.* **55**:73–78.

Brodde, O. E., 1982, Vascular dopamine receptors: Demonstration and characterization by *in vitro* studies, *Life Sci.* **31**:289–306.

Brown, E. M., Carroll, R. J., and Aurbach, G. D., 1977, Dopaminergic stimulation of cyclic AMP accumulation and parathyroid hormone release from dispersed bovine parathyroid cells, *Proc. Natl. Acad. Sci. U.S.A.* **74**:4210–4213.

Brown, E. M., Attie, M. F., Reen, S., Gardner, D. G., Kebabian, J., and Aurbach, G. D., 1980, Characterization of dopaminergic receptors in dispersed bovine parathyroid cells, *Mol. Pharmacol.* **18**:335–340.

Carey, R. M., Thorner, M. O., and Ortt, E. M., 1979, Effects of metoclopramide and bromocriptine on the renin–angiotensin–aldosterone system in man. Dopaminergic control of aldosterone, *J. Clin. Invest.* **63**:727–735.

Carlsson, A., and Lindqvist, M., 1963, Effect of chlorpromazine or haloperidol or formation of 3-methoxytyramine and normetanephrine in mouse brain, *Acta Pharmacol. Toxicol.* (*Kbh.*) **20**:140–144.

Cavero, I., Massingham, R., and Lefevre-Borg, F., 1982a, Peripheral dopamine receptors, potential targets for a new class of antihypertensive agents. Part I. Subclassification and functional description, *Life Sci.* **31**:939–948.

Cavero, I., Massingham, R., and Lefevre-Borg, F., 1982b, Peripheral dopamine receptors, potential targets for a new class of antihypertensive agents. Part II. Sites and mechanisms of action of dopamine receptor agonists, *Life Sci.* **31**:1059–1069.

Collins, G. G., and West, G. B., 1968, The release of ^{3}H-dopamine from the isolated rabbit ileum, *Br. J. Pharmacol.* **34**:514–522.

Commissiong, J. W., and Neff, N. H., 1979, Current status of dopamine in the mammalian spinal cord, *Biochem. Pharmacol.* **28**:1569–1573.

Commissiong, J. W., Galli, C. L., and Neff, N. H., 1978, Differentiation of dopaminergic and noradrenergic neurons in rat spinal cord, *J. Neurochem.* **30**:1095–1099.

Costa, E., and Neff, H. H., 1966, Isotopic and non-isotopic measurements of the rate of catecholamine biosynthesis, in: *Biochemistry and Pharmacology of the Basal Ganglia* (E. Costa, L. J. Cote, and M. D. Yahr, eds.), Raven Press, New York, pp. 141–156.

Dahlstrom, A., and Fuxe, K., 1965, Evidence of the existence of an outflow of noradrenaline nerve fibers in the ventral roots of the rat spinal cord, *Experientia* **21**:409–410.

Dinerstein, R. J., Vannice, J., Henderson, R. C., Roth, L. J., Goldberg, L. I., and Hoffmann, P. C., 1979, Histofluorescence techniques provide evidence for dopamine-containing neuronal elements in canine kidney, *Science* **205**:497–499.

Dunn, M. G., and Bosmann, B. H., 1981, Peripheral dopamine receptor identification: Properties of a specific dopamine receptor in the rat adrenal zona glomerulosa, *Biochem. Biophys. Res. Commun.* **99**:1081–1087.

Edvinsson, L., Hardebo, J. E., McCulloch, J., and Owman, C., 1978, Effects of dopaminergic agonists and antagonists on isolated cerebral blood vessels, *Acta. Physiol. Scand.* **104:**349–359.

Eranko, O., and Harkonen, M., 1963, Histochemical demonstration of fluorogenic amines in the cytoplasm of sympathetic ganglion cells of the rat, *Acta Physiol. Scand.* **58:**285–286.

Furuta, Y., Hashimoto, K., Iwatsuki, K., and Takeuchi, O., 1973, Effects of enzyme inhibitors of catecholamine metabolism and of haloperidol on the pancreatic secretion induced by L-DOPA and by dopamine in dogs, *Br. J. Pharmacol.* **47:**77–84.

Gentleman, S., Parenti, M., Commissiong, J. W., and Neff, N. H., 1981, Dopamine-activated adenylate cyclase of spinal cord: Supersensitivity following transection of the cord, *Brain Res.* **210:**271–275.

George, D. T., and Rayfield, E. J., 1974, L-Dopa induced plasma glucagon release, *J. Clin. Endocrinol. Metab.* **39:**618–621.

Goldberg, L. I., 1972, Cardiovascular and renal actions of dopamine: Potential clinical applications, *Pharmacol. Rev.* **24:**1–29.

Goldberg, L. I., Volkman, P. H., and Kohli, J. D., 1978, A comparison of the vascular dopamine receptor with other dopamine receptors, *Annu. Rev. Pharmacol. Toxicol.* **18:**57–79.

Hadjiconstantinou, M., Potter, P. E., and Neff, N. H., 1982, Transsynaptic modulation via muscarinic receptors of serotonin-containing SIF cells of superior cervical ganglion, *J. Neurosci.* **2:**1836–1839.

Head, R. J., and Berkowitz, B. A., 1979, Concentration and function of dopamine in normal and diseased blood vessels, in: *Peripheral Dopamine Receptor* (J. L. Imbs and J. Schwartz, eds.), Pergamon Press, Oxford, pp. 173–181.

Head, R. J., Hjelle, J. T., Jarrott, B., Berkowitz, B., Cardinale, G., and Spector, S., 1980, Isolated brain microvessels: Preparation, morphology, histamine and catecholamine contents, *Blood Vessels* **17:**173–186.

Heilman, R. D., and Lum, B. K., 1971, Studies on the intestinal relaxation produced by dopamine, *J. Pharmacol. Exp. Ther.* **178:**63–72.

Hokfelt, T., Kellerth, J. O., Nilsson, G., and Pernow, B., 1975, Experimental immunohistochemical studies on the localization and distribution of substance P in cat primary sensory neurons, *Brain Res.* **100:**232–252.

Iwatsuki, K., and Chiba, S., 1980, Comparative study of the secretory response to dopamine and seven amino acid conjugated derivatives on the blood-perfused canine pancreas, *Jpn. J. Pharmacol.* **30:**621–627.

Karoum, F., Garrison, C. K., Neff, N. H., and Wyatt, R. J., 1977, Transsynaptic modulation of dopamine metabolism in the rat superior cervical ganglion, *J. Pharmacol. Exp. Ther.* **201:**654–661.

Karoum, F., Speciale, S. G., Jr., and Neff, N. H., 1980, 3,4-Dihydroxyphenylacetic acid content of sympathetic ganglia as a possible biochemical indicator of small intensely fluorescent cell participation in ganglionic transmission, *Biochem. Pharmacol.* **29:**118–119.

Katz, D. M., Markey, K. A., Goldstein, M., and Black, I. B., 1982, Expression of catecholaminergic characteristic by peripheral sensory ganglion cells in the normal adult rat in vivo, *Soc. Neurosci. Abstr.* **8:**8.

Kebabian, J. W., and Calne, D. B., 1979, Multiple receptors for dopamine, *Nature* **277:**93–96.

Kojima, H., Suetake, K., Yokoo, H., Anraku, S., Inanago, K., Higashi, H., Nishi, S., Yamamoto, T., and Ochi, J., 1981, Dopamine-containing cells in rabbit nodose ganglia, *Experientia* **37:**1332–1333.

Koslow, S. H., Bjegovic, M., and Costa, E., 1975, Catecholamines in sympathetic ganglia of rat: Effects of dexamethasone and reserpine, *J. Neurochem.* **24**:277–281.

Lackovic, Z., and Neff, N. H., 1980, Evidence for the existence of peripheral dopaminergic neurons, *Brain Res.* **193**:289–292.

Lackovic, Z., Kleinman, J., Karoum, F., and Neff, N. H., 1981, Dopamine and its metabolites in human peripheral nerves: Is there a widely distributed system of peripheral dopaminergic nerves? *Life Sci.* **29**:917–922.

Lackovic, Z., Relja, M., and Neff, N. H., 1982, Catabolism of endogenous dopamine in peripheral tissues: Is there an independent role for dopamine in peripheral neurotransmission? *J. Neurochem.* **38**:1453–1458.

Libet, B., 1977, The role SIF-cells play in ganglionic transmission, *Adv. Biochem. Psychopharmacol.* **16**:541–546.

Libet, B., and Owman, C., 1974, Concomitant changes in formaldehyde-induced fluorescence of dopamine interneurons and in slow inhibitory postsynaptic potentials of the rabbit superior cervical ganglion, induced by stimulation of the preganglionic nerve or by a muscarinic agent, *J. Physiol. (Lond.)* **237**:635–662.

Libet, B., and Tosaka, T., 1970, Dopamine as a synaptic transmitter and modulator in sympathetic ganglia: a different mode of synaptic action, *Proc. Natl. Acad. Sci. U.S.A.* **67**:667–673.

Lokhandwala, M. F., 1979, Presynaptic receptor systems on cardiac sympathetic nerves, *Life Sci.* **24**:1823–1832.

Long, J. P., Heintz, S., Cannon, J. G., and Kim, J., 1975, Inhibition of the sympathetic nervous system by 5,6-dihydroxy-2-dimethylamino tetralin (M-7), apomorphine and dopamine, *J. Pharmacol. Exp. Ther.* **192**:336–342.

Lutold, B. E., Karoum, F., and Neff, N. H., 1979, Activation of rat sympathetic ganglia SIF cell dopamine metabolism by muscarinic agonists, *Eur. J. Pharmacol.* **54**:21–26.

Matthews, M. R., 1980, Ultrastructural studies relevant to the possible functions of small granule-containing cells in the rat superior cervical ganglion, *Adv. Biochem. Psychopharmacol.* **25**:77–86.

McKenna, T. J., Island, D. P., Nicholson, W. E., and Liddle, G. W., 1979, Dopamine inhibits angiotensin-stimulated aldosterone biosynthesis in bovine adrenal cells, *J. Clin. Invest.* **64**:287–291.

Morgunov, N., and Baines, A. D., 1981, Renal nerves and catecholamine excretion, *Am. J. Physiol.* **240**:F75–F81.

Mukhopadhyay, A. K., and Weisbrodt, N., 1977, Effect of dopamine on esophageal motor function, *Am. J. Physiol.* **232**:E19–E24.

Murthy, V. V., Gilbert, J. C., Goldberg, L. I., and Kuo, J. F., 1976, Dopamine-sensitive adenylate cyclase in canine renal artery, *J. Pharm. Pharmacol.* **28**:567–571.

Nagy, J. I., and Hunt, S. P., 1982, Fluoride-resistant acid phosphatase-containing neurones in dorsal root ganglia are separate from those containing substance P or somatostatin, *Neuroscience* **7**:89–97.

Nakajima, T., Naitoh, F., and Kuruma, I., 1977, Dopamine-sensitive adenylate cyclase in the rat kidney particulate preparation, *Eur. J. Pharmacol.* **41**:163–169.

Nielsen, K. C., and Owman, C., 1967, Adrenergic innervation of pial arteries related to the circle of Willis of the cat, *Brain Res.* **6**:773–776.

Norbiato, G., Bevilacqua, M., Raggi, U., Micossi, P., and Moroni, C., 1977, Metoclopramide increases plasma aldosterone concentration in man, *J. Clin. Endocrinol. Metab.* **45**:1313–1316.

Noth, R. H., McCallum, R. W., Contino, C., and Havelick, J., 1980, Tonic dopaminergic suppression of plasma aldosterone, *J. Clin. Endocrinol. Metab.* **51**:64–69.

Owman, C., and Santini, M., 1966, Adrenergic nerves in spinal ganglia of the cat, *Acta Physiol. Scand.* **68:**127-128.

Price, J., and Mudge, A. W., 1983, A subpopulation of rat dorsal root ganglion neurones in catecholaminergic, *Nature* **301:**241-243.

Relja, M., Lackovic, Z., and Neff, N. H., 1982, Evidence for the presence of dopaminergic receptors in vas deferens, *Life Sci.* **31:**2571-2575.

Rolewicz, T. F., and Zimmerman, B. G., 1972, Peripheral distribution of cutaneous sympathetic vasodilator system, *Am. J. Physiol.* **223:**939-943.

Shima, S., Kawashima, Y., Hirai, M., and Asakura, M., 1980, Effect of adrenergic stimulation on adenylate cyclase activity in rat prostate, *Biochem. Biophys. Acta* **628:**255-262.

Simon, A., and Van Maanen, E. F., 1976, Dopamine receptors and dopaminergic nerves in vas deferens of the rat, *Arch. Int. Pharmacodyn. Ther.* **222:**4-15.

Sowers, J. R., Stern, N., and Taylor, I. L., 1982, Evidence for dopaminergic modulation of pancreatic polypeptide secretion in man, *Life Sci.* **31:**2971-2975.

Spitz, I. M., Zylber, E., Jersky, J., and Leroith, D., 1979, Atropine suppression of basal and metoclopramide-induced human pancreatic polypeptide secretion in man, *Metabolism* **28:**527-530.

Stephenson, R. K., Sole, M. J., and Baines, A. D., 1982, Neural and extraneural catecholamine production by rat kidneys, *Am. J. Physiol.* **242:**F261-F266.

Suzuki, Y., Okada, T., Shibuya, M., Mutsuga, N., Kageyama, N., and Hidaka, H., 1983, Regional distribution of dopamine and norepinephrine in canine cerebral arteries—Effect of pre- or postganglionic sympathetic denervation, *Brain Res.* **258:**53-58.

Tayo, F. M., 1979, Potentiation of dopamine-induced contractions of the rat vas deferens by low concentrations of its antagonists, *Arch. Int. Pharmacodyn. Ther.* **241:**190-196.

Tayo, F. M., 1981, Prejunctional inhibitory dopamine receptors in the rat isolated vas deferens, *Arch. Int. Pharmacodyn. Ther.* **254:**28-37.

Valenzuela, J. E., 1976, Dopamine as a possible neurotransmitter in gastric relaxation, *Gastroenterology* **71:**1019-1022.

Verhofstad, A. A. J., Steinbusch, H. W. M., Penke, B., Varga, J., and Joosten, H. W. J., 1981, Serotonin-immunoreactive cells in the superior cervical ganglion of the rat. Evidence for the existence of separate serotonin- and catecholamine-containing small ganglionic cells, *Brain Res.* **212:**39-49.

Wamsley, J. K., Black, A. C., Jr., Redick, J. A., West, J. R., and Williams, T. H., 1978, SIF cells, cyclic AMP responses, and catecholamines of guinea pig superior cervical ganglion, *Brain Res.* **156:**75-82.

Williams, T. H., Chiba, T., Black, A. C., Jr., Bhalla, R. C., and Jew, J., 1976, Species variation in SIF cells of superior cervical ganglia: Are there two functional types? in: *SIF Cells: Structure and Function of the Small Intensely Fluorescent Sympathetic Cells* (O. Eranko, ed.), Fogarty International Center Proceedings No. 30, pp. 143-162. DHEW Publication No (NIH) 76-942, Washington, D. C.

8

Vascular Dopamine and Dopamine Receptor Agonists

BARRY A. BERKOWITZ, ROBERT ERICKSON,
BODGAN ZABKO-POTAVPOVICH, and ELIOT H. OHLSTEIN

1. Introduction

Regulation and modulation of the sympathetic nervous system have been and remain cornerstone strategies for the treatment of cardiovascular disease. Whereas stimulating, mimicking or antagonizing norepinephrine and epinphrine have been the most frequently utilized approach to cardiovascular renal therapeutics, the possibility that dopamine and dopamine receptors serve as useful target sites for drug action has received less attention.

In this chapter, we review as well as present new data concerning the roles of dopamine and dopamine receptors in the vasculature. From a drug discovery point of view, we have examined two distinct approaches: (1) dopamine-β-hydroxylase (DBH) inhibition as a means to increase the dopamine/norepinephrine ratio in blood vessels, and (2) the use of SK&F 82526 as a selective dopamine receptor agonist.

2. Can Endogenous Dopamine Concentrations Be Regulated for Therapeutic Advantage?

The possibility of altering the cardiovascular dopamine/norepinephrine ratio in favor of dopamine remains an attractive but as yet an unrealized possibility. Inhibition of DBH, which catalyzes con-

BARRY A. BERKOWITZ, ROBERT ERICKSON, BODGAN ZABKO-POTAVPOVICH, and ELIOT H. OHLSTEIN • Smith Kline & French Laboratories, Philadelphia, Pennsylvania 19101.

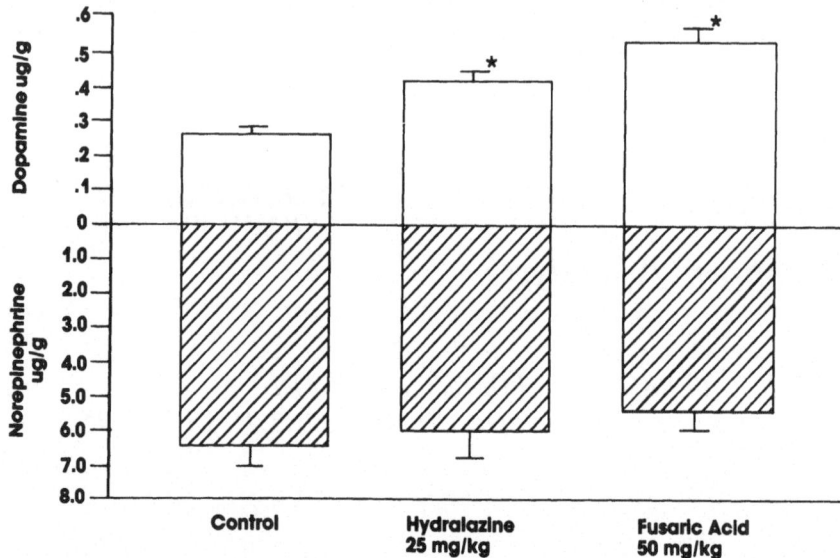

Figure 1. Dopamine and norepinephrine levels in the mesenteric artery of the spontaneously hypertensive rat. Hydralazine (25 mg/kg) or fusaric acid (50 mg/kg) were given twice in oral doses 18 hr apart, and rats were killed 2 hr later. Results are the average of at least three experiments ± the standard error of the mean for this and subsequent figures. * indicates a statistically significant difference compared to control rats ($P < 0.05$). Catecholamines were measured by a radioenzymatic assay (Head and Berkowitz, 1979).

version of dopamine to norepinephrine, is the most direct approach towards this goal. Two drugs that have been suggested as owing at least some of their antihypertensive action to DBH inhibition are hydralazine ($IC_{50} = 2 \times 10^{-4}$ M) and the investigational drug fusaric acid ($IC_{50} = 8 \times 10^{-7}$ M) (for review, see Berkowitz, 1983).

To examine directly the possibility that antihypertensive doses of hydralazine or fusaric acid alter vascular dopamine, these compounds were administered to spontaneously hypertensive rats (SHR). The endogenous concentration of dopamine in the mesenteric artery of the rats in these experiments averaged 0.26 ± 0.04 μg/g, whereas the norepinephrine concentration averaged 6.6 ± 0.04 μg/g (Fig. 1). Following administration of hydralazine (25 mg/kg) or fusaric acid (50 mg/kg), the norepinephrine concentration decreased slightly but not significantly. However, the dopamine concentration significantly increased to 0.42 ± 0.03 μg/g in hydralazine-treated animals and doubled to 0.52 ± 0.05 μg/g following treatment with fusaric acid. Data showing that both drugs markedly increased the dopamine/norepinephrine ratio are shown in Fig. 2. It

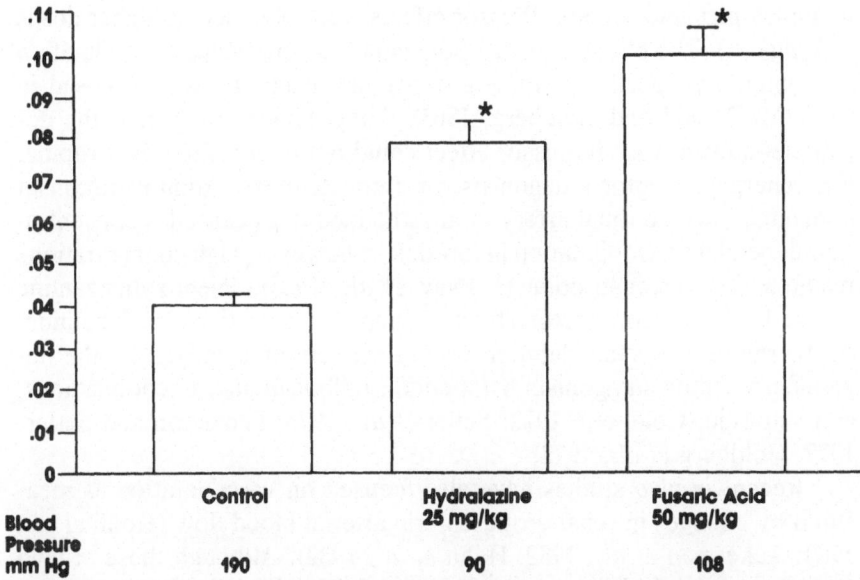

Figure 2. Dopamine/norepinephrine ratio in the mesenteric artery of the SHR. Experimental details are as in Fig. 1. Blood pressure was determined by a tail cuff method.

can also be seen that both hydralazine and fusaric acid lowered blood pressure in SHR at these doses.

It cannot be concluded from these results that fusaric acid and hydralazine lower blood pressure because they are DBH inhibitors and raise the vascular dopamine/norepinephrine ratio at these doses. Both compounds are also able to relax vascular smooth muscle directly, and this property is likely to be important in their antihypertensive action. However, the data do show that alterations of the vascular dopamine content may be a valuable adjunct to the vasodilator properties of these drugs. Nevertheless, the promise of a clinically effective DBH inhibitor with a high therapeutic index still remains to be realized.

3. Characterization of Dopamine Receptor Agonists in the Vasculature

3.1. In Vivo

The first report demonstrating the *in vivo* vasodilating activity of dopamine appeared in 1942 (Holtz and Credner, 1942). Dopamine, in contrast to norepinephrine and epinephrine, produced a vasodepressor effect in guinea pigs and rabbits. Pressor effects were obtained at higher doses (>1 mg i.v.). The hypothesis that dopamine was producing vasodilatation by stimulating specific peripheral dopamine receptors was proposed in 1963 (McDonald and Goldberg, 1963). They demonstrated that the dopamine-induced vasodepressor effect could not be inhibited by atropine, β-adrenergic receptor antagonists, or antihistamines. Administration of dopamine into the renal artery of anesthetized dogs caused a concentration-dependent vasodilatation in low doses; however, high concentrations resulted in vasoconstriction (McNay et al., 1965). Phenoxybenzamine blocked the vasoconstrictor effect of high concentrations of dopamine. Furthermore, the vasodilatation was selectively antagonized by the dopamine receptor antagonists haloperidol, bulbocapnine, phenothiazines, and sulpiride (Goldberg, 1972; Setler et al., 1975; Pendleton and Setler, 1977; Goldberg et al., 1978).

Recent *in vivo* studies have also focused on vasodilatation as measured by changes in renal or mesenteric arterial blood flow (Kohli et al., 1980; Ackerman et al., 1982; Hahn et al., 1982). Although these *in vivo* studies are a critical component in the understanding of the vascular actions of dopamine agonists, they are subject to several major criticisms. First, *in vivo* metabolism may modify the compounds, complicating events thought to occur at the receptor. Second, Lokhandwala and Jandhyala (1979) have shown that some dopamine agonists may produce vasodilator action both directly on the vasculature and via a prejunctional neurogenic inhibitory mechanism. These authors demonstrated that dopamine can increase renal blood flow through either ganglionic or prejunctional dopamine receptor action, leading to decreased norepinephrine release and diminished sympathetic neuronal discharge to blood vessels.

3.2. In Vitro

Demonstration of dopamine-mediated relaxation in isolated blood vessels has been a more recent development. Dopamine-mediated vascular relaxation *in vitro* was reported in 1973 by Toda and Goldberg. Isolated canine mesenteric and renal arteries pretreated with phenoxybenzamine (10^{-5} M) and contracted with KCl (10 to 30 mM) were relaxed by dopamine (10^{-6} to 5×10^{-4} M) in a concentration-responsive manner. In a subsequent study, they reported an improvement of this technique by using $PGF_{2\alpha}$ instead of KCl as the contracting agent (Goldberg and Toda, 1975). Dopamine (10^{-6} M to 5×10^{-4} M) caused consistent and reproducible relaxations in isolated canine renal, mesenteric, and small femoral arteries. However, antagonism of dopamine's relaxant effect by dopamine receptor antagonists could not be demonstrated.

Antagonism of dopamine-induced relaxation in an isolated organ system was later demonstrated by Toda (1978, 1979). In arteries preincubated with phenoxybenzamine (10^{-5} M) and contracted with $PGF_{2\alpha}$, the relaxation produced by dopamine was antagonized by the neuroleptic drug droperidol (10^{-5} to 10^{-4} M). Brodde and co-workers were also able to demonstrate antagonism of dopamine-mediated relaxation in the isolated rabbit mesenteric artery using droperidol (Brodde and Meyer, 1979), metoclopramide (Brodde and Schemuth, 1979), and (+)-butaclamol (Brodde *et al.*, 1981a). The antagonism by metoclopramide, (+)-butaclamol, and droperidol was competitive.

The isolated rabbit splenic artery has been used by several investigators to study the vascular dopamine receptor *in vitro* (Crooks and Martin, 1979). In vessels pretreated with phenoxybenzamine (5×10^{-6} M) and contracted with $PGF_{2\alpha}$ (10^{-7} to 10^{-5} M), dopamine (3×10^{-8} to 3 $\times 10^{-5}$ M) caused dose-related vascular relaxation. Bulbocapnine (10^{-6} to 3×10^{-5} M) competitively antagonized the dopamine-induced relaxation. Hilditch and Drew (1981) also employed the isolated rabbit splenic artery to demonstrate dopamine-induced vascular relaxation. In their preparation, after treatment with phenoxybenzamine (3×10^{-5} M) and contraction with $PGF_{2\alpha}$, dopamine (10^{-8} to 10^{-4} M)-induced relaxation was specifically and competitively antagonized.

The isolated human basilar artery has also been utilized for studying dopamine-mediated relaxation *in vitro* (Forster and Whalley, 1981; Forster *et al.*, 1983). After tissue pretreatment with phenoxybenzamine (10^{-5} M) and contraction with $PGF_{2\alpha}$ (10^{-8} to 10^{-4} M), dopamine elicited a concentration-dependent vascular relaxation. (+)-Butaclamol, *cis*-α-flupenthixol, fluphenazine, and haloperidol competitively antagonize the relaxant effects of dopamine.

Schmidt and Imbs and Schmidt *et al.* (1979, 1980, 1982, 1983) used the isolated perfused rat kidney as a model for the demonstration of vascular dopamine receptors. The vascular relaxant effect of dopamine was studied in the presence of phenoxybenzamine (10^{-5} M) and sotalol (10^{-5} M) while renal vasoconstriction was induced with $PGF_{2\alpha}$. The ED_{50} value for dopamine-induced renal vasodilation was 2.53×10^{-6} M. (+)-Butaclamol, flupenthixol, haloperidol, and sulpiride competitively antagonized the dopamine-induced vasodilation without affecting relaxation produced by papaverine.

Brown *et al.* (1983) have recently described an *in vitro* method for the evaluation of the effects of dopamine receptor agonists at postjunctional vascular dopamine receptors. They measured the vasodilation response under constant-flow perfusion to various dopamine receptor agonists in an isolated rabbit mesenteric–ileal vascular bed contracted by KCl.

Pretreatment with phenoxybenzamine (5×10^{-6} M) was necessary to block α-adrenergic receptors. Dopamine (3×10^{-10} to 3×10^{-7} M) caused concentration-related decreases in perfusion pressure. cis-α-Flupenthixol, but not sulpiride, selectively and competitively inhibited the vasodilator effect of dopamine.

Unfortunately, procedures for receptor binding studies that are readily applicable to the tissues of the central nervous system do not easily lend themselves to studies of the vasculature, since the muscle and connective tissue components resist gentle tissue disruption. Thus, only recently has there been success in utilizing receptor binding approaches.

Brodde and Gross (1980) and Brodde (1982) demonstrated the presence of vascular dopamine receptors by direct radioligand binding studies in membrane preparations from the isolated rabbit mesenteric artery with [^{3}H]-spiroperidol. Binding was of high affinity (K_D = 13 nM), saturable, rapid, and readily reversible, with both dopamine agonists and antagonists selectively competitive in displacing the labeled ligand.

The classification of peripheral dopamine receptors has been a controversial subject. There appears to be a heterogeneous population of peripheral dopamine receptors. In order to be consistent with the terminology for other receptors, the receptors have been classified as DA_1 and DA_2 (Goldberg and Kohli, 1979; Langer, 1980; Cavero et al., 1982; Goldberg and Kohli, 1983). In general, the DA_1 dopamine receptor occurs postjunctionally, and its stimulation directly mediates vascular smooth muscle relaxation. In contrast, the DA_2 dopamine receptor occurs on postganglionic sympathetic neurons, and its stimulation leads to a reduction of neuronal release of norepinephrine. It should be emphasized that the association of these receptors with a specific anatomic location does not necessarily preclude different subpopulations of dopamine receptors within the same tissue type.

The existence of DA_1 dopamine receptors in the peripheral vasculature is now generally accepted, since there is a well-defined relationship in vivo between the structure and activities of various dopamine receptor agonists (Goldberg et al., 1978). In vitro correlation of a rank order of potency for DA_1 receptor agonists was not apparent until reproducible in vitro systems for demonstrating dopamine-mediated vascular relaxation were established.

SK&F 38393 has been reported to be a partial agonist in the isolated rabbit mesenteric (Brodde et al., 1981b) and splenic artery (Hilditch and Drew, 1981) and isolated perfused rat kidney (Schmidt et al., 1982), whereas it is a full agonist in the isolated human basilar artery (Forster et al., 1983). SK&F 38393 exhibits partial agonist activity in vivo in the dog, but it is also a relatively selective DA_1 dopamine receptor agonist

Table I. Comparison of SK&F 82526, R-82526, S-82526, and Dopamine on Renal
Vascular Resistance and Rat Adenylate Cyclase

Drug	ED_{15} renal vascular resistance (i.v.) ($\mu g/kg^a$)	ED_{50} rat striatal adenylate cyclase $(nM)^b$	Percent of $DA_{max}{}^c$
SK&F 82526 (racemate)	0.56	57	70
SK&F R-82526	0.31	37	70
SK&F S-82526	>1	1500	43
Dopamine	3.5	3500	100

[a] Determined in anesthetized dogs (Ackerman *et al.*, 1982).
[b] H. Sarau, SK&F Labs. (personal communication).
[c] Percent of maximum stimulation of adenylate cyclase by dopamine.

(Hahn and Wardell, 1980). However, SK&F 82526, a close chemical analogue to SK&F 38393, appears to be a full agonist because it is a more potent renal vasodilator than dopamine and produces maximal effects greater than those of dopamine (Ackerman *et al.*, 1982; Hahn *et al.*, 1982). The *in vitro* activity of SK&F 82526 is described in this chapter.

4. Isolated Rabbit Blood Vessels as Model Systems for the Study of Vascular Dopamine and Dopamine Receptor Agonists: SK&F 82526

We have previously utilized SK&F 82526 and its optical isomers in *in vivo* studies as a renal vasodilator in conscious and anesthetized dogs and have also characterized these compounds on rat striatal adenylate cyclase (Table I). In general, the potency is *R*-isomer > *R,S*-isomer > *S*-isomer (Ackerman *et al.*, 1983). Among the most widely used vascular preparations to analyze dopaminomimetic substances are the blood vessels of the arterial tree of the rabbit. We have further studied SK&F 82526 in these vascular beds.

Initial studies were undertaken using ring segments of rabbit splenic arterial rings as described in the classical protocol of Toda and Goldberg (1973). Tissues were pretreated with phenoxybenzamine and contracted with KCl. Relaxation was only observed at high doses of SK&F 82526 ($>10^{-4}$ M), with the rank order of *S*-isomer > *R,S*-isomer > *R*-isomer (Fig. 3). Moreover, dopamine receptor antagonists did not produce any large shifts in the dose-response curves. These data differed substantially from those found in other systems with respect to rank order (see above)

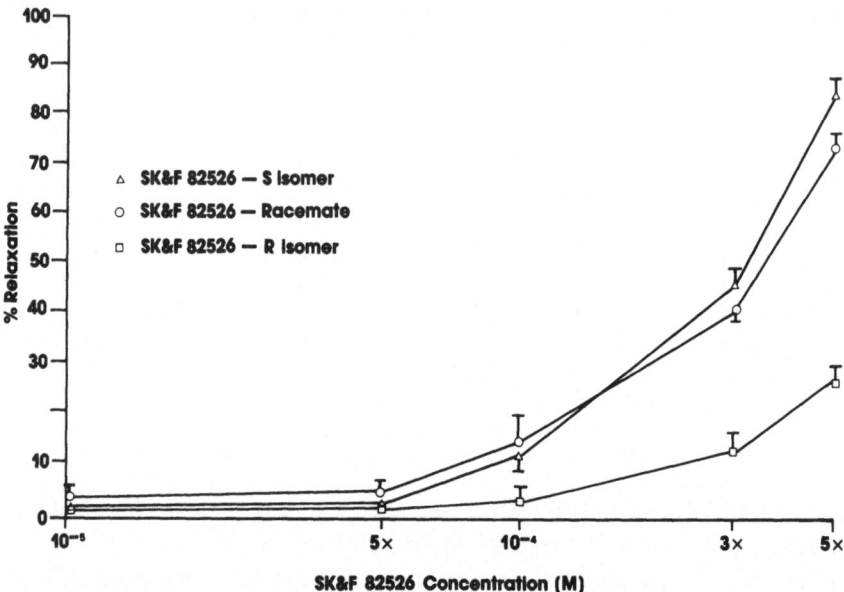

Figure 3. Relaxation of potassium chloride-contracted rabbit splenic arterial rings by SK&F 82526. Potassium chloride (30 mM) was utilized to contract the vessels, which had previously been pretreated with phenoxybenzamine (10^{-5} M) for 60 min.

and *in vivo* antagonism (Hahn *et al.*, 1982), and further studies were required to resolve these findings.

Others have found the sensitivity of KCl-contracted preparations to be low (Toda and Goldberg, 1973; Goldberg and Toda, 1975). It has been suggested that $PGF_{2\alpha}$-contracted vascular preparations pretreated with phenoxybenzamine may be a more useful system. However, we have found that the contractile response is too variable, a limitation also noted by Hilditch and Drew (1981).

SK&F 82526 has a distinct advantage compared to most other dopaminergic agents in that it lacks α-adrenoreceptor agonist activity. It is this action of dopamine that necessitates the use of phenoxybenzamine in the analysis of dopaminergic agents in most vascular preparations. This blocking drug also prevents use of norepinephrine as a contractile agonist. Moreover, phenoxybenzamine has been reported to inhibit ligand binding to dopamine receptors (Hamblin and Creese, 1982) and prevent stimulation of dopamine-sensitive adenylate cyclase (Walton *et al.*, 1978). These limitations are not necessary with SK&F 82526, and the lack of α-agonist activity of this drug has permitted examination of dopamine receptors in the vasculature for the first time without the presence of phen-

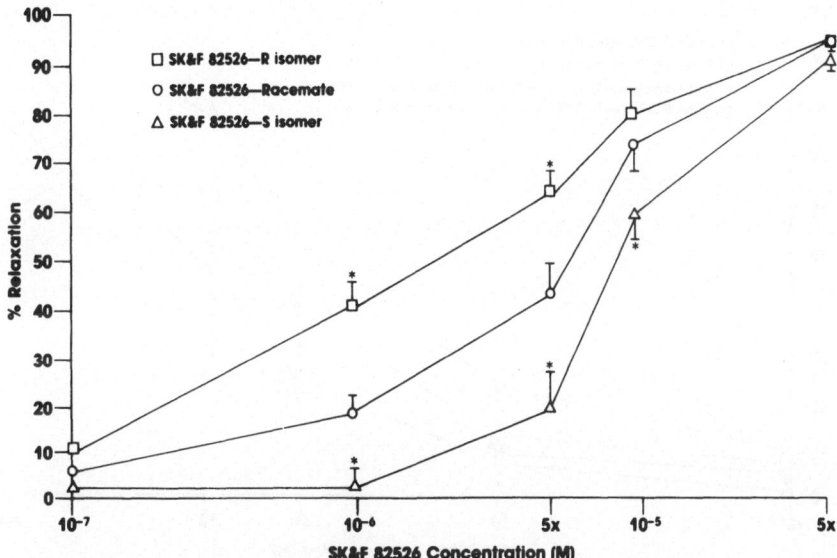

Figure 4. Relaxation of norepinephrine-contracted rabbit splenic arterial rings by SK&F 82526. * indicates a statistically significant difference compared to relaxation produced by the racemate of SK&F 82526 ($P < 0.05$).

oxybenzamine while employing the natural endogenous contractile agonist, norepinephrine.

SK&F 82526 was found to be a potent relaxant compound when norepinephrine was used to contract a phenoxybenzamine-free splenic arterial ring preparation (Fig. 4). As *in vivo*, the rank order of potency was R-isomer > R,S-isomer > S-isomer, and relaxation began at quite low doses (10^{-7} M).

The evidence that we were dealing with a specific receptor of the dopamine class would be strengthened by antagonism with a selective dopamine receptor antagonist. This was accomplished with metoclopramide, as shown in Fig. 5. Doses of 10^{-5} to 8×10^{-5} M caused a parallel shift in the relaxant dose–response curve produced by SK&F 82526. The pA_2 value of metoclopramide was approximately 5.2. This value is extremely close to that reported by others in the inhibition of dopamine relaxation by metoclopramide (Brodde *et al.*, 1981b).

One concern that should be addressed is the possibility that SK&F 82526 is an α-receptor antagonist of sufficient potency to interfere in the above assays. SK&F 82526 is not an α_1-adrenergic receptor antagonist since it does not readily relax the norepinephrine-contracted rat or rabbit aortic preparation, the classical α_1-antagonist response. SK&F 82526 is

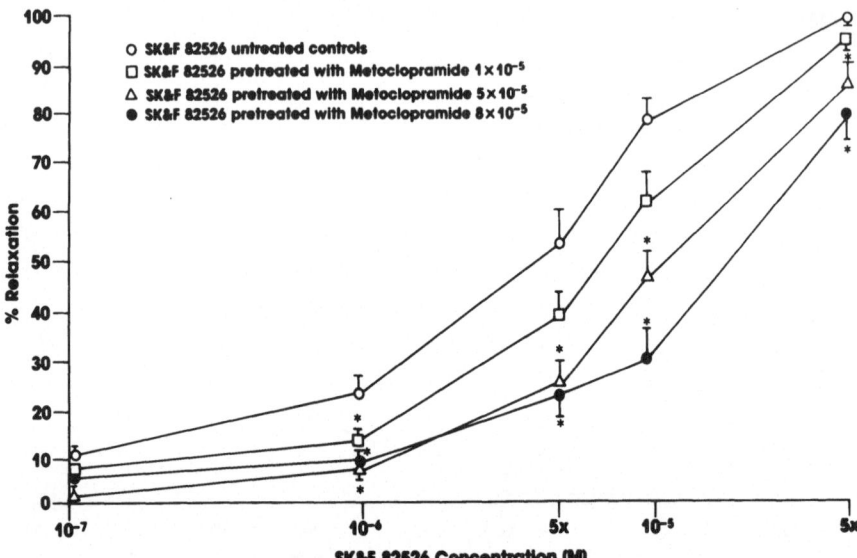

Figure 5. Antagonism of SK&F 82526-induced vascular relaxation by the dopamine receptor antagonist metoclopramide. Splenic arterial rings were contracted with norepinephrine (10^{-6} M). * indicates a statistically significant difference compared to relaxation produced by SK&F 82526 alone ($P < 0.05$).

also unlikely to be a potent α_2-receptor antagonist since we find no evidence for α_2 receptors in the rabbit splenic arterial ring preparation.

5. What is the Location of Vascular Dopamine Receptors?

It has been generally accepted that there must be two types of dopamine receptors in blood vessels. One type is located on vascular smooth muscle, and the second is located prejunctionally, probably on the sympathetic nerves innervating the vasculature. Recently, Furchgott and Zawadzki (1980) have proposed that the response of the endothelium may be important in determining vascular relaxation produced by certain drugs and hormones. We have begun to assess whether dopaminergic agents may relax blood vessels through mechanisms that may involve the endothelium.

SK&F 82526-mediated relaxation was maximal in vessels with an intact endothelium (Fig. 6). This is not a generalized finding for all relaxant drugs, since nitroglycerin-mediated relaxation is not enhanced in blood vessels with a damaged endothelial layer (unpublished observations). If

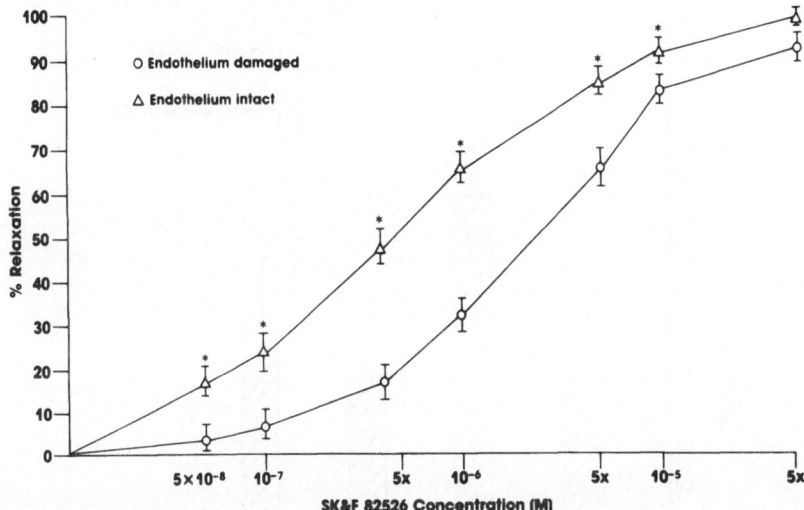

Figure 6. Enhanced relaxation of the vasculature produced by SK&F 82526 in vessels with intact endothelium. Endothelial damage was produced by gentle rubbing and confirmed by lack of relaxation to acetylcholine (Furchgott and Zawadzki, 1980). * indicates statistically significant difference compared to endothelial intact vessels ($P < 0.05$).

these studies can be extended to other vessels and other dopamine agonists, they would suggest that the endothelium is a target site for dopamine agonists. Moreover, endothelial cells should be examined directly for the presence of dopamine receptors. Positive results would have important therapeutic and research implications.

6. Are Dopamine Vascular Receptors Subserved by a Dopaminergic Innervation?

As demonstrated in this and other studies (Brodde, 1982), the abdominal vessels of the rabbit can be shown to possess dopamine receptors by several criteria. However, it is unclear if these receptors are the target sites of an endogenous dopaminergic nervous system. There has been considerable debate concerning the role of dopamine as a peripheral neurotransmitter, with data from the kidney vasculature and dog hindpaw providing the bulk of the affirmative evidence (Bell and Lang, 1982). In the rabbit aorta and the celiac, splenic, mesenteric, and renal arteries, as shown in Fig. 7, the dopamine concentration was low compared to that of norepinephrine and did not exceed 10% of the total catecholamine content. These values are consistent with those found in other blood ves-

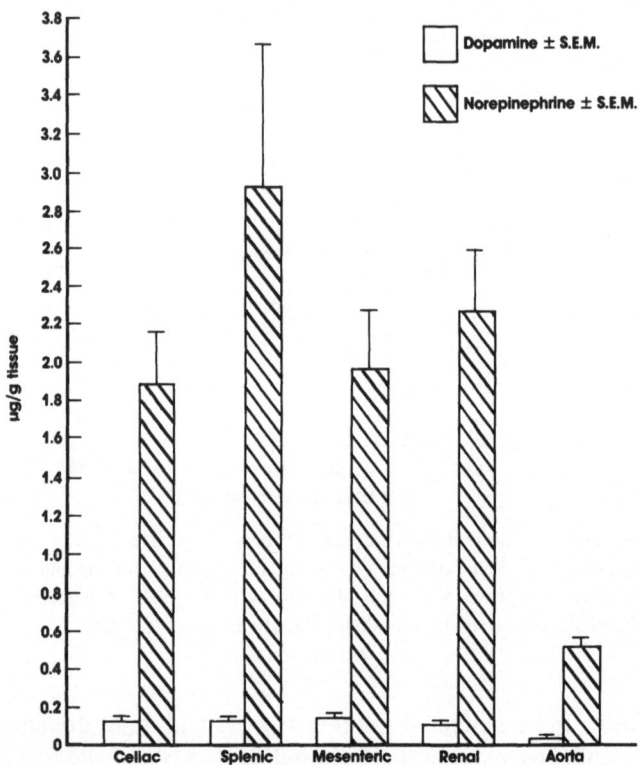

Figure 7. Dopamine and norepinephrine concentrations in rabbit vasculature. Results are the mean ± S.E.M. obtained from the vessels of three rabbits. Catecholamines were measured by a radioenzymatic assay as previously described (Head and Berkowitz, 1979).

sels (Head and Berkowitz, 1979; Berkowitz, 1983) and are best explained by a precursor rather than neurotransmitter role for endogenous dopamine under normal circumstances. Compelling evidence that dopamine receptors subserve a dopaminergic innervation is not yet at hand.

References

Ackerman, D. M., Weinstock, J. Wiebelhaus, V. D., and Berkowitz, B., 1982, Renal vasodilators and hypertension, *Drug Dev. Res.* **2**:283–297.

Bell, C., and Lang, W., 1982, Is there a place for dopamine in autonomic neuromuscular transmission: in: *Trends in Autonomic Pharmacology*, Volume 2 (Stanley Kalsner, ed.), Urban & Schwarzenberg, Baltimore, pp. 263–282.

Berkowitz, B. A., 1983, Dopamine and dopamine receptors as target sites for cardiovascular drug action, *Fed. Proc.* **42**:3019–3021.

Brodde, O.-E., 1982, Vascular dopamine receptors: Demonstration and characterization by *in vitro* studies, *Life Sci.* **31**:289–306.

Brodde, O.-E., and Gross, G., 1980 (^{3}H]-Spiroperidol labels dopamine receptors in membranes from rabbit mesenteric artery, *Naunyn Schmiedebergs Arch. Pharmacol.* **311**:249–254.

Brodde, O.-E., and Meyer, F.-J., 1979, On the existence of vascular dopamine receptors on the isolated rabbit mesenteric artery, *Naunyn Schmiedebergs Arch Pharmacol.* **308**(Suppl):R56.

Brodde, O.-E., and Schemuth, W., 1979, Specific antagonism by metoclopramide of dopamine induced relaxation on isolated rabbit mesenteric arteries contracted with prostaglandin $F_{2\alpha}$, *Life Sci.* **25**:23–30.

Brodde, O.-E., Freistühler, J., and Meyer, F.-J., 1981a, Stereospecific antagonism by d-Butaclamol of dopamine-induced relaxation of the isolated rabbit mesenteric artery, *J. Cardiovasc. Pharmacol.* **3**:828–837.

Brodde, O.-E., Meyer, F.-J., Schemuth, W., and Freistühler, J., 1981b, Demonstration of specific vascular dopamine receptors mediating vasodilation on the isolated rabbit mesenteric artery, *Naunyn Schmiedebergs Arch. Pharmacol.* **316**:24–30.

Brown, R. A., O'Connor, S. E., Smith, G. W., and Verity, A., 1983, The rabbit isolated arterially perfused intestinal segment preparation: A model for vascular dopamine receptors, *J. Pharmacol. Methods.* **9**:137–145.

Cavero, J., Massingham, R., and Lefevre-Borg, F., 1982, Peripheral dopamine receptors, potential targets for a new class of antihypertensive agents, Part I: Subclassification and functional description. *Life Sci.* **31**:939–948.

Crooks, R. J., and Martin, G. R., 1979, An isolated vascular tissue preparation showing a specific relaxant effect of dopamine, *Br. J. Pharmacol.* **67**:474P.

Forster, C., and Whalley, E. T., 1981, Dopamine receptors mediating relaxation of the human basilar artery *in vitro*, *Br. J. Pharmacol.* **74**:944P–945P.

Forster, C., Drew, G. M., Hilditch, A., and Whalley, E. T., 1983, Dopamine receptors in human basilar arteries, *Eur. J. Pharmacol.* **87**:227–235.

Furchgott, R. F., and Zawadzki, J. V., 1980, The obligatory role of endothelial cells in the relaxation of arterial smooth muscle by acetylcholine, *Nature* **288**:373–376.

Goldberg, L. I., 1972. Cardiovascular and renal actions of dopamine: Potential clinical application, *Pharmacol. Rev.* **24**:1–29.

Goldberg, L. I., and Kohli, J. D., 1979, Peripheral pre- and post-synaptic dopamine receptors: Are they different from dopamine receptors in the central nervous system? *Commun. Psychopharmacol.* **3**:447–456.

Goldberg, L. I., and Kohli, J. D., 1983, Peripheral dopamine receptors: A classification based on potency series and specific antagonism, *Trends Pharmacol.* **4**:64–66.

Goldberg, L. I., and Toda, N., 1975, Dopamine induced relaxation of isolated canine renal, mesenteric and femoral arteries contracted with prostaglandin $F_{2\alpha}$, *Circ. Res.* **36**(Supp. I):97–102.

Goldberg, L. I., Volkman, P. H., and Kohli, J. D., 1978, A comparison of the vascular dopamine receptor with other dopamine receptors, *Annu. Rev. Pharmacol. Toxicol.* **18**:57–79.

Hahn, R. A., and Wardell, J. R., Jr., 1980, Renal vascular activity of SK&F 38393 and dopamine in anesthetized dogs, *J. Cardiovasc. Pharmacol.* **2**:583–593.

Hahn, R. A., Wardell, J. R., Jr., Sarau, H. M., and Ridley, P. T., 1982, Characterization of the peripheral and central effects of SK&F 82526, a novel dopamine receptor agonist, *J. Pharmacol. Exp. Ther.* **223**:305–313.

Hamblin, M. W., and Creese, I., 1982, Phenoxybenzamine treatment differentiates dopaminergic ^{3}H-ligand binding sites in bovine caudate membranes, *Mol. Pharmacol.* **21**:44–51.

Head, R. J., and Berkowitz, B. A., 1979, Radioenzymatic determination of the dopamine, epinephrine and norepinephrine content of the rabbit ear artery, *Blood Vessels* **16**:320–324.

Hilditch, A., and Drew, G., 1981, Characteristics of the dopamine receptors in the rabbit isolated splenic artery, *Eur. J. Pharmacol.* **72**:287–296.

Holtz, P., and Credner, K., 1942, Die enzymatische Entstebung von Oxytyramin im Organismus und die physiologische Bedeutung der Dopadecarboxylase, *Naunyn Schmiedebergs Arch Pharmakol. Exp. Pathol.* **200**:356–388.

Kohli, J. D., Weder, A. B., Goldberg, L. I., and Ginos, J. Z., 1980, Structure activity relationships of N-substituted dopamine derivatives as agonists of the dopamine vascular and other cardiovascular receptors, *J. Pharmacol. Exp. Ther.* **213**:370–374.

Langer, S. Z., 1981, Presynaptic regulation of the release of catecholamines, *Pharmacol. Rev.* **32**:337–362.

Lokhandwala, M. F., and Jandhyala, B. S., 1979, The role of sympathetic nervous system in the vascular actions of dopamine, *J. Pharmacol. Exp. Ther.* **210**:120–126.

McDonald, R. H., and Goldberg, L. I., 1963, Analysis of the cardiovascular effects of dopamine in the dog, *J. Pharmacol. Exp. Ther.* **140**:60–66.

McNay, J. L., McDonald, R. H., and Goldberg, L. I., 1965, Direct renal vasodilation produced by dopamine in the dog, *Circ. Res.* **16**:510–517.

Pendleton, R. G., and Setler, P. E., 1977, Peripheral cardiovascular dopamine receptors, *Gen. Pharmacol.* **8**:1–5.

Schmidt, M., and Imbs, J. L., 1980, Pharmacological characterization of renal vascular dopamine receptors, *J. Cardiovasc. Pharmacol.* **2**:595–605.

Schmidt, M., Imbs, J.-L., and Schwartz, J., 1979, Effets renaux de la bromocriptine, *J. Pharmacol. (Paris)* **10**:525–532.

Schmidt, M., Imbs, J. L., Giesen, E. M., and Schwartz, J., 1982, Vasodilator effects of dopaminomimetics in the perfused rat kidney, *Eur. J. Pharmacol.* **84**:61–70.

Schmidt, M., Imbs, J. L., Giesen, E. M., and Schwartz, J., 1983, Blockade of dopamine receptors in the renal vasculature by isomers of flupenthixol and sulpiride, *J. Cardiovasc. Pharmacol.* **5**:86–89.

Setler, P. E., Pendleton, R. G., and Finlay, E., 1975, The cardiovascular actions of dopamine and the effects of central and peripheral catecholaminergic receptor blocking drugs, *J. Pharmacol. Exp. Ther.* **192**:702–712.

Toda, N., 1978, Heterogeneity in the relaxation of vascular smooth muscle, in: *Mechanisms of Vasodilation* (P. M. Vanhoutte and J. Leusen, eds.), Karger, Basel, pp. 129–136.

Toda, N., and Goldberg, L. I., 1973, Dopamine induced relaxation of isolated arterials strips, *J. Pharm. Pharmacol.* **25**:587–589.

Toda, N., and Hatano, Y., 1979, Antagonism by droperidol of dopamine-induced relaxation in isolated arteries, *Eur. J. Pharmacol.* **57**:231–238.

Walton, K. G., Liepmann, P., and Baldessarini, R. J., 1978, Inhibition of dopamine stimulated adenylate cyclase activity by phenoxybenzamine, *Eur. J. Pharmacol.* **52**:231–234.

9

Dopamine Receptor Agonists and Hypertension

MUSTAFA F. LOKHANDWALA and RICHARD J. BARRETT

1. Introduction

Dopamine receptor agonists exert pronounced cardiovascular actions that result from activation of specific dopamine receptors located at various sites within the cardiovascular system (Clark, 1981; Cavero *et al.*, 1982a,b; Lokhandwala and Barrett, 1981, 1982, 1983). Although dopamine is the prototype of dopamine receptor agonists, in addition to the activation of dopamine receptors, this catecholamine also possesses agonistic actions at α and β adrenoceptors (Goldberg, 1972; Lokhandwala and Barrett, 1982). Therefore, attempts have been made to develop compounds that are selective at dopamine receptors and do not exert significant actions at other adrenoceptors. As discussed in several chapters of this volume, one of the major aims in developing these compounds is for the therapeutic potential they offer in the treatment of various cardiovascular and renal disorders.

The ergot alkaloids, commonly referred to as ergolines, have multiple actions at several different receptors. However, some of these ergolines, such as bromocriptine, lergotrile, and pergolide, are more selective at dopamine receptors, and their cardiovascular actions resulting from dopamine receptor stimulation have been extensively studied (Clark, 1979; Lokhandwala, 1979; Lokhandwala *et al.*, 1979; Barrett and Lokhandwala,

MUSTAFA F. LOKHANDWALA and RICHARD J. BARRETT • Department of Pharmacology and Institute for Cardiovascular Studies, College of Pharmacy, University of Houston Central Campus, Houston, Texas 77004. *Present address of R.J.B.*: Department of Biomedical Research, ICI Americas, Inc., Wilmington, Delaware 19897.

1981a; Hahn, 1981; Hahn and Farrell, 1981; Yen *et al.*, 1979). These studies have revealed that although ergolines act on the neurotropic or DA_2 receptors located at various sites within the sympathetic nervous system, they do not activate the postsynaptic dopamine (DA_1) receptors (Lokhandwala, 1979; Lokhandwala *et al.*, 1979). Bromocriptine is also found to exert antihypertensive action in hypertensive patients (Greenacre *et al.*, 1976; Kaye *et al.*, 1976). Both lergotrile and pergolide lower blood pressure in normotensive as well as spontaneously hypertensive rats by activating peripheral presynaptic dopamine receptors (Yen *et al.*, 1979; Sved and Fernstrom, 1980; Hahn, 1981; Hahn and Farrell, 1981).

We have performed experiments to study the mechanism of antihypertensive action of the dopaminergic ergoline pergolide in neurogenic hypertensive dogs. In this chapter we discuss experimental evidence that suggests that activation of neurotropic dopamine receptors located in the periphery as well as in the central nervous system is responsible for the antihypertensive action of pergolide. In addition, we also present regional hemodynamic changes associated with the antihypertensive action of pergolide in neurogenic hypertensive dogs.

2. Cardiovascular Actions of Pergolide in Neurogenic Hypertensive Dogs

Mongrel dogs of either sex weighing between 15 and 25 kg were anesthetized with sodium pentobarbital (35 mg/kg, i.v.) and prepared for the recording of blood pressure and heart rate as previously described (Barrett and Lokhandwala, 1981a). The left renal, superior mesenteric, and left iliac arteries were isolated, and Statham electromagnetic flow probes were placed around them to measure blood flows utilizing Statham electromagnetic flowmeters. All signals were displayed on a Grass Model-7 polygraph. Vascular resistances of the respective organs were calculated by dividing mean blood pressure by flow and are expressed as mm Hg/ ml per min.

Neurogenic hypertension was produced by sinoaortic deafferentation (SAD). In order to accomplish this, carotid sinus nerves were bilaterally sectioned at their origins at the carotid bifurcations, and both vagosympathetic trunks were sectioned in the cervical region. A stabilization period of 30–60 min was allowed after SAD before administering any drugs.

Sinoaortic deafferentation produced marked and sustained hypertension and tachycardia (Fig. 1). Regional hemodynamic studies revealed that the hypertension was associated with a significant increase in iliac vascular resistance, whereas vascular resistances in the kidney and the

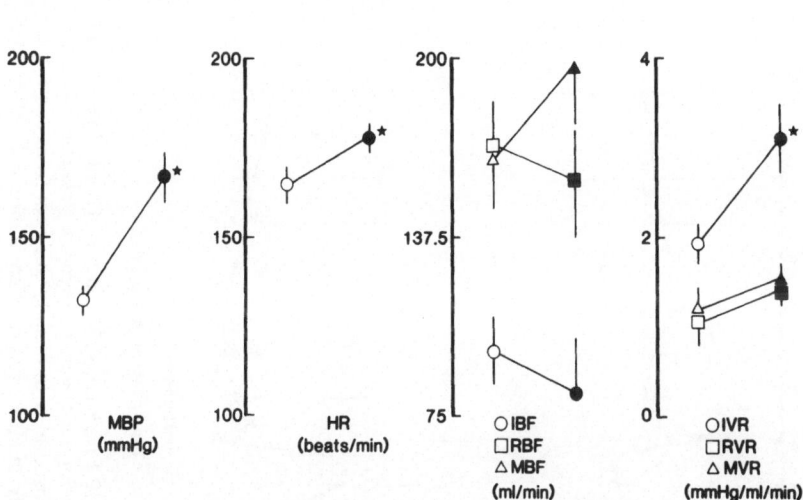

Figure 1. Effect of sinoaortic deafferentation (SAD) on mean blood pressure (MBP), heart rate (HR), iliac blood flow (IBF), iliac vascular resistance (IVR), renal blood flow (RBF), renal vascular resistance (RVR), mesenteric blood flow (MBF), and mesenteric vascular resistance (MVR) in pentobarbital-anesthetized dogs. The data represent mean values from all the different groups of experiments performed in neurogenic hypertensive dogs. The hypertension, tachycardia, and increase in the iliac vascular resistance caused by sinoaortic deafferentation were sustained for a 2-hr observation period in a group of three dogs (*$P <$ 0.05).

mesentery were not significantly altered (Fig. 1). In a control group of three dogs, all measured and calculated parameters remained stable for at least 2 hr following SAD. Therefore, we considered this preparation a stable model of neurogenic hypertension for analyzing the cardiovascular actions of pergolide.

Intravenous administration of pergolide (2.5 μg/kg per min for 5 min, 12.5 μg/kg total dose) to a separate group of seven neurogenic hypertensive dogs produced a significant decrease in mean blood pressure, which was immediate in onset and was sustained for the duration of the experiment (Fig. 2). Pergolide also produced a decrease in heart rate, which was evident for up to 30 min (Fig. 2). Although blood flow to renal and mesenteric beds decreased below control, resistance in both the beds was not altered. Pergolide administration caused a significant increase in iliac blood flow, which was associated with a significant decrease in iliac vascular resistance (Fig. 2). The iliac vasodilatory effect of pergolide was sustained for up to 2 hr.

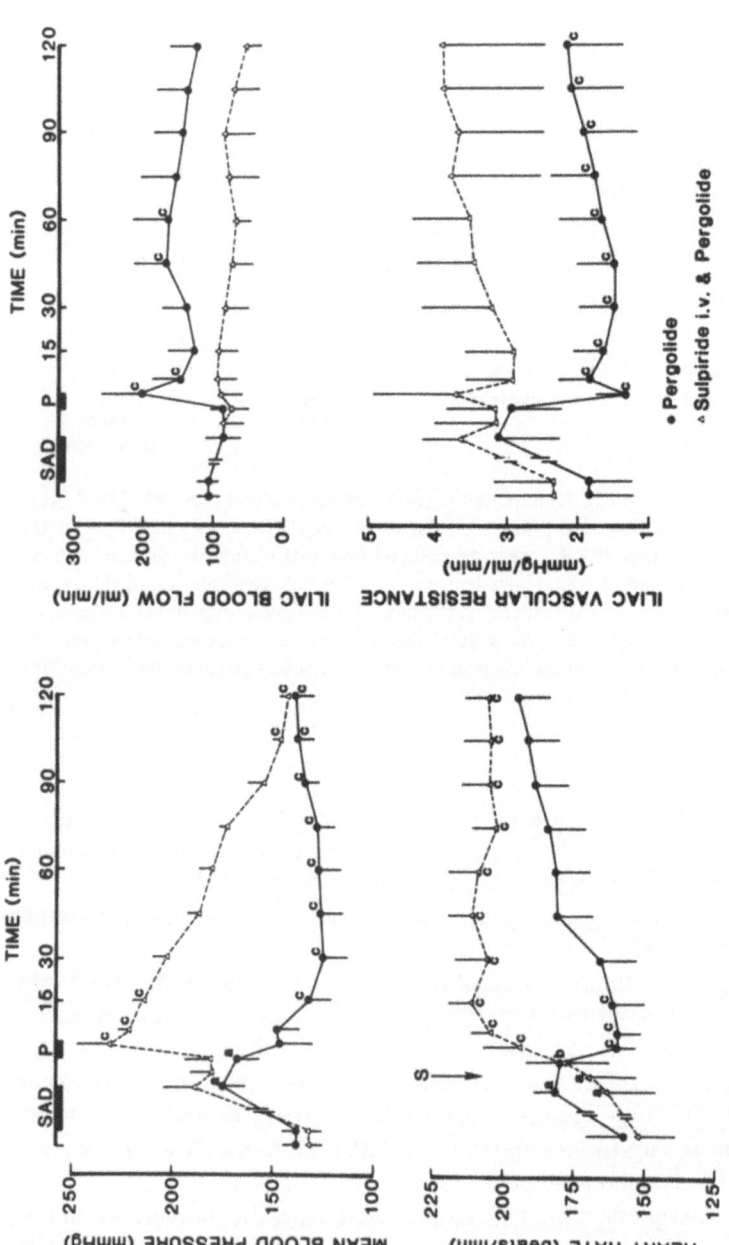

Figure 2. Antihypertensive, bradycardic, and iliac vasodilatory actions of pergolide (12.5 μg/kg, i.v.) in a group of control neurogenic hypertensive dogs ($N = 7$) and in neurogenic hypertensive dogs ($N = 5$) treated with the dopamine receptor antagonist sulpiride (S) (0.5 mg/kg, i.v.). In sulpiride-treated dogs, pergolide produced a pressor response. (a) Significantly different from control; (b) Significantly different from postdeafferentation control; (c) Significantly different from either postdeafferentation control or post-sulpiride control.

In order to determine the involvement of dopamine receptors in the antihypertensive, bradycardic, and iliac vasodilatory actions of pergolide, a separate group of dogs was treated with the dopamine receptor antagonist sulpiride (Barrett *et al.*, 1982). Administration of sulpiride (0.5 mg/kg, i.v.) to a group of four neurogenic hypertensive dogs did not result in changes in any of the measured or calculated parameters. In a separate group of five dogs, pergolide was administered 5 min after sulpiride. Pergolide failed to lower blood pressure, heart rate, or iliac vascular resistance; instead, it produced an increase in mean blood pressure in these sulpiride-treated dogs (Fig. 2). This pressor effect of pergolide was similar to that previously reported in normotensive dogs (Barrett and Lokhandwala, 1981b).

Since sulpiride prevented the antihypertensive, bradycardic, and iliac vasodilatory actions of pergolide, it can be suggested that dopamine receptor stimulation was responsible for these actions of pergolide. However, dopamine receptors are located at several sites within the cardiovascular system, and since pergolide does not activate postsynaptic dopamine (DA_1) receptors (Barrett and Lokhandwala, 1981b), it is likely that activation of neurotropic dopamine (DA_2) receptors produced the observed cardiovascular actions. Additional experiments were carried out to determine actions of pergolide at presynaptic dopamine receptors located on postganglionic sympathetic nerves.

3. Presynaptic Dopaminergic Inhibition of Sympathetic Nerve Function by Pergolide

Experiments were performed to study the effects of pergolide on cardiac and renal sympathetic nerve function by utilizing procedures described previously (Lokhandwala, 1979; Barrett and Lokhandwala, 1981a).

In a group of five pentobarbital-anesthetized dogs, pergolide (12.5 μg/kg infused over a 10-min period) caused significant impairment of cardioacceleration elicited during stimulation of the right postganglionic cardiac sympathetic nerves. The inhibition of responses to nerve stimulation was seen 30 and 60 min after administration of pergolide (Fig. 3). When sulpiride (0.5 mg/kg, i.v.) was administered to a group of five dogs, it did not produce any changes in the positive chronotropic effect of cardiac nerve stimulation (Fig. 3). However, in these sulpiride-treated dogs, pergolide failed to exert any effect on the tachycardia elicited during cardiac nerve stimulation (Fig. 3). Therefore, these results suggest that the inhibition of cardiac sympathetic nerve function caused by pergolide oc-

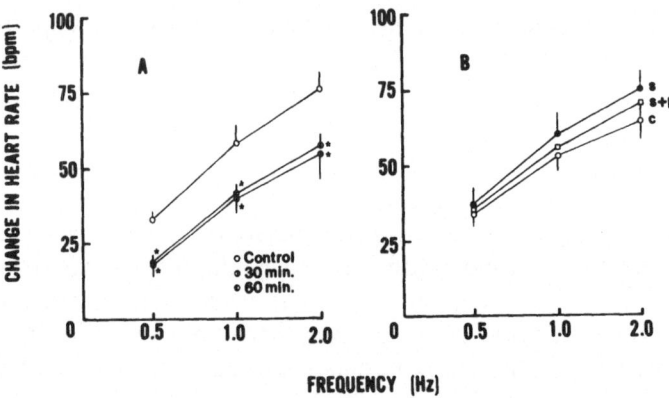

Figure 3. Effect of pergolide (12.5 μg/kg infused over a 10-min period) on the positive chronotropic effect of cardiac nerve stimulation in a group of five pentobarbital-anesthetized dogs (A). The influence of sulpiride (S) (0.5 mg/kg, i.v.) on the effect of pergolide (P) on responses to cardiac nerve stimulation is shown in B in a separate group of five dogs.

curred through activation of presynaptic dopamine receptors. It should be noted that this dose of sulpiride is shown to be effective in selectively antagonizing presynaptic dopamine receptors but not presynaptic α adrenoceptors (Barrett *et al.*, 1982).

Pergolide (12.5 μg/kg infused over a 10-min period) also caused significant impairment of renal vasoconstriction elicited during stimulation of renal sympathetic nerves (Table I). The inhibitory action of pergolide on renal sympathetic nerve function was antagonized in a separate group of five dogs treated with sulpiride (0.5 μg/kg), which suggests that activation of presynaptic dopamine receptors was responsible for this action of pergolide.

Table I. Effect of Pergolide on the Renal Vasoconstrictor Responses to Renal Nerve Stimulation in Control Animals and in a Separate Group of Dogs Treated with Sulpiride[a]

Treatment	Decrease in renal blood flow (ml/min)		
	1 Hz	2 Hz	4 Hz
None	-21 ± 3	-47 ± 4	-78 ± 15
Pergolide	$- 8 \pm 3^b$	-22 ± 6^b	-42 ± 9^b
Sulpiride	-18 ± 4	-42 ± 6	-65 ± 16
Sulpiride plus pergolide	-16 ± 6	-39 ± 11	-67 ± 14

[a] Pergolide (12.5 μg/kg) was infused i.v. over a 10-min period; sulpiride (0.5 mg/kg) was also administered i.v. Results are means ± S.E.M. (N = 5 per group).
[b] Significantly different from control at $P < 0.05$ level.

These results show that pergolide can activate presynaptic dopamine receptors located on cardiac and renal sympathetic nerves. It is likely that activation of presynaptic dopamine receptors and subsequent inhibition of sympathetic neuronal function to these and other organs were responsible for the antihypertensive and bradycardic actions of pergolide. However, in addition to sympathetic nerve terminals, neurotropic or DA_2 receptors are also located at the cardiovascular control centers within the central nervous system (Kondo *et al.*, 1981). Therefore, it is likely that pergolide may also act on these receptors to exert its cardiovascular actions. We carried out additional experiments to determine the central cardiovascular actions of pergolide.

4. Centrally Mediated Cardiovascular Actions of Pergolide

Separate groups of normotensive dogs were prepared for the measurements of blood pressure, heart rate, and renal, mesenteric, and iliac blood flow. A 21-gauge, $1\frac{1}{2}$-inch needle filled with saline was introduced into the fourth cerebral ventricle by penetrating the atlanto–occipital membrane overlying the cisterna magna. Following a 30-min stabilization period, drugs were administrated via this needle in volumes of 0.2 ml or less and flushed with a small amount of animal's own cerebrospinal fluid.

Pergolide (12.5 μg/kg) administered intracisternally (i.c.) to a group of five normotensive dogs produced decreases in mean blood pressure, heart rate, and iliac vascular resistance (Table II). These actions of pergolide persisted for the entire 60-min observation period. In a second group of four dogs sulpiride (0.5 mg, i.c.) was administered. Although sulpiride by itself did not produce changes in any of the parameters, it antagonized the hypotensive, bradycardic, and iliac vasodilatory actions of pergolide (Table II). In order to establish further that these actions of pergolide resulted from the activation of central dopamine receptors and not α adrenoceptors, a third group of four dogs was treated with yohimbine (0.5 mg i.c.). When pergolide was administered to these yohimbine-treated dogs, it still produced all of the cardiovascular changes that were seen in control dogs (Table II). These results suggest that the central actions of pergolide were mediated by the stimulation of central dopamine receptors and not α adrenoceptors. It should be noted that in a separate group of dogs, this dose of yohimbine (0.5 mg, i.c.), which failed to prevent the central actions of pergolide, significantly antagonized the hypotensive and bradycardic actions of clonidine (1 μg/kg, i.c.).

Table II. The Effects of Intracisternal Administration of Pergolide (12.5 µg/kg) on Mean Blood Pressure, Heart Rate, and Iliac Vascular Resistance of Pentobarbital-Anesthetized Normotensive Dogs[a]

Agonist	Antagonist[b]	Mean blood pressure (mm Hg)		Heart rate (beats/min)		Iliac vascular resistance (mm Hg/ml per min)	
		Control	Change	Control	Change	Control	Change
Pergolide	None	130 ± 10	-40 ± 11[c]	152 ± 7	-31 ± 8[c]	2.18 ± 0.52	-1.24 ± 0.44[c]
Pergolide	Sulpiride	148 ± 7	-6 ± 2	160 ± 5	-11 ± 4	2.75 ± 0.53	0.48 ± 0.47
Pergolide	Yohimbine	164 ± 6	-41 ± 4[c]	178 ± 2	-18 ± 5[c]	1.60 ± 0.17	-0.51 ± 0.26[c]

[a] Pergolide was given alone and then in separate groups of dogs treated with either sulpiride (0.5 mg, i.c.) or yohimbine (0.5 mg, i.c.). The values given represent maximum changes following the administration of pergolide (mean ± S.E.M.; four to five dogs per group).

[b] Pergolide was given 15 min after administration of the antagonist.

[c] Significantly different from control ($P < 0.05$).

5. Involvement of Central Nervous System Dopamine Receptors in the Antihypertensive Action of Pergolide

Since pergolide was found to activate central dopamine receptors selectively and to cause lowering of blood pressure, heart rate, and iliac vascular resistance, it is possible that the antihypertensive action of this compound in neurogenic hypertensive dogs may also have resulted from the stimulation of central dopamine receptors. In order to test this hypothesis, in a separate group of six neurogenic hypertensive dogs sulpiride (0.5 mg i.c.) was administered. It should be noted that this dose of intracisternally administered sulpiride antagonized the centrally mediated hypotensive, bradycardic, and iliac vasodilatory actions of pergolide. When pergolide (12.5 μg/kg, i.v.) was administered to these sulpiride-treated neurogenic hypertensive dogs, its antihypertensive, bradycardic, and iliac vasodilatory actions were significantly attenuated (Fig. 4). These results demonstrate that blockade of central dopamine receptors significantly antagonized the cardiovascular actions of pergolide in neurogenic hypertensive dogs and provide evidence in support of the suggestion that stimulation of central dopamine receptors by intravenously administered pergolide was responsible, at least in part, for the antihypertensive action of this compound. However, before we could accept this postulation, it was important to show that centrally administered sulpiride was restricted within the central nervous system and did not antagonize peripheral presynaptic dopamine receptors.

In a separate group of four dogs, cardioaccelerator nerve stimulation was performed, and frequency-dependent increases in heart rate were recorded (Table III). Sulpiride (0.5 mg i.c.) was then administered, and cardioaccelerator nerve stimulation was repeated. Sulpiride did not alter responses to nerve stimulation (Table III). Pergolide was infused (1.25 μg/kg per min for 10 min), and cardioaccelerator nerve stimulation was repeated 30 and 60 min after termination of pergolide infusion. Pergolide caused significant impairment of the positive chronotropic effect of cardioaccelerator nerve stimulation in these dogs (Table III). The degree of inhibition was similar to that exerted by pergolide in a group of control dogs, as previously described in Section 3. These results demonstrate that intracisternally administered sulpiride did not leak into the peripheral circulation to antagonize peripheral presynaptic dopamine receptors. This is based on the observation that pergolide was still able to cause a presynaptic dopaminergic inhibition of cardiac sympathetic nerve function in these animals. Therefore, these results provide further evidence that stimulation of central dopamine receptors contributes to the antihypertensive action of pergolide in neurogenic hypertensive dogs. Although

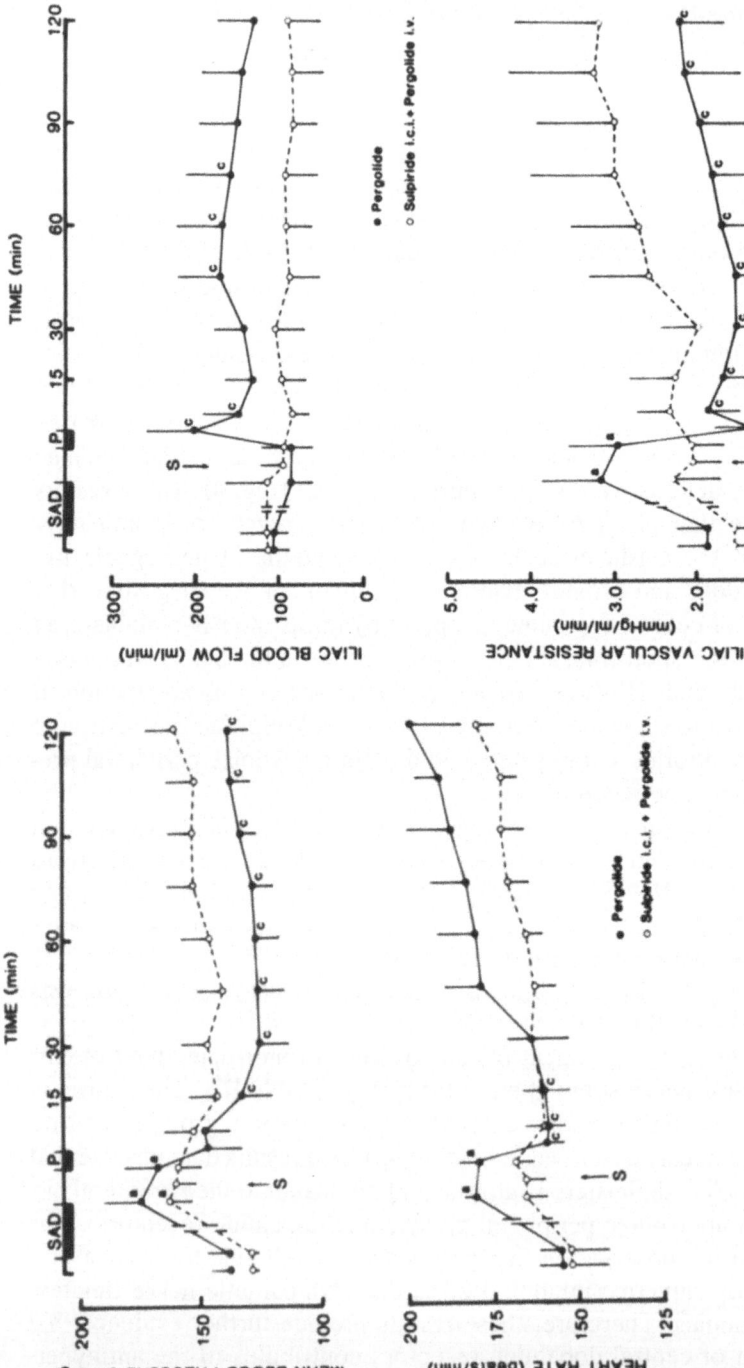

Figure 4. Antihypertensive, bradycardic, and iliac vasodilatory actions of pergolide (12.5 μg/kg, i.v.) in neurogenic hypertensive dogs (same as in Fig. 2). These effects of pergolide were significantly attenuated in a separate group of neurogenic hypertensive dogs (*N* = 6) in which central nervous system dopamine receptors were selectively antagonized with intracisternal sulpiride (S) (0.5 mg, i.c.i.).

Table III. Failure of Intracisternally Administered Sulpiride (0.5 mg) to Antagonize the Impairment of the Positive Chronotropic Effect of Cardioaccelerator Nerve Stimulation Produced by Intravenous Pergolide (12.5 μg/kg)

Treatment	Increase in heart rate (beats/min)[a]		
	0.5 Hz	1 Hz	2 Hz
None	28 ± 2	54 ± 3	76 ± 5
Sulpiride	26 ± 3	53 ± 2	74 ± 4
Sulpiride plus pergolide[b]	15 ± 2*	34 ± 4*	56 ± 3*
Sulpiride plus pergolide[c]	16 ± 1*	36 ± 3*	60 ± 4*

[a] Mean ± S.E.M. (N = 4). * $P < 0.05$ versus control and sulpiride.
[b] Cardioaccelerator nerve stimulation 30 min after administration of pergolide.
[c] Cardioaccelerator nerve stimulation 60 min after administration of pergolide.

these results do not necessarily rule out the involvement of peripheral presynaptic dopamine receptors in the action of pergolide, they suggest that the antihypertensive action of pergolide results from simultaneous stimulation of both central and peripheral presynaptic dopamine receptors.

6. Cardiovascular Dopamine Receptors and Antihypertensive Drug Action

It is proposed by us, as well as others in this volume and elsewhere, that stimulation of cardiovascular dopamine receptors by dopamine receptor agonists may represent a novel approach for the development of antihypertensive agents (Lokhandwala and Barrett, 1981, 1982, 1983; Cavero *et al.*, 1982a,b; Langer, 1980; Ackerman *et al.*, 1982). Therefore, it is important first to demonstrate antihypertensive action of these compounds in models of experimental hypertension and then to assess the relative contribution of cardiovascular dopamine receptors located at different sites in such an action.

Pergolide was found to exert a marked antihypertensive action in neurogenic hypertensive dogs. It is reported that sinoaortic deafferentation results in the disinhibition of sympathetic discharge, leading to increases in peripheral vascular resistance and blood pressure (Kirchheim, 1976; Laubie and Schmitt, 1979). The increase in vascular resistance is noted primarily in the skeletal muscle regions rather than in the renal or mesenteric circulation (Snyder *et al.*, 1978; Cox and Bagshaw, 1980). We also noted a similar pattern in that the iliac vascular resistance was significantly elevated in neurogenic hypertensive dogs, whereas resistance in the kidney and the mesentery was only slightly affected. Since neurogenic hypertension in our model resulted primarily from an increase in sympathetic discharge to the iliac vascular bed and subsequent increase in iliac vascular resistance, pergolide produced a lowering of blood pressure in these hypertensive animals by reducing the elevated iliac vascular resistance, while was responsible for the production of neurogenic hypertension.

The involvement of dopamine receptors in the cardiovascular actions of pergolide was established when it was observed that the dopamine receptor antagonist sulpiride prevented the antihypertensive, bradycardic, and iliac vasodilatory actions of pergolide. Experiments performed to determine the action of pergolide on presynaptic dopamine receptors revealed that the compound activates these receptors on cardiac and renal sympathetic nerves. Presynaptic dopamine receptors are also reported to be located on lumbar sympathetic nerves innervating the hindlimb (Laubie *et al.*, 1977). Therefore, it is possible that the iliac vasodilatory action of pergolide may have resulted from activation of these presynaptic dopamine receptors and subsequent inhibition of sympathetic vasoconstrictor tone to this vasculature in the hypertensive dogs.

The role of central nervous system dopamine receptors in the action of pergolide was established in additional experiments when it was observed that sulpiride, in a dose small enough to antagonize only central dopamine receptors, also significantly attenuated the antihypertensive action of intravenously administered pergolide in neurogenic hypertensive dogs. Therefore, these results suggest that central dopamine receptor activation also contributes to the antihypertensive action of pergolide.

Our study shows that pergolide, a dopaminergic ergoline, decreases blood pressure and heart rate in neurogenic hypertensive dogs, actions attributable to activation of cardiovascular dopamine receptors located on the sympathetic nerve terminals and within the central nervous system. Studies reported in this volume as well as those reported previously have demonstrated that dopamine receptor agonists also exert a potent antihypertensive action in spontaneously hypertensive rats. Therefore, these studies have provided experimental evidence in support of the concept that cardiovascular dopamine receptor stimulation represents a novel and effective approach in lowering blood pressure in hypertensive animals. Future research in this area should be directed towards determining the clinical effectiveness and tolerability of dopamine receptor agonists in hypertensive patients.

7. Summary

We have performed experiments to determine whether pergolide, a dopaminergic ergoline, would exert antihypertensive action in neurogenic hypertensive dogs and to elucidate further the role of cardiovascular dopamine receptors in the action of pergolide. Sinoaortic deafferentation resulted in sustained hypertension and tachycardia, which was associated with a significant elevation of iliac vascular resistance but not renal or mesenteric resistance. Intravenous administration of pergolide (12.5 µg/kg) to these neurogenic hypertensive dogs produced significant decreases in blood pressure, heart rate, and iliac vascular resistance. These actions of pergolide were prevented by the dopamine receptor antagonist sulpiride (0.5 mg/kg, i.v.), suggesting that dopamine receptor activation was responsible for the antihypertensive action of pergolide.

Pergolide caused significant impairment of cardioacceleration as well as renal vasoconstriction elicited during the stimulation of cardiac and renal sympathetic nerves, respectively. This action of pergolide was antagonized by sulpiride, suggesting that activation of presynaptic dopamine receptors was responsible for the inhibition of sympathetic nerve function caused by pergolide. In normotensive dogs, pergolide (12.5 µg/kg) administration directly into the fourth cerebral ventricle via the cisterna magna resulted in hypotension, bradycardia, and iliac vasodilatation. These actions were prevented by sulpiride but not by yohimbine, suggesting that specific activation of central dopamine receptors by pergolide produces lowering of blood pressure and heart rate.

In a separate group of neurogenic hypertensive dogs, the antihypertensive, bradycardic, and iliac vasodilatory actions of intravenous pergolide were significantly attenuated by a small dose of sulpiride administered directly within the brain via the cisterna magna. It was established that this dose of sulpiride antagonized central dopamine receptors but not peripheral presynaptic dopamine receptors. These results demonstrate that pergolide is an effective antihypertensive agent in neurogenic hypertensive dogs. Activation of neurotropic dopamine (DA$_2$) receptors located within the brain as well as on the peripheral postganglionic sympathetic nerve terminals is responsible for the antihypertensive action of pergolide. Dopamine receptor agonists may well offer a novel pharmacological approach in the treatment of hypertension.

ACKNOWLEDGMENTS. This study was supported by NIH grant HL-26262 from NHLBI. Richard J. Barrett was supported by NIH Predoctoral Training Grant GM-07405 from NIGMS. We are grateful to Mrs. Sanober M. Lokhandwala of the Word Processing Center for the preparation of this manuscript.

References

Ackerman, D. M., Weinstock, J., Weibelhaus, V. D., and Berkowitz, B., 1982, Renal vasodilators and hypertension, *Drug Dev. Res.* 2:283–297.

Barrett, R. J., and Lokhandwala, M. F., 1981a, Presynaptic dopamine receptor stimulation in the cardiovascular actions of lergotrile, *J. Pharmacol. Exp. Ther.* **217**:660–665.

Barrett, R. J., and Lokhandwala, M. F., 1981b, The role of *alpha* adrenergic and dopamine receptor activation in the cardiovascular effects of pergolide, *Fed. Proc.* **40**:315.

Barrett, R. J., Ginos, J. Z., and Lokhandwala, M. F., 1982, Evaluation of peripheral dopamine receptor and α-adrenoceptor blocking activity of sulpiride, *Eur. J. Pharmacol.* **79**:273–281.

Cavero, I., Massingham, R., and Lefevre-Borg, F., 1982a, Peripheral dopamine receptors, potential targets for a new class of antihypertensive agents: Subclassification and functional description, *Life Sci.* **31**:939–948.

Cavero, I., Massingham, R., and Lefevre-Borg, F., 1982b, Peripheral dopamine receptors, potential targets for a new class of antihypertensive agents: Sites and mechanisms of action of dopamine receptor agonists, *Life Sci.* **31**:1059–1069.

Clark, B. J., 1979, Cardiovascular effects of ergot alkaloids, *J. Pharmacol. (Paris)* **10**:439–453.

Clark, B. J., 1981, Dopamine receptors and the cardiovascular system, *Postgrad. Med. J.* **57**(Suppl 1):45–54.

Cox, R. H., and Bagshaw, R. J., 1980, Effects of anesthesia on carotid sinus reflex control of arterial hemodynamics in the dog, *Am. J. Physiol.* **239**:H681–H691.

Goldberg, L. I., 1972, Cardiovascular and renal actions of dopamine: Potential clinical applications, *Pharmacol. Rev.* **24**:1–29.

Greenacre, J. K., Teychenne, P. F., Petrie, A., Calne, D. B., Leigh, P. N., and Reid, J. L., 1976, The cardiovascular effects of bromocriptine in parkinsonism, *Br. J. Clin. Pharmacol.* **3**:571–574.

Hahn, R. A., 1981, Inhibitory effects of pergolide on peripheral adrenergic neurotransmission in spontaneously hypertensive rats, *Life Sci.* **29**:2501–2509.

Hahn, R. A., and Farrell, S. K., 1981, Inhibition of peripheral adrenergic neurotransmission by lergotrile in spontaneously hypertensive rats, *Life Sci.* **28**:2497–2504.

Kaye, S. B., Shaw, K. M., and Ross, E. J., 1976, Bromocriptine and hypertension, *Lancet* **1**:1176–1177.

Kirchheim, H. R., 1976, Systemic arterial baroreceptor reflexes, *Physiol. Rev.* **56**:100–176.

Kondo, S., Ebihara, A., Suzuki, H., and Saruta, T., 1981, Role of dopamine in the regulation of blood pressure and the renin–angiotensin–aldosterone system in conscious rats, *Clin. Sci.* **61**:235s–237s.

Langer, S. Z., 1980, Presynaptic regulation of the release of catecholamines, *Pharmacol. Rev.* **32**:337–362.

Laubie, M., and Schmitt, H., 1979, Destruction of nucleus tractus solitari in the dog: Comparison with sinoaortic denervation, *Am. J. Physiol.* **236**:H736–H743.

Laubie, M., Schmitt, H., and Falq, E., 1977, Dopamine receptors in the femoral vascular bed of the dog as mediators of a vasodilator and sympathoinhibitory effect, *Eur. J. Pharmacol.* **42**:307–310.

Lokhandwala, M. F., 1979, Analysis of the effects of bromocriptine on blood pressure and sympathetic nerve function, *Eur. J. Pharmacol.* **56**:253–256.

Lokhandwala, M. F., and Barrett, R. J., 1981, Pharmacological role of presynaptic dopamine receptors in the cardiovascular actions of dopaminergic agents, in: *Central Nervous System Mechanisms in Hypertension* (J. P. Buckley and C. M. Ferrario, eds.), Raven Press, New York, pp. 203–213.

Lokhandwala, M. F., and Barrett, R. J., 1982, Cardiovascular dopamine receptors: Physiological, pharmacological and therapeutic implications, *J. Autonom. Pharmacol.* **3**:189–215.

Lokhandwala, M. F., and Barrett, R. J., 1983, Dopamine receptor agonists in cardiovascular therapy, *Drug Dev. Res.* **3**:299–310.

Lokhandwala, M. F., Tadepalli, A. S., and Jandhyala, B. S., 1979, Cardiovascular actions of bromocriptine: Evidence for a neurogenic mechanism, *J. Pharmacol. Exp. Ther.* **211**:620–625.

Snyder, D. W., Doba, N., and Reis, D. J., 1978, Regional distribution of blood flow during arterial hypertension produced by lesions of the nucleus tractus solitarii in rats, *Circ. Res.* **42**:87–91.

Sved, A. F., and Fernstrom, J. D., 1980, Evidence for a peripheral dopaminergic mechanism in the antihypertensive action of lergotrile, *Life Sci.* **27**:349–354.

Yen, T. T., Stamm, N. B., and Clemens, J. A., 1979, Pergolide, a potent dopaminergic antihypertensive, *Life Sci.* **25**:209–216.

III

CRITICAL CONCEPTS OF PHYSIOLOGICAL AND MOLECULAR MECHANISMS OF CARDIOVASCULAR AND RENAL FUNCTION

10

Role of Inflammatory Cells in Metabolic and Cellular Alterations Underlying the Exaggerated Renal Prostaglandin and Thromboxane Synthesis in Ureter Obstruction

PHILIP NEEDLEMAN

1. Exaggerated Arachidonate Metabolism in the Perfused Hydronephrotic Kidney

Perfused normal rabbit kidney releases modest amounts of prostaglandin (PG) E_2 in response to vasoactive peptides (bradykinin and angiotensin II) (Needleman *et al.*, 1973). In microsomes prepared from the normal kidney, the medulla is the primary site of arachidonic acid metabolism; much less PG production occurs in the cortex (Larsson and Anggard, 1974). Unilateral ureter obstruction (hydronephrosis) for several days results in a marked facilitation of (1) PGE_2 release from an isolated perfused kidney (Nishikawa *et al.*, 1977), (2) cortical microsomal arachidonate metabolism (Morrison *et al.*, 1977; Needleman *et al.*, 1979), and (3) cortical slice PG release (Currie *et al.*, 1981). In addition, the perfused hydronephrotic kidney (HNK) has been demonstrated to release thromboxane A_2 (TxA_2). The thromboxane synthetase activity is clearly evident in HNK cortical microsomes, whereas this enzyme is not detectable in normal or contralateral unobstructed rabbit kidneys (CLK) (Morrison *et al.*,

PHILIP NEEDLEMAN • Department of Pharmacology, Washington University School of Medicine, St. Louis, Missouri 63110.

1977, 1978). Measurement of prostaglandins by radioimmunoassay demonstrated that PGE_2, 6-keto-$PGF_{1\alpha}$, and TxB_2 levels are increased in the venous effluent of the hydronephrotic kidney in both the basal and hormone-stimulated states (e.g., bradykinin and angiotensin) (Reingold et al., 1981). The release of these substances could be blocked with indomethacin treatment.

Other models of renal damage in rabbits, such as renal venous constriction (Zipser et al., 1980) and glycerol-induced renal failure (Benabe et al., 1980), are also associated with an unmasking of renal thromboxane biosynthesis. Thus, there are quantitative and qualitative changes occurring simultaneously in renal arachidonate metabolism associated with renal damage. The renal thromboxane production resulting from ureter obstruction has been associated with renal vasoconstriction and the reduced glomerular filtration rate that also occurs with hydronephrosis (Yarger et al., 1980).

We demonstrated that OKY-1581 was effective in the intact perfused hydronephrotic kidney at selectively inhibiting thromboxane synthesis without altering renal PGE_2 or PGI_2 production (Kawasaki et al., 1982). OKY-1581 infusion into the hydronephrotic kidney simultaneously reversed the renal thromboxane synthesis and the associated vasoconstriction produced by bradykinin or the second-phase increase in renal resistance produced by angiotensin II. The vascular tone in the hydronephrotic kidney seems to be balanced between the vasoconstrictor effect of TxA_2 and the vasodilatory effect of PGE_2 and PGI_2.

2. Sites of Enhanced Prostaglandin Synthesis

Locating the site of enhanced biosynthesis of prostaglandins and thromboxane in the hydronephrotic kidney might clarify the role of arachidonic acid metabolism in renal pathological states. We have used multiple approaches to determine the site(s) of altered prostaglandin biosynthesis associated with the hydronephrotic kidney.

2.1. Qualitative Changes in Renal Arachidonate Metabolism

Cortical and medullary microsomes from hydronephrotic and normal kidneys were incubated with [^{14}C]-arachidonic acid. These radiochemical experiments revealed that the enhancement of prostaglandin synthesis and the unmasking of thromboxane production occur in both the cortex and the medulla, with the most dramatic change occurring in the cortical region (Needleman et al., 1979). Hydronephrotic cortical microsomes converted arachidonate to prostaglandins, primarily PGE_2, and thromboxane B_2. Normal cortical microsomes converted arachidonate to prostaglandins to a lesser degree than did cortical microsomes from the hydronephrotic kidney and did not form thromboxane B_2. Medullary microsomes from the hydronephrotic kidney had a slight enhancement of activity when compared to microsomes from normal medulla and formed a considerable amount of thromboxane. These experiments reveal the regions of the kidney that have increased capacity to produce prostaglandins; however, they do not provide insight into the regions of the kidney that are sensitive to hormonal stimulation.

2.2. Kinetic Comparison of Renal Microsomal Arachidonate Metabolism in Normal and Ureter-Obstructed Rabbit Kidneys

Unilateral ureteral obstruction of rabbit kidney results, after 3 days, in an exaggerated release of prostaglandin E_2 and thromboxane A_2 by the *ex vivo* perfused hydronephrotic kidney (HNK) but not by the surgically unaltered contralateral kidney (CLK) (Wu *et al.*, 1983). Both cyclooxygenase (PG endoperoxide synthetase) and thromboxane synthetase activities increased 20- to 40-fold in cortical microsomes prepared from HNK compared with microsomes from CLK, but the highly active PG-endoperoxide–E_2 isomerase rate did not change. In medullary microsomes, the high rate of cyclooxygenase activity was increased two- to threefold, whereas the thromboxane synthetase activity increased 15-fold in the HNK compared to CLK. In the 6-day HNK cortex, the cyclooxygenase (V_{max} ~1000 pmole/mg protein per min) was clearly the rate-limiting step, proceeding at only about one-fifth the rate of thromboxane synthetase (V_{max} ~5000 pmole/mg per min) and only 1/40 the rate of the extremely rapid prostaglandin endoperoxide–E_2 isomerase (V_{max} = 40–60,000 pmole/mg per min).

Hydronephrotic cortical and medullary microsomes convert arachidonate into equivalent amounts of prostaglandin E_2 and thromboxane A_2. However, when the renal microsomes were incubated in the presence of reduced glutathione, the primary product was prostaglandin E_2, and the ratio of prostaglandin E_2 to thromboxane A_2 was about 10:1. Similarly, there was an 8–12:1 ratio of PG-endoperoxide–E_2 isomerase:thromboxane synthetase in the HNK. The ratio of PGE_2 to thromboxane A_2 obtained in the renal venous effluent from a stimulated hydronephrotic kidney was also 8:1, suggesting that the intact tissue is dominated by the PG-endoperoxide–E_2 isomerase and that reduced glutathione may be a key influence on the *in vivo* synthesis of prostaglandins in hydronephrosis.

2.3. Slice Experiments for Localization of the Metabolic Changes in the HNK

Utilizing a slice technique permits a more thorough localization of the renal site of exaggerated prostaglandin synthesis to be accomplished. In this study, cortical or medullary slices were incubated in Krebs–Henseleit buffer either in the presence or absence of hormone; the resulting PGE_2 and TxB_2 released by the tissue into the medium was measured by radioimmunoassay. Hydronephrotic cortical slices produce ten times more PGE_2 (basal and bradykinin-stimulated) than the contralateral cortical slices (Currie et al., 1981). The hydronephrotic medullary slices also exhibit increased PGE_2 synthesis but do not exhibit a time-dependent recovery of PG endoperoxide synthetase (cyclooxygenase) after aspirin treatment, whereas HNK cortical slices recover after aspirin (Schwartzman and Raz, 1981). Therefore, the PGE_2 response of the hydronephrotic cortical slices most closely resembles the response obtained with the intact perfused hydronephrotic kidney. A more complete localization of the enhanced prostaglandin synthesis associated with ureter obstruction was accomplished by studying slices from the outer cortex, inner cortex, outer medulla, and inner medulla (Currie et al., 1981). Normal kidneys were unresponsive to bradykinin in all regions except the inner medulla. The hydronephrotic kidney exhibited an enhanced prostaglandin and thromboxane A_2 synthesis in response to bradykinin stimulation in all the regions.

2.4. Quantitative Comparison of PGE_2 and TxB_2 Released from the Isolated Intact Perfused Hydronephrotic Rabbit Kidney

Administration of the vasoactive peptide bradykinin to an intact HNK activates a renal acyl hydrylase that releases intrinsic arachidonic acid (Isakson et al., 1976). Therefore, the released PGE_2 and TxB_2 following bradykinin administration reflects the preferred pathway in intrinsic renal arachidonate conversion with maintained cell separation and endogenous cofactors. Bradykinin, administered to a perfused unobstructed normal kidney, released 132 ± 43 ng ($n = 4$) of PGE_2 and no detectable thromboxane into the renal venous effluent. Administration of bradykinin to perfused 3-day hydronephrotic kidneys releases 5650 ± 300 ng of PGE_2 ($n = 3$) and 250 ± 70 ng of TxB_2 (Kawasaki et al., 1982). The ratio of $PGE_2:TxB_2$ released from the isolated intact perfused hydronephrotic kidney was therefore $8:1$, which compares favorably with the ratio of the PGE_2/TxB_2 formed when hydronephrotic renal microsomes were incubated with arachidonate as substrate in the presence of

GSH (Wu *et al.*, 1983). Similarly, there was an 8–12:1 ratio of PG-endoperoxide-E_2 isomerase:thromboxane synthetase in the 3-day hydronephrotic kidney. These kinetic data therefore suggest that the response of the intact kidney is dictated by its GSH concentration. The normal kidney has very high concentrations of GSH, especially in the cortex (Brehe *et al.*, 1976).

3. Role of Mononuclear Cells in the Exaggerated Arachidonate Metabolism in Renal Injury

The mechanism that produces such major metabolic changes within an organ when a pathological situation is induced is difficult to determine; however, an attractive possible explanation has been suggested from morphological examination of hydronephrosis in rabbits. Nagle *et al.* (1973, 1976) found that complete unilateral obstruction in the rabbit produced a diffuse fibrosis and parenchymal atrophy. Twenty-four hours after obstruction, there were marked histological changes in the rabbit cortex that became exaggerated with time. There was a pronounced widening of the interstitial space, an increase of fibroblasts, and the presence of mononuclear cells. The initial proliferative stimulus may be the increase in intrarenal pressure, which causes an enlargement of the interstitial space and decreases the contact of the few normally present fibroblasts with their environment, resulting in the promotion of fibroblast proliferation. Contact inhibition of fibroblast proliferation has previously been demonstrated (Martz and Steinberg, 1972).

The demonstration of mononuclear cells in close contact with the cytoplasmic processes of the cortical fibroblasts (Nagle *et al.*, 1973) may have profound implications in the progression of the histological and metabolic changes involved in the renal injury. Leibovich and Ross (1975, 1976) found that abolition of circulating blood monocytes by the use of antimacrophage serum and steroids substantially delayed the appearance of fibroblasts at sites of tissue injury and suppressed the fibroblast proliferation rate. The macrophages also appear to actively modulate fibroblast PG biosynthesis. Several investigators have reported that conditioned media obtained from adherent mononuclear cell cultures contain a factor that is mitogenic for fibroblasts, and in several instances it has been correlated to a marked (50- to 200-fold) stimulation of PGE_2 biosynthesis by dermal fibroblasts (Korn *et al.*, 1980), by gingival fibroblastlike cells (D'Souza *et al.*, 1981), and by synovial cells (Dayer *et al.*, 1977). Of course, the presence of a substantial number of macrophages in the damaged tissue introduces the possibility that these mononuclear cells themselves contribute to the arachidonic acid metabolites released by the hydronephrotic kidney. Macrophages have a high arachidonic acid metabolic potential and have been demonstrated to synthesize PGE_2, TxA_2, PGI_2, and a number of lipoxygenase products (Humes *et al.*, 1982; Hsueh *et al.*, 1979).

In our studies, unilateral ureter obstruction in rabbits produced profound changes in endogenous and exogenous renal arachidonic acid metabolism. Isolated perfused hydronephrotic kidney (removed after 3 or 10 days of ureter obstruction) responded to bradykinin stimulation with a markedly enhanced release of prostaglandin E_2 and thromboxane A_2 from the perfused hydronephrotic kidney. Histological analysis of the renal cortex in rabbits with ureteral obstruction revealed a proliferation of fibroblastlike cells and the presence of mononuclear cells; removal of the obstruction did not result in the disappearance of cortical fibroblasts but did result in a decrease of monocytes (Okegawa *et al.*, 1983).

The critical involvement of mononuclear cells in the exaggerated arachidonate metabolism that occurs during hydronephrosis was exhibited by the demonstration that (1) only the perfused hydronephrotic rabbit kidney responded to administration of endotoxin with a sustained release of prostaglandin E_2 and thromboxane A_2, (2) the contralateral rabbit kidney, which is devoid of mononuclear cells, did not respond to endotoxin, and (3) the hydronephrotic cat kidney, which exhibits a fibroblast proliferation with a low number of mononuclear cells, did not respond to endotoxin (Okegawa *et al.*, 1983). Thus, proliferation of fibroblastlike cells and the presence of mononuclear cells appear to be involved in the exaggerated prostaglandin and thromboxane production underlying hydronephrosis. The mononuclear cells (possibly via monokines) seem to be critical for the markedly enhanced prostaglandin and thromboxane release induced by endotoxin and bradykinin.

Thus, in our studies we took advantage of the demonstration that endotoxin stimulates cultured peritoneal macrophages to synthesize PGE_2 and TxA_2 (Kurland and Bockman, 1978; Humes *et al.*, 1982). We found that the perfused rabbit HNK, but not the rabbit CLK, responded to a bolus injection of endotoxin with a slowly initiated but sustained release of PGE_2 and TxB_2 (Okegawa *et al.*, 1983). The time course of the release of arachidonic metabolites, especially thromboxane, from the perfused kidney compared favorably with the time course of metabolite production from cultured macrophages in response to endotoxin (Halushka *et al.*, 1981). We could observe macrophages only in the HNK, not in the CLK or normal kidney; thus, the endotoxin induction of intrinsic arachidonate metabolism only by the obstructed rabbit kidney suggests preferential stimulation of the macrophage cell type. In addition, endotoxin has not been shown to stimulate PG production by the cultured fibroblast. However, endotoxin stimulation of PGE_2 release may in part be caused by the release of factors by the macrophage, which in turn stimulates fibroblast PGE_2 production, as has been demonstrated for synovial fibroblastlike cells (Dayer *et al.*, 1980). Furthermore, we previously showed that unilateral ureter obstruction of the cat kidney only modestly increased peptide-induced PGE_2 release, and no thromboxane production was demonstrable (Reingold *et al.*, 1981). Histological examination of the cat HNK indicated only the modest presence of macrophages. Now we have found that endotoxin does not stimulate PGE_2 or TxA_2 release from the perfused ureter-obstructed cat kidney.

We propose the sequence of events that could encompass many of the observations obtained in studies of hydronephrosis in the rabbit. Ureter obstruction causes a mechanical disruption and/or an immunologic (e.g., via the entrapped urine) stimulus in the cortex that triggers a regional inflammatory response resulting in stimulation of the interstitial cell and the presence of mononuclear cells. The macrophages, which are in direct contact with the fibroblasts, are capable of releasing a factor that stimulates (1) fibroblast proliferation, (2) cortical microsomal cyclooxygenase activity, and (3) PGE_2 release (i.e., intrinsic arachidonate metabolism). The enhanced thromboxane synthetase levels and the TxA_2 release may come from the macrophages directly or from the activated fibroblasts.

References

Benabe, J. E., Klahr, S., Hoffman, M. H., and Morrison, A. R., 1980, Production of thromboxane A₂ by the kidney in glycerol-induced acute renal failure, *Prostaglandins* **19**:333–347.

Brehe, J. C., Chan, A. W. K., Alvey, T. R., and Burch, H. B., 1976, Effect of methionine sulfoximine on glutathione and amino acid levels in the nephron, *Am. J. Physiol.* **231**:1536–1540.

Currie, M. G., Davis, B. B., and Needleman, P., 1981, Localization of exaggerated prostaglandin synthesis associated with renal damage, *Prostaglandins* **22**:933–944.

D'Souza, S. M., Englis, D. J., Clark, A., and Russell, R. G., 1981, Stimulation of production of prostaglandin E in gingival cells exposed to products of human blood mononuclear cells, *Biochem. J.* **198**:391–396.

Dayer, J.-M., Passwell, J. H., Schneeberger, E. E., and Krane, S. M., 1980, Interactions among rheumatoid synovial cells and monocyte-macrophages: production of collagenase-stimulating factor by human monocytes exposed to concanavalin A or immunoglobulin Fc fragments, *J. Immunol.* **124**:1712–1720.

Dayer, J.-M., Robinson, D. R., and Krane, S. M., 1977, Prostaglandin production by rheumatoid synovial cells. Stimulation by a factor from human mononuclear cells, *J. Exp. Med.* **145**:1399–1404.

Halushka, P. V., Cook, J. A., and Wise, W. C., 1981, Thromboxane A_2 and prostacyclin production by lipopolysaccharide-stimulated peritoneal macrophages, *J. Reticuloendothel. Soc.* **30**:445–450.

Hsueh, W., Kuhn, C., and Needleman, P., 1979, Relationship of prostaglandin secretion by rabbit alveolar macrophages to phagocytosis and lysosomal enzyme release, *Biochem. J.* **184**:345–354.

Humes, J. L., Sadowski, S., Galavage, M., Goldenberg, M., Subers, E., Bonney, R. J., and Kuehl, F. A., 1982, Evidence for two sources of arachidonic acid for oxidative metabolism by mouse peritoneal macrophages, *J. Biol. Chem.* **257**:1591–1595.

Isakson, P. C., Raz, A., and Needleman, P., 1976, Selective incorporation of ^{14}C-arachidonic acid into the phospholipids of intact tissues and subsequent metabolism to ^{14}C-prostaglandins, *Prostaglandins* **12**:739–748.

Kawasaki, A., and Needleman, P., 1982, Contribution of thromboxane to renal resistance changes in the isolated perfused hydronephrotic rabbit kidney, *Circ. Res.* **50**:486–490.

Korn, J. H., Halushka, P. V., and LeRoy, E. C., 1980, Mononuclear cell modulatin of connective tissue function. Suppression of fibroblast growth by stimulation of endogenous prostaglandin production, *J. Clin. Invest.* **65**:543–554.

Kurland, J. I., and Bockman, R., 1978, Prostaglandin E production by human blood monocytes and mouse peritoneal macrophages, *J. Exp. Med.* **147**:952–956.

Larsson, C., and Anggard, E., 1974, Regional differences in the formation and metabolism of prostaglandins in the rabbit kidney, *Eur. J. Pharmacol.* **25**:326–334.

Leibovich, S. J., and Ross, R., 1975, The role of macrophage in wound repair. A study with hydrocortisone and antimacrophage serum, *Am. J. Pathol.* **78**:71–91.

Leibovich, S. J., and Ross, R., 1976, A macrophage-dependent factor that stimulates the proliferation of fibroblasts *in vitro, Am. J. Pathol.* **84**:501–513.

Martz, E., and Steinberg, M. S., 1972, The role of cell–cell contact in "contact" inhibition of cell-division: A review and new evidence, *J. Cell. Physiol.* **79**:189–210.

Morrison, A. R., Nishikawa, K., and Needleman, P., 1977, Unmasking of thromboxane A_2 synthesis by ureter obstruction in the rabbit kidney, *Nature* **267**:259–260.

Morrison, A. R., Nishikawa, K., and Needleman, P., 1978, Thromboxane A_2 biosynthesis in the ureter obstructed isolated perfused kidney of the rabbit, *J. Pharmacol. Exp. Ther.* **205**:1–8.

Nagle, R. B., Bulger, R. E., Cutter, R. E., Jervis, H. R., and Benditt, E. P., 1973, Unilateral obstructive nephropathy in the rabbit. I. Early morphologic, physiologic, and histochemical changes, *Lab. Invest.* **28**:456–467.

Nagle, R. B., Johnson, M. E., and Jervis, H. R., 1976, Proliferation of renal interstitial cells following injury induced by ureteral obstruction, *Lab. Invest.* **35**:18–22.

Needleman, P., Kauffman, A. H., Douglas, J. R., Johnson, E. M., and Marshall, G. R., 1973, Specific simulation and inhibition of renal prostaglandin release by angiotensin analogs, *Am. J. Physiol.* **224**:1415–1419.

Needleman, P., Wyche, A., Bronson, S. D., Holmberg, S., and Morrison, A. R., 1979, Specific regulation of peptide-induced renal prostaglandin synthesis, *J. Biol. Chem.* **254**:9772–9777.

Nishikawa, K., Morrison, A. R., and Needleman, P., 1977, Exaggerated prostaglandin biosynthesis and its influence on renal resistance in the isolated hydronephrotic rabbit kidney, *J. Clin. Invest.* **59**:1143–1150.

Okegawa, T., Jonas, P. E., DeSchryver, K., Kawasaki, A., and Needleman, P., 1983, Metabolic and cellular alterations underlying the exaggerated renal prostaglandins and thromboxane synthesis in ureter obstruction in rabbits. Inflammatory response involving fibroblasts and mononuclear cells, *J. Clin. Invest.* **71**:81–90.

Reingold, D. F., Waters, K., Holmberg, S., and Needleman, P., 1981, Differential biosynthesis of prostaglandins by hydronephrotic rabbit and cat kidneys, *J. Pharmacol. Exp. Ther.* **216:**510–515.

Schwartzman, M., and Raz, A., 1981, Selective induction of *de novo* prostaglandin biosynthesis in rabbit kidney cortex, *Biochim. Biophys. Acta* **664:**469–474.

Wu, Y.S., Lysz, T. A., Wyche, A., and Needleman, P., 1983, Kinetic comparison and regulation of the cascade of microsomal enzymes involved in renal arachidonate and endoperoxide metabolism, *J. Biol. Chem.* **258:**2188–2192.

Yarger, W. E., Schocken, D. D., and Harris, R. H., 1980, Obstructive nephrophathy in the rat. Possible roles for the renin–angiotensin system, prostaglandins, and thromboxanes in postobstructive renal function, *J. Clin. Invest.* **65:**400–412.

Zipser, R., Myers, S., and Needleman, P., 1980, Exaggerated prostaglandin and thromboxane synthesis in the rabbit with renal vein constriction. *Circ. Res.* **47:**231–237.

11

The Kidney and Hypertension

ARTHUR C. GUYTON, R. DAVIS MANNING,
THOMAS E. LOHMEIER, and JOHN E. HALL

1. Introduction

From the earliest studies on kidney disease it was already apparent that the kidneys play a very important role in controlling arterial pressure. However, the mechanism or mechanisms by which the kidney affects pressure have remained unclear even to the present. All research workers have known of the obvious possibility that renal disease might cause retention of water and salt in the body and that excess volume could drive the circulatory system toward a higher level of activity, thus causing hypertension. Yet, even Bright (1836) in his classical studies on "Bright's disease" noted vasospastic phenomena associated with renal hypertension, leading to the suggestion that renal hypertension might result from some circulating vasoconstrictor agent.

We now know that abnormal renal function can at times lead to retention of water and salt and at other times cause secretion of vasoactive agents, especially the renal hormone renin, and these two effects can occur independently of each other or together. Furthermore, both can raise the arterial pressure. Therefore, the present problem is not whether both effects occur but instead what is the quantitative significance of each. Furthermore, can either or both of them cause chronic hypertension? Or is either of them limited to causing only acute hypertension? These are some of the questions that we explore in this chapter.

Another important question is: What is the relationship of the renal pressure control mechanisms to the many nonrenal mechanisms for con-

ARTHUR C. GUYTON, R. DAVIS MANNING, THOMAS E. LOHMEIER, and JOHN E.
HALL • Department of Physiology and Biophysics, University of Mississippi Medical Center, Jackson, Mississippi 39216.

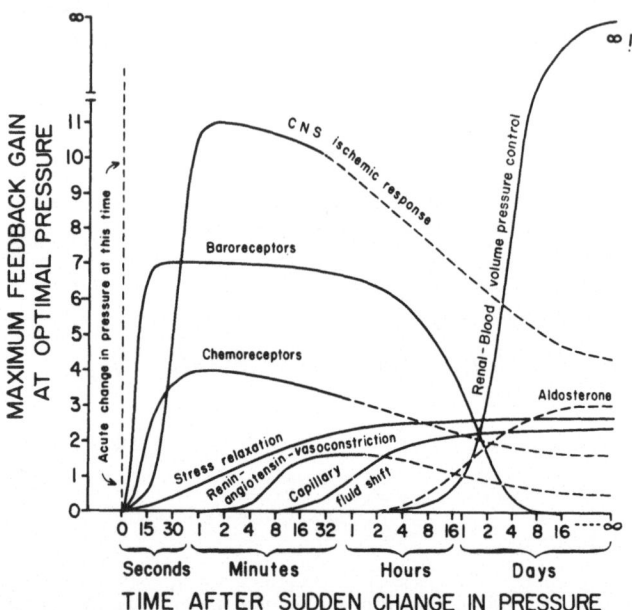

Figure 1. Degree of activation, expressed in terms of feedback gain, of different pressure control mechanisms following a sudden change in arterial pressure. Note the rapid activation of the three nervous control mechanisms, the moderately rapid activation of several intermediate pressure control mechanisms, and the slow but extremely powerful activation of the renal blood volume–pressure control system. (Reprinted from Guyton, 1980.)

trolling pressure? In recent years, the effectiveness of the different pressure control mechanisms has been quantitated in two different ways. (1) The potency of each pressure control mechanism has been measured in terms of *feedback gain*. For instance, a pressure control mechanism that has a feedback gain of 5 is capable of correcting an abnormal arterial pressure 5/6th of the way back toward the control value. (2) The time course of the response of each pressure control mechanism has been studied to determine how rapidly it can correct the pressure abnormality and also whether or not the correction can last indefinitely. Figure 1 illustrates an approximate summary of what is known about the effectiveness of each of eight different important pressure control mechanisms. Several of these are related to kidney function, and others are nonrenal. Some of their characteristics are described the following.

1.1. Nervous Feedback Mechanisms

The most rapidly acting of the pressure control mechanisms are the nervous controls. That is, an abnormal pressure elicits signals from several different nervous receptors including (1) the *baroreceptors* located in the carotid sinuses and in the aortic arch, (2) the *chemoreceptors* in the carotid and aortic bodies, and (3) *receptors in the vasomotor center* in the brainstem. These signals then feed back through the autonomic nervous system to the heart, the arterioles, and the veins to help correct the abnormal pressure. All of these mechanisms react within seconds and reach full response within 10 sec to a minute. Therefore, they are the first line of defense when some factor tends to cause an abnormal systemic arterial pressure.

Though these nervous control mechanisms have extreme potency for controlling arterial pressure, it is also known that many of the nervous receptors that excite the nervous feedback mechanisms adapt—that is, lose their responsiveness—within hours or days (McCubbin *et al.*, 1958; Kreiger, 1970). For this reason, most of the nervous feedback control mechanisms are of importance in controlling arterial pressure only during the first few minutes or hours after an abnormality occurs, and it still has not been proven that the nervous system is of major significance in normal long-term pressure control.

1.2. The Intermediate-Term Pressure Control Mechanisms

Several pressure control mechanisms begin to act within minutes and usually reach full activity within a few hours. These include the following. (1) The *stress relaxation mechanism*: When the pressures increase in the different blood vessels, the vessels themselves gradually stretch, which allows the pressure to fall. Conversely, when the pressure falls below normal, the vessels have a tendency to constrict slowly, a phenomenon called "reverse stress relaxation." These effects generally take place over a period of minutes; (2) The *renin–angiotensin–vasoconstrictor mechanism*: When the arterial pressure falls below normal, the kidneys secrete renin, and this causes the formation of angiotensin in the blood; the angiotensin in turn constricts the peripheral blood vessels, thus raising the arterial pressure back toward normal. This mechanism generally reaches its peak action in 20 to 30 min (Brough, 1975); (3) The *capillary fluid shift mechanism*: This functions by transferring fluid through the capillary membranes. When the capillary pressure falls too low, which often occurs when the arterial pressure falls below normal, fluid is pulled by osmosis from the tissue spaces into the blood, thus increasing both the blood volume and the arterial pressure. This mechanism usually achieves its full effect within a few hours.

1.3. The Long-Term Mechanisms

Several of the pressure-controlling mechanisms respond hardly at all during the first few hours after a pressure abnormality occurs but become very important over many hours or days. Two of these are (1) the *aldosterone mechanism* and (2) the *renal blood volume–pressure control mechanism*.

The aldosterone pressure control mechanism helps to control pressure by controlling extracellular fluid volume, but as shown in Fig. 1, it has almost no effect for the first few hours, partly because aldosterone requires 45 min to an hour to act on the tubular cells of the kidneys and partly because still many hours are required to change the fluid volume enough to affect the pressure. However, this is an important long-term pressure control mechanism.

Finally, note the curve to the far right in Fig. 1 depicting the response of the renal blood volume–pressure control mechanism. This mechanism controls both blood volume and arterial pressure as a direct result of the hemodynamic effect of arterial pressure on renal output of fluid. However, as illustrated in the figure, it responds very little during the first few hours after some abnormality of the circulation causes an abnormal pressure. Yet, over a period of many days its controlling capability progressively accumulates until its feedback gain is tremendous, actually, under most conditions, a feedback gain of infinity. Because of the extreme potency of this mechanism for long-term pressure control, and because hypertension is a long-term pressure abnormality, this is the mechanism that we principally address.

2. The Renal Blood Volume–Pressure Control System

2.1. Basic Mechanism and Infinite Gain Characteristic

The basic mechanism of the renal blood volume–pressure control system is very simple: the renal output of water and salt is directly related to the arterial pressure level. Therefore, when the arterial pressure becomes too great, loss of water and salt from the body decreases both the extracellular fluid volume and blood volume. In turn, the decrease in blood volume decreases the arterial pressure back to its control level. Conversely, when the pressure falls too low, the kidneys retain water and salt until the pressure eventually rises back to its control level.

The function of the renal blood volume–pressure control system is depicted graphically in Fig. 2, which shows two curves, one giving the relationship between arterial pressure and sodium intake, and the other

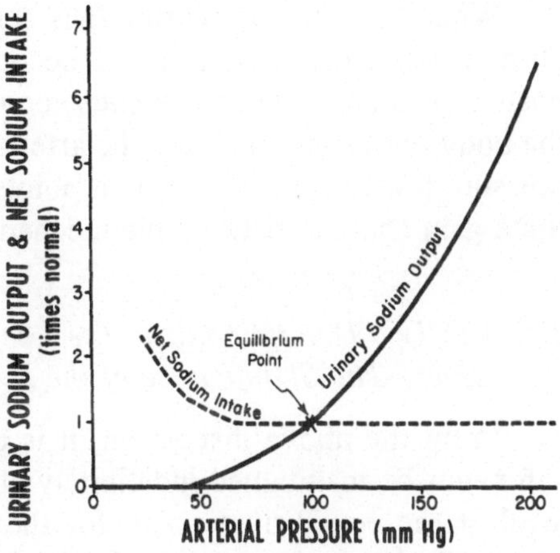

Figure 2. A pressure-analysis diagram; this shows the acute renal function curve for urinary sodium output equating with a curve relating arterial pressure to net sodium intake. The "equilibrium point" is the operating point of the system. (Reprinted from Guyton, 1980.)

the relationship between arterial pressure and urinary sodium output. The second of these curves, the urinary output curve, is called the "renal function curve." For many reasons, which have been well documented, the extracellular fluid volume is determined mainly by the quantity of sodium in the body. Therefore, the balance between sodium intake and output as depicted in this figure can also be considered to represent the balance between fluid volume intake and output as well.

Note in Fig. 2 that the urinary sodium output decreases to zero when the arterial pressure falls into the range between 40 and 60 mm Hg. At the other extreme, sodium output is some six to seven times normal when the arterial pressure rises to about 200 mm Hg. The sodium intake, on the other hand, remains relatively constant, as dictated mainly by a person's dietary habits, except when the pressure falls quite low, where it is said that the shocklike state that develops causes a person to have an increased appetite for salt.

The most important feature of Fig. 2 is that sodium output and sodium intake are in exact balance at only a single arterial pressure level. When the kidneys are functioning normally and the person has a normal intake of salt, this pressure level averages approximately 100 mm Hg, as illustrated in the figure by the point where the two curves intersect, called the "equilibrium point." If the arterial pressure rises above the pressure level of the equilibrium point, the urinary sodium output (and volume output) becomes greater than the intake. Furthermore, this negative sodium balance continues indefinitely until the arterial pressure falls all the way back to the level of the equilibrium point. The fact that the pressure falls all the way back is what is meant by the infinite gain characteristic of the renal blood volume–pressure control system.

When the arterial pressure falls below the pressure level of the equilibrium point, the sodium intake becomes greater than the output. This position sodium balance will cause continued accumulation of sodium in the body until such time that the arterial pressure rises all the way to the pressure level of the equilibrium point. Again, this demonstrates the infinite gain characteristic of the mechanism.

2.2. The Two Determinants of the Long-Term Arterial Pressure Level—The Significance of the Infinite Gain Characteristic

From the above discussion, it is obvious that the arterial pressure can never be maintained indefinitely at a level greater than the pressure level of the equilibrium point, for the continued loss of sodium would eventually bring the pressure back to this level. Likewise, the arterial pressure cannot remain indefinitely at a pressure level below that of the equilibrium point, or otherwise the body would eventually accumulate so much sodium and fluid that the person would die of edema. Therefore, the point of intersection of the two curves in Fig. 2—that is, the equilibrium point—describes absolutely the long-term pressure level that will be attained. From this concept, one can see that there are two basic determinants of the long-term arterial pressure level (Guyton, 1980). These are: (1) the level of salt intake and (2) the degree of shift of the renal function curve along the arterial pressure axis. Thus, if some abnormality of the kidney develops that causes its renal function curve to shift to the right in Fig. 2, then obviously the body sodium, the extracellular fluid volume, the blood volume, and the function of the circulatory system will all change progressively until the pressure rises high enough to achieve sodium balance. However, remember that it takes a number of days and sometimes even several weeks to reach exactly the new pressure level. Therefore, it is easy to understand that this mechanism of pressure control has little to do with hour-by-hour or even day-by-day pressure regulation. Its extreme potency as a pressure controller is manifested in long-term pressure regulation, not in short-term regulation.

2.3. Volume-Loading Hypertension and the Role of "Autoregulation" to Increase Total Peripheral Resistance

When the kidneys retain excess amounts of water and salt, a type of hypertension eventually occurs called "volume-loading hypertension" (Langston et al., 1963; Coleman and Guyton, 1969; Manning et al., 1979). The mechanism of this is the following: first, the extracellular fluid volume increases, and a portion of this increased extracellular fluid remains in the circulation, thus increasing the blood volume as well. The increased blood volume in turn leads to increased venous return and increased cardiac output. The increase in cardiac output obviously increases the pressure.

One might expect from the above sequence of events that volume-loading hypertension would be associated with considerably increased blood volume and cardiac output. However, once the hypertension has become fully established, neither of these two effects is found. Instead, both the blood volume and cardiac output are within the normal ranges; on the other hand, the total peripheral resistance is greatly increased. How could this be possible if the basic reason for the hypertension is retention of sodium and water by the kidneys? To answer this question, let us consider the phenomenon called blood flow "autoregulation."

Blood flow autoregulation means the ability of the local tissues everywhere in the body to control their own blood flows. Studies in individual tissues in almost all parts of the body have demonstrated that when the blood flow in any area of the body becomes too little, the local blood vessels dilate and return the flow back toward normal (Guyton, 1980). Conversely, when the flow becomes too great, the vessels constrict, and this also returns the flow back toward normal. However, like the blood-pressure-regulating mechanisms, blood flow autoregulation does not occur instantaneously. Instead, it occurs in stages, occurring part way within minutes but requiring weeks or months to develop fully.

The first stage of autoregulation, which occurs within minutes, results from contraction or relaxation of the smooth muscle of the arteriolar walls. Local factors such as tissue oxygenation, pH, carbon dixoide concentration, and concentrations of other local substances have all been shown to affect the degree of smooth muscle contraction when they become abnormal. However, the amount of autoregulation that occurs within the first few minutes is probably very small compared to the degree of autoregulation that can occur over a period of weeks or months.

The autoregulation that occurs over weeks or months is called "long-term autoreguation." The best studies on this phenomenon have involved blood flow measurements in patients with coarctation of the aorta (Wakim, 1948; Patterson, 1957). In different studies, the blood flows in the upper extremities of patients with coarctation have been measured to be almost exactly the same as the blood flows in normal persons. Likewise, the blood flows in the lower extremities have also been measured to be almost exactly the same as in normal persons. Yet, the mean arterial pressure in the upper extremities may average as much as 50 to 60% more than the pressure in the lower extremities. Except for this pressure difference, the blood vessels of both the upper and lower extremities are exposed to exactly comparable conditions for all other factors such as oxygenation of the blood, electrolytes in the blood, circulating hormones, and degree of nervous stimulation.

Therefore, we must ask the question, what is it in coarctation of the aorta that causes the blood flows in the local tissues to be so very exactly regulated even though there are marked pressure differences between the upper and lower extremities? At present, the only answer to this is some powerful mechanism of long-term regulation. The best studies on the way that this autoregulation occurs have been those of Folkow and his colleagues (1970, 1971), who have shown in the rat that structural changes in the vascular walls can account for most of the long-term autoregulation. That is, if the pressure is too high, with correspondingly high blood flow, the walls of the arterioles increase in thickness, and their lumens decrease in diameter. At low pressure, exactly the opposite structural changes occur. These structural changes take place over a period of 3 weeks to several months.

Now let us apply the principles of long-term autoregulation to volume-loading hypertension. Figure 3 illustrates typical results from volume-loading hypertension experiments, showing composite curves drawn from data that we have accumulated in a number of experiments over a period of 20 years (Guyton, 1980). Several weeks prior to the onset of the experiment, 70% of the kidney mass had been removed, so that only a portion of one kidney remained. After recovery from the surgery, beginning on day zero in Fig. 3, the animals were placed on a high intake of salt and water, given either by mouth or intravenously. The immediate effect was a marked increase in extracellular fluid volume, blood volume, and cardiac output. The rise in arterial pressure was somewhat slow because the total peripheral resistance decreased during the first few days of the experiment. However, after the first few days, the extracellular fluid volume, blood volume, and cardiac output all began to return back toward normal while the arterial pressure continued to rise to still higher levels. Also, the total peripheral resistance now reversed itself and instead of remaining below normal began to rise far above normal. At the end of 2 weeks, the arterial pressure had increased approximately 40%, and the total peripheral resistance was increased almost as much. On the other hand, the extracellular fluid volume, blood volume, and cardiac output had all returned very near to normal.

But, how does the phenomenon of long-term autoregulation apply to the experiment of Fig. 3? During the first few days of the experiment, the cardiac output rose far above normal while the total peripheral resistance fell below normal. This initial decrease in peripheral resistance was caused mainly by the baroreceptor feedback mechanism that dilated

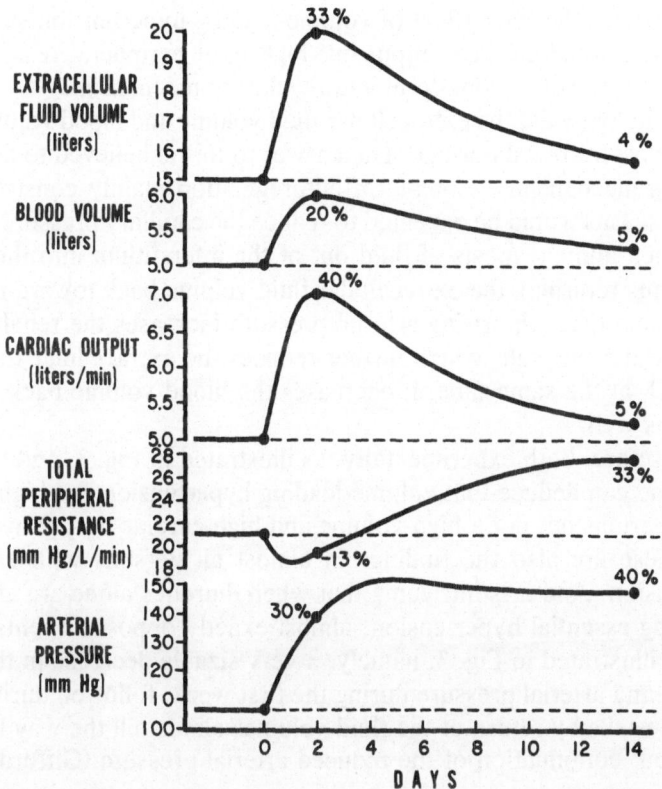

Figure 3. Composite results from a series of volume-loading hypertension experiments show-ing acute increases in extracellular fluid volume, blood volume, and cardiac output but decreased total peripheral resistance at the onset of the hypertension, yet followed by con-version to high total peripheral resistance and normal values for extracellular fluid volume, blood volume, and cardiac output within 2 weeks. (Modified from Guyton, 1980.)

the peripheral arterioles in an attempt to reduce the pressure back toward normal. (In a separate series of experiments the baroreceptors were de-nervated, and the initial decrease in total peripheral resistance did not occur.) At 2 days into the experiment, the cardiac output averaged about 40% above normal. Therefore, the blood flows through the peripheral tissues also average 40% above normal. Since high tissue blood flow is the potent stimulus for activating the long-term autoregulation mecha-nisms, one would expect this to cause a progressive increase in total peripheral resistance, which is what happened. Also, one would expect this increase in resistance to decrease the local blood flows throughout the body back toward normal, thus decreasing the cardiac output back toward normal as well, which is also what happened in the experiments.

Consequently, the final effect of volume-loading hypertension should be an almost normal cardiac output but high total peripheral resistance if there is a very potent long-term autoregulatory mechanism.

Finally, why did the extracellular fluid volume and blood volume also decrease back toward normal? The answer to this is believed to lie in the following mechanisms. Long-term autoregulation mainly constricts the arterioles. This would be expected to reduce the capillary pressure, which would then allow osmosis of fluid out of the interstitium into the circulation, thus returning the extracellular fluid volume back toward normal. At the same time, the rising arterial pressure increases the renal output of both water and salt, which further reduces the extracellular fluid volume, and, at the same time, it decreases the blood volume back toward normal as well.

Therefore, both experimentally, as illustrated in Fig. 3, and theoretically, one can deduce that volume-loading hypertension is a high-resistance hypertension, not a high-volume and high-cardiac-output hypertension. These are also the findings in almost all persons with essential hypertension. And it is intriguing that when diuretics alone are effective in treating essential hypertension, almost exactly opposite events ensue to those illustrated in Fig. 3, namely, a very sizable decrease in the fluid volumes and arterial pressure during the first week, followed during subsequent weeks by return of the fluid volumes almost all the way back to normal but continuation of the reduced arterial pressure (Gifford *et al.*, 1961).

3. The Noncauses of Hypertension: Increased Total Peripheral Resistance, Increased Heart Strength, and Decreased Vascular Capacitance

If one acutely increases the total peripheral resistance or the heart strength, or if one decreases vascular capacitance, any one of these interventions will cause a sudden rise in arterial pressure. Therefore, each of these three interventions has been credited with the capability of causing chronic hypertension. Yet, from our discussions in this chapter, it appears that it is impossible to cause chronic hypertension in any way except by increasing the salt intake or by shifting the renal function curve toward higher pressure levels on the pressure axis. No one of the above three interventions normally affects either the salt intake or the chronic renal function curve. Therefore, the acute elevation of blood pressure caused by any one of these interventions should eventually be corrected by the renal blood volume–pressure control system.

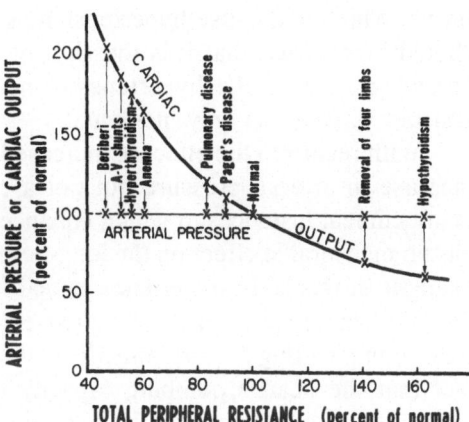

Figure 4. Effect of primary changes in total peripheral resistance on arterial pressure and cardiac output, based on studies in different circulatory abnormalities that change the total peripheral resistance but do not affect the renal function curve. (Reprinted from Guyton, 1980.)

The main question is whether or not this principle is really true. Figure 4 illustrates a test of the principle in the case of total peripheral resistance. This figure shows the effect on both arterial pressure and cardiac output caused by long-term increases or decreases in total peripheral resistance in clinical conditions that do not alter the renal function curve (Guyton, 1980). Note that the arterial pressure remains at the normal level in all of the conditions regardless of the abnormal total peripheral resistances. On the other hand, the cardiac output in each condition is inversely proportional to the total peripheral resistance. Thus, long-term changes in total peripheral resistance (when these do not cause a simultaneous change in the renal function curve) affect the cardiac output, not the arterial pressure.

If an increase in total peripheral resistance does not cause hypertension, why is it that almost all patients with hypertension have increased total peripheral resistance? We have already discussed one of the reasons for this, namely, the effect of the autoregulatory mechanism to convert a volume-loading type of hypertension from a high-cardiac-output hypertension to a high-total-resistance hypertension. In this case, the increase in total peripheral resistance is secondary to the development of the hypertension and not the primary cause of the hypertension. But still another mechanism that can cause a high total peripheral resistance in hypertension is the following: when generalized vasoconstriction occurs everywhere in the body, as might occur with increased sympathetic nervous tone or a circulating vasoconstrictor agent, the vasoconstriction often increases both the total peripheral resistance and the intrarenal vascular resistance at the same time. In turn, the increased intrarenal resistance will usually shift the renal function curve toward higher pressure levels, which will cause hypertension as already explained. However, it should be realized that it is the shift of the renal function curve that is crucial in causing the hypertension, not the increased total peripheral resistance, which is only incidental.

With regard to the effect of increased heart strength to cause an acute increase in arterial pressure but not a chronic increase, there are also many clinical instances in which enhanced pumping strength of the heart has no measurable effect on the long-term arterial pressure level. A prime example of this is the experience gained from cardiac operations in which the heart pumping capacity is increased greatly. Except when there are other complicating factors, this does not cause hypertension despite the fact that the heart's pumping capacity might be increased as much as several hundred percent by the operation.

Finally, a clinical example in which total vascular capacitance is greatly decreased is surgical removal of extensive varicose veins or even the putting of tight binders on the legs to occlude great masses of varicose veins. Neither of these procedures causes chronic hypertension. Nor does delivery of a baby from a pregnant mother cause hypertension, which is another instance in which the vascular capacitance is greatly diminished.

In essence, therefore, some of the circulatory interventions that are well known to cause acute elevation of blood pressure will not cause chronic hypertension if they do not affect the pressure level of the renal function curve. The reason for this is that the renal blood volume–pressure control system can fully compensate for the acute hypertension caused by these factors. Therefore, perhaps the most significant importance of the infinite gain characteristic of the renal blood volume–pressure control system is that, over the long term, it can compensate fully for the pressure effects of changes in total peripheral resistance, heart strength, and vascular capacitance.

4. The Chronic Salt-Loading Renal Function Curve

From the above discussion of the renal blood volume–pressure control system, one would expect that a greatly increased salt intake would lead to greatly increased blood volume and therefore also cause greatly increased arterial pressure. However, in a normal person this does not occur. Let us explain this, beginning with the results illustrated in Fig. 5. This figure shows two different renal function curves, (1) the *acute renal function curve*, which is the same as the curve illustrated in Fig. 2, and (2) the "chronic salt-loading renal function curve." The chronic salt-loading renal function curve was determined in the following way (DeClue

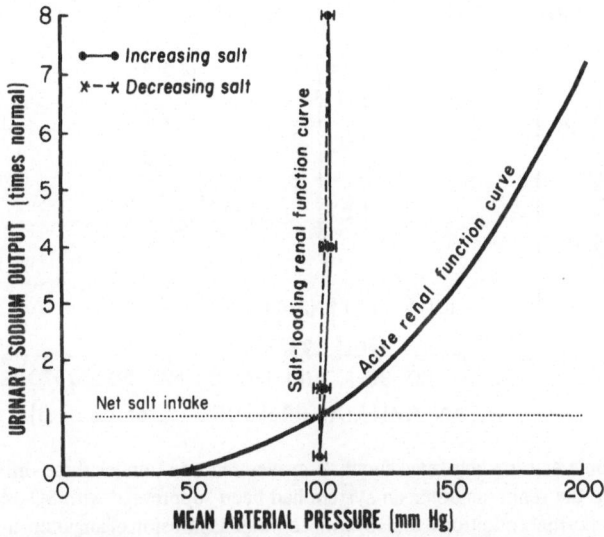

Figure 5. Comparison of the acute renal function curve and the chronic salt-loading renal function curve determined by loading an animal with salt at different rates of intake for several days at a time. (Explained in the text.) (Modified from Guyton, 1980.)

et al., 1978): dogs were given salt solution by intravenous infusion at different rates, beginning at a very low rate equivalent to about one-eighth the normal daily rate of sodium intake and increasing in steps to about ten times the normal intake, a total change of about 80-fold. The rate of salt intake was maintained at each step for approximately 3 days, at the end of which time both the arterial pressure and the urinary output had reached stable values. At the end of the experiment, arterial pressure and sodium outputs were plotted for all of the separate levels of salt intake to determine the chronic salt-loading renal function curve. The two almost parallel curves were for (1) increasing levels of salt intake followed by (2) decreasing levels. The almost exact correspondence between the two curves illustrates the stability of the results.

The question raised by the results of Fig. 5 is the following: Why is the chronic salt-loading renal function curve so vastly different from the acute renal function curve? In the case of the acute renal function curve, all other factors besides arterial pressure were exactly controlled, and arterial pressure was the only independent variable in determining the curve. In the case of chronic salt loading, the arterial pressure rose very little, so that the rise in pressure was only part of the cause of the increased sodium output. Instead, several other effects of the increased salt intake undoubtedly were responsible for most of the increase in sodium output.

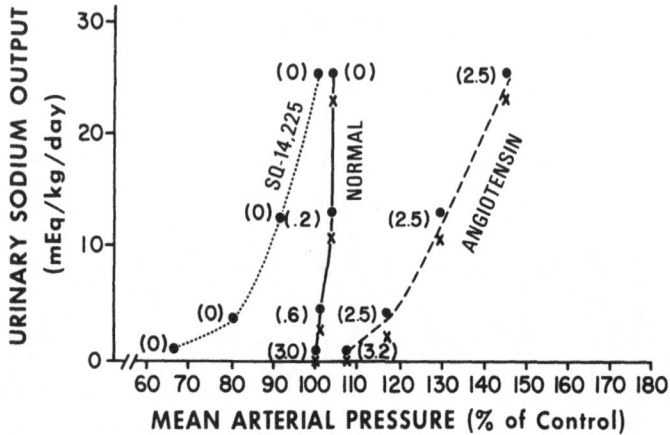

Figure 6. Chronic salt-loading renal function curves recorded under three different conditions: (1) when the renin–angiotensin system had been suppressed with SQ-14,225 (captopril), (2) under normal conditions, and (3) with continuous infusion of angiotensin. The values in parentheses are calculated levels of circulating angiotensin in relation to a normal value of 1.0. (Reprinted from Guyton, 1980.)

Therefore, the steepness of the chronic salt-loading renal function curve is determined not only by the direct relationship of urinary sodium output to arterial pressure but also by several other simultaneously occurring factors as well. One of these is the effect of the renin–angiotensin system to shift the acute renal function curve along the arterial pressure axis, as is explained in the next section.

4.1. Role of the Renin–Angiotensin System to Shift the Acute Renal Function Curve and to Steepen the Chronic Salt-Loading Renal Function Curve

Figure 6 illustrates three different salt-loading renal function curves recorded under different conditions. The quantitative values in parentheses represent calculated levels of circulating angiotensin, with the normal circulating level considered to have a value of 1.0. The centralmost curve is the same as the chronic salt-loading renal function curve of Fig. 5. The curve to the right was recorded in exactly the same manner as the central curve except that during the several weeks required to record this curve the animals received a continuous infusion of angiotensin at a rate equal to approximately two and one-half times the normal rate of angiotensin formation in the circulation (DeClue *et al.*, 1978). The left-hand curve was also measured in the same way except that this time the dogs were subjected to continuous infusion of the converting enzyme inhibitor captopril (SQ-14,225) to block the renal effects of the angiotensin system (Hall *et al.*, 1980). Note specifically that while the converting enzyme inhibitor was being infused, the level of circulating angiotensin was calculated to be zero and to remain at that level for the entire curve. Conversely, when angiotensin was infused continuously, the circulating level of angiotensin was calculated to remain near 2.5 times normal. In either instance, the level of angiotensin did not change significantly during the course of recording each curve. In the case of each of these curves, a considerable increase in arterial pressure was associated with the rising sodium output. In other words, when the angiotensin did not change, salt loading had a considerable effect on arterial pressure.

Now, let us compare the centralmost curve with the other two curves. In the normal animals, massive salt loading greatly depressed the renin–angiotensin system, so that no circulating renin could be measured at the top point on the "normal" curve. Therefore, the angiotensin was calculated to be zero at that point because the renin measurements were too low to measure. Note also that the top point on the "normal" curve coincides almost exactly with the top point on the SQ-14,225 curve, for which the calculated angiotensin was also zero. On the other hand, at the very lowest sodium output level, the animals secreted considerable amounts of renin, and from these measured levels, the circulating angiotensin was calculated to be approximately three times normal. Now, note that the bottom point of the "normal" curve coincides very closely with the bottom point of the "angiotensin" curve, for which the level of circulating angiotensin was also calculated to be very near to three times normal.

Therefore, one can see that much of the effect to steepen the normal renal function curve is caused by a feedback effect of the renin–angiotensin system to shift the acute renal function curve along the pressure axis. That is, at high salt intake levels, the turn-off of the renin–angiotensin system shifts the top of the normal renal function curve far to the left. At low salt intakes, on the other hand, the strong stimulation of the renin–angiotensin system shifts the bottom of the renal function curve far to the right. Thus, the feedback effects of the renin–angiotensin system seem to be the major factor that makes the chronic salt-loading renal function curve very steep in comparison with the acute renal function curve.

4.2. Other Factors That Steepen the Chronic Salt-Loading Renal Function Curve

Still other factors besides the renin–angiotensin system can shift the bottom of the chronic renal function curve to the right and the top to the left. One of these is the effect of aldosterone on renal function (Pan *et al.*, 1982). When sodium intake is low, aldosterone is secreted in increased quantities. This causes the kidneys to retain increased quantities of salt and water, which therefore shifts the low end of the chronic salt-loading renal function curve to the right. Conversely, when the person eats large quantities of salt, the rate of aldosterone secretion decreases to very little. Then the kidneys retain far less salt and water, so that the top of the curve shifts to the left.

Likewise, feedback mechanisms involving the sympathetic nervous system, the vasopressin system, and perhaps still other yet uncharted factors might become activated with changing salt intakes to steepen the renal function curve. The obvious advantage of having a very steep chronic salt-loading renal function curve is that this allows a person to subsist on either a very low salt intake or a very high salt intake without this having a significant effect on the arterial pressure. In fact, experiments on human beings have shown that so long as the kidneys function normally, changes in salt intake of more than 100-fold affect the arterial pressure no more than 10 to 20 mm Hg (Murray *et al.*, 1978). This is not true, however, when the various feedback control mechanisms discussed above that steepen the chronic salt-loading renal function curve are no longer operative, and it also is not true in certain pathological conditions of the kidneys, as we shall see in the following section.

4.3. Use of the Chronic Salt-Loading Renal Function Curve to Analyze Different Types of Hypertension

Although it would be desirable to measure the acute renal function curve in each type of renal abnormality and then to use this acute curve in predicting the effect of the abnormality on the arterial pressure, this is not feasible because it is almost impossible to measure the acute renal function curve in the intact animal or human being. On the other hand, measuring the chronic salt-loading renal function curve is a very simple procedure, requiring only that the animal or person ingest salt at different levels of intake for several days at each level and then to plot the rates of intake (which, after several days, equals the output) against the measured values of arterial pressure.

Figure 7 illustrates a "pressure-analysis diagram" from which arterial pressures can be predicted in different conditions of abnormal renal function and at different levels of salt intake. It shows a number of different patterns of chronic salt-loading renal function curves that have been determined in different conditions, and it also shows two different levels of

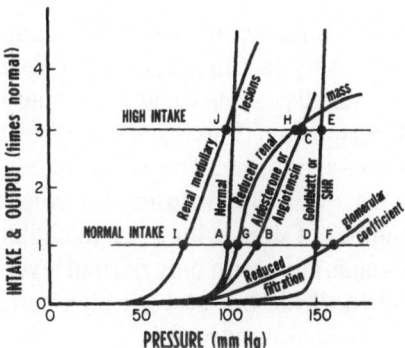

Figure 7. A pressure-analysis diagram showing chronic salt-loading renal function curves for several different abnormal functional states of the kidneys and also showing these curves equating at different equilibrium points with both normal and high sodium intake curves. (Reprinted from Guyton, 1980.)

salt intake, (1) normal intake and (2) high intake (Guyton, 1980). Some of the specific analyses using this diagram are the following.

When the kidneys are normal, as represented by the "normal" curve, and the salt intake level is also normal, the long-term arterial pressure equilibrates at point A, which represents the normal pressure. If one then follows the "normal" curve upward to the high salt intake level, he sees that increasing the salt intake has little effect on the pressure.

Some of the abnormal renal function curves are shifted along the pressure axis, and some of them have greatly reduced slopes. In two conditions, Goldblatt hypertension and spontaneous hypertension in the rat, the renal function curve is shifted to very high pressure levels along the pressure axis, but the slope remains mainly unchanged. Thus, in Fig. 7 it is shown that in either of these types of hypertension, when the animal has a normal salt intake, the pressure might be about 150 mm Hg, as represented by point D in the curve. If the curve is traced upward to the high intake level, the pressure level now is represented by point E, which is hardly any further increase in pressure. Thus, these two types of hypertension are said to be "non-salt-sensitive."

On the other hand, many types of hypertension are very "salt sensitive." This occurs when the slope of the chronic salt-loading renal function curve is diminished, as illustrated by the curve labeled "aldosterone or angiotensin" and even more so by the curve labeled "reduced glomerular filtration coefficient." In each of these instances, increasing the salt intake causes marked increase in arterial pressure. In other words, the homeostatic feedback mechanisms that steepen the chronic salt-loading function curve are mainly inoperative in these conditions.

With reduced renal mass but normal salt intake, the arterial pressure is predicted by point G in Fig. 7, which depicts only a slight rise in pressure above the normal. Yet, when the subject is exposed to high salt intake, the pressure rises to point H, which represents a large increase in pressure. Thus, a combination of reduced renal mass plus high salt intake is very likely to cause serious hypertension.

Finally, some renal abnormalities can cause hypotension rather than hypertension. For instance, renal medullary lesions can lead to a salt-losing syndrome. The renal function curve labeled "renal medullary lesions" was drawn from anecdotal data recorded in our laboratory in a number of dogs with renal medullary lesions. It is difficult to keep these animals alive with only normal levels of salt intake because their pressures fall too low, but at very high salt intakes their pressures can often be maintained at normal levels.

In summary, chronic salt-loading renal function curves measured in abnormal renal states can be used in pressure-analysis diagrams of the type illustrated in Fig. 7 to predict the long-term arterial pressure level by equating the function curves with lines representing the salt intake levels.

5. Role of the Kidneys in Essential Hypertension

It is often stated that the kidneys play little role in the genesis of essential hypertension. The principal reason for this contention has been that in the early to midstages of essential hypertension renal excretory function is usually quite normal. However, critical measurements have shown several renal hemodynamic abnormalities in essential hypertension even though urinary output is not at all compromised (Kolsters *et al.*, 1975). Some of the abnormalities are the following. First, the vascular resistance is increased several times as much in the kidneys as in the other areas of the body. Second, the filtration fraction is greatly increased in almost all patients who have essential hypertension; this suggests that the renal resistance is increased in both pre- and postglomerular renal vessels. Third, by the time the patient develops severe essential hypertension, the renal blood flow is usually decreased to less than 60% of normal. Fourth, when the arterial pressure in a person who has essential hypertension is decreased to a normal level, as frequently occurs during surgical operations or following blood loss, the urinary output is greatly decreased. To state this another way, the kidneys of the patient with essential hypertension require a very high renal arterial pressure if they are to provide normal urinary output.

Therefore, there is much reason to believe that from the very beginning in essential hypertension the kidneys function abnormally. However, we do not know what causes the abnormal function. This could result from pathology in the kidneys themselves, especially pathological in-

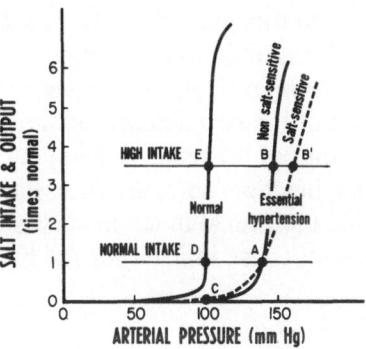

Figure 8. Chronic salt-loading function curves in "non-salt-sensitive" essential hypertension and in "salt-sensitive" essential hypertension compared with the normal salt-loading renal function curve. Note that both of the essential hypertension curves are shifted to higher pressure levels. (Reprinted from Guyton, 1980.)

crease in preglomerular vascular resistance or reduced glomerular filtration coefficient. Both of these effects have been found in the spontaneously hypertensive rat in which the hypertension has characteristics very similar to those in essential hypertension (Evan *et al.*, 1979; Gothberg *et al.*, 1979). Yet, it is also possible that the abnormal renal function results from some factor extrinsic to the kidneys, which might include vasoconstrictor agents, agents that cause increased tubular reabsorption of electrolytes and water, or nervous stimulation of the renal vasculature. Thus far, none of these factors has been proved to exist in the great majority of essential hypertension patients, which leads one to suspect that essential hypertension is basically caused by intrinsic renal pathology.

To illustrate once again the principle of analyzing long-term pressure regulation, Fig. 8 illustrates a pressure-analysis diagram for essential hypertension. Two different chronic salt-loading renal function curves are illustrated to represent different types of essential hypertensive patients. One of these is a steep curve, and the other is more of a sloping curve, but both are shifted far to the right along the pressure axis. In both instances, the mean arterial pressure is shown to be approximately 135 mm Hg when the salt intake is normal, as illustrated by equilibrium point A in the diagram. At high salt intake, the essential hypertensive patient with the steep salt-loading renal function curve has a pressure designated by point B, which is hardly changed from the pressure at point A. Therefore, this person is said to have "non-salt-sensitive" essential hypertension. On the other hand, in the hypertensive patient whose renal function curve has a decreased slope, the pressure increases about 20 mm Hg during salt loading, representing a "salt-sensitive" type of essential hypertension. The principles illustrated in Fig. 8 are approximately the same as those demonstrated with actual measurements by Bartter and his colleagues (Kawasaki *et al.*, 1978) in essential hypertensive patients whose pressures were studied at different levels of salt loading.

In summary, the chronic salt-loading renal function curves of patients with essential hypertension are shifted far to the right along the arterial pressure axis. Remembering from earlier discussions in this chapter that one of the two determinants of arterial pressure regulation is the degree of shift of the renal function curve, one can conclude that the kidneys do not function normally in essential hypertension. Furthermore, the fact that their renal function curves are shifted toward higher pressure is sufficient cause in itself for the hypertension.

6. Summary

The kidney has two primary mechanisms for pressure control, the renin–angiotensin–vasoconstrictor mechanism and the kidney blood volume–pressure control system. The second of these has a special feature called the "infinite gain" characteristic. This characteristic gives the kidney blood volume–pressure control system extreme potency for controlling the long-term arterial pressure level. In fact, it allows this mechanism to override, over the long term, the pressure effects caused by changes in heart strength, total peripheral resistance, or vascular capacitance, for which reason these factors have no effect on the long-term arterial pressure level unless some parallel effect simultaneously alters the function of the kidney blood volume–pressure control system. Instead, the long-term arterial pressure level is determined mainly by the degree of shift of the chronic salt-loading renal function curve (that relates urinary sodium output to arterial pressure) along the pressure axis.

Studies on volume-loading hypertension have shown that the acute phase of this type of hypertension is characterized by high blood volume, high cardiac output, and low total peripheral resistance. However, after about 2 weeks, the characteristics convert to high total peripheral resistance but essentially normal cardiac output and blood volume. The only mechanism presently know that could cause these conversions is the long-term blood flow autoregulation mechanism.

Recent studies in patients with essential hypertension have shown a number of renal abnormalities, including (1) extremely great increase in renal vascular resistance, (2) very high filtration fraction, and (3) especially a marked shift of the chronic salt-loading renal function curve toward high pressure levels.

References

Bright, R., 1836, Tabular view of the morbid appearances in 100 cases connected with albuminous urine. With observations, *Guys Hosp. Rep.* **1**:380.

Brough, R. B., Cowley, A. W., and Guyton, A. C., 1975, Quantitative analysis of the acute response to hemorrhage of the renin–angiotensin–vasoconstrictor feedback loop in areflexic dogs, *Cardiovasc. Res.* **9**:722.

Coleman, T. G., and Guyton, A. C., 1969, Hypertension caused by salt loading in the dog. III. Onset transients of cardiac output and other circulatory variables. *Circ. Res.* **25**:153.

DeClue, J. W., Guyton, A. C., Cowley, A. W., Jr., Coleman, T. G., Norman, R. A., Jr., and McCaa, R. E., 1978, Subpressor angiotensin infusion, renal sodium handling, and salt-induced hypertension in the dog. *Circ. Res.* **43**:503.

Evan, A. P., Luft, F. C., Gattone, V., Connors, B. A., McCarron, D. A., and Willis, L. R., 1981, The glomerular filtration barrier in the spontaneously hypertensive rat, *Hypertenion* **3**:I-154.

Folkow, B., Hallback, M., Lundgren, Y., and Weiss, L., 1970, Structurally based increase of flow resistance in spontaneously hypertensive rats, *Acta Physiol. Scand.* **79**:373.

Folkow, B., Gurevich, M., Hallback, M., Lundgren, Y., and Weiss, L., 1971, The hemodynamic consequences of regional hypotension in spontaneously hypertensive and normotensive rats, *Acta Physiol. Scand.* **83**:532.

Gifford, R. W., Jr., Mattox, V. R., Orvis, A. L., Sones, D. A., and Rosevear, J. U., 1961, Effect of thiazide diuretics on plasma volume, body electrolytes, and excretion of aldosterone in hypertension, *Circulation* **24**:1197.

Göthberg, G., Lundin, S., Ricksten, S. E., and Folkow, B., 1979, Apparent and true vascular resistances to flow in SHR and NCR kidneys as related to the pre/post-glomerular resistance ratio, *Acta Physiol. Scand.* **105**:282.

Guyton, A. C., 1980, *Arterial Pressure and Hypertension*, W. B. Saunders, Philadelphia.

Hall, J. E., Guyton, A. C., Smith, M. J., Jr., and Coleman, T. G., 1980, Long-term regulation of arterial pressure, glomerular filtration, and renal sodium reabsorption by angiotensin II in dogs, *Clin. Sci.* **59**(Suppl.):87.

Kawasaki, T., Delea, C. S., Bartter, F. C., and Smith, H., 1978, The effect of high-sodium and low-sodium intakes on blood pressure and other related variables in human subjects with idiopathic hypertension, *Am. J. Med.* **64**:193.

Kolsters, G., Schalekamp, M. A. D. H., Birkenhager, and Lever, A. F., 1975, Renin and renal function in benign essential hypertension: Evidence for a renal abnormality, in *Pathophysiology and Management of Arterial Hypertension* (G. Berglund, L. Hansson, and L. Werko, eds.), A. Lindgren & Soner AB, Molndal, Sweden, p. 54.

Kreiger, E. M., 1970, Time course of baroreceptor resetting in acute hypertension, *Am. J. Physiol.* **218**:486.

Langston, J. B., Guyton, A. C., Douglas, B. H., and Dorsett, P. E., 1963, Effect of changes in salt intake on arterial pressure and renal function in nephrectomized dogs, *Circ. Res.* **12**:508.

Manning, R. D., Jr., Coleman, T. G., Guyton, A. C., Norman, R. A., Jr., and McCaa, R. E., 1979, Essential role of mean circulatory filling pressure in salt-induced hypertenion, *Am. J. Physiol.* **236**:R40.

McCubbin, J. W., Green, J. H., and Page, I. H., 1956, Baroreceptor function in chronic renal hypertension, *Circ. Res.* **4**:205.

Murray, R. H., Luft, F. C., Bloch, R., and Weyman, A. E., 1978, Blood pressure responses to extremes of sodium intake in normal man, *Proc. Soc. Exp. Biol. Med.* **159**:432.

Pan, Y.-J., and Young, D. B., 1982, Experimental aldosterone hypertension in the dog, *Hypertension* **4**:279.

Patterson, G. C., Shepherd, J. T., and Whelan, R. F., 1957, The resistance to blood flow in the upper and lower limb vessels in patients with coarctation of the aorta, *Clin. Sci.* **16**:627.

Selkurt, E. E., Hall, P. W., and Spencer, M. P., 1949, Influence of graded arterial pressure decrement on renal clearance of creatinine, p-amino hippurate and sodium, *Am. J. Physiol.* **159**:369.

Shipley, R. E., and Study, R. S., 1951, Changes in renal blood flow, extraction of inulin, glomerular filtration rate, tissue pressure, and urine flow with acute alterations of renal artery blood pressure, *Am. J. Physiol.* **167**:676.

Thompson, D. D., and Pitts, R. F., 1952, Effects of alterations of renal arterial pressure on sodium and water excretion, *Am. J. Physiol.* **168**:490.

Wakim, K. G., Slaughter, O., and Clagett, O. T., 1948, Studies on the blood flow in the extremities in cases of coarctation of the aorta: Determination before and after excision of the coarctate region, *Proc. Mayo Clin.* **23**:347.

12

Molecular Mechanisms of Vasodilatation

LOUIS J. IGNARRO, CARL A. GRUETTER,
ALBERT L. HYMAN, and PHILIP J. KADOWITZ

1. Introduction

The mechanisms by which chemical substances relax vascular smooth muscle have received considerable attention in recent years. These vasodilators include β-adrenergic receptor agonists, muscarinic receptor agonists, dopamine receptor agonists, certain autacoids, calcium antagonists, nucleosides, nucleotides, and nitrogen oxide-containing agents. This chapter deals primarily with the latter agents, which include organic nitrates and nitrites, inorganic nitrites, nitroso compounds, S-nitrosothiols, and nitric oxide.

The likely involvement of cAMP in modulating the vasodilatory action of β-adrenoceptor agonists stems from the experimental fulfillment of the original criteria suggested by Sutherland and his colleagues for establishing a second messenger role for cAMP in a given cellular function. Recent studies in this laboratory have provided evidence that cAMP is also involved in the relaxant responses of intrapulmonary artery and vein to isoproterenol (Edwards et al., 1984). Cyclic AMP is also linked to the relaxant actions of adenosine (Kukovetz et al., 1978, 1979a) and prostacyclin (Kukovetz et al., 1979b). Moreover, cAMP itself directly relaxes vascular smooth muscle (Robison et al., 1968; Schultz et al., 1979; Napoli et al., 1980).

LOUIS J. IGNARRO, CARL A. GRUETTER, ALBERT L. HYMAN, and PHILIP J. KADOWITZ • Departments of Pharmacology and Surgery, Tulane University School of Medicine, New Orleans, Louisiana 70112. Present address of C.A.G.: Department of Pharmacology, Marshall University School of Medicine, Huntington, West Virginia 25701.

Until recently, the vasodilatory effects of organic nitrates and nitrites had been widely attributed to a "direct" interaction with smooth muscle. This knowledge, or lack of it, epitomized our paucity of information on these drugs. We have recently referred to this class of so-called "direct acting" vasodilators as nitrogen oxide-containing vasodilators (Ignarro *et al.*, 1981a). The latter chemical classification is more appropriate because the term "direct acting" implies an interaction between vasodilator and some unknown receptor, which is no longer considered to be the case. Prior to recent reports from this laboratory that methylene blue specifically antagonizes the relaxant effect of nitrogen oxide-containing drugs, no antagonist of these drugs was known (Gruetter *et al.*, 1979, 1980, 1981b).

The first clue that cGMP might be involved in smooth muscle relaxation developed in 1975, when sodium azide, hydroxylamine, and sodium nitrite were reported to elevate tissue levels of cGMP and to activate soluble guanylate cyclase (Kimura *et al.*, 1975a,b; Katsuki *et al.*, 1977). Subsequently, Diamond and colleagues showed that nitroglycerin elevated cGMP levels in rat myometrium and canine femoral artery (Diamond and Holmes, 1975; Diamond and Blisard, 1976). Schultz *et al.* (1977) reported that sodium nitroprusside markedly increased cGMP levels in rat ductus deferens independently of calcium. Similarly, Katsuki and Murad (1977) showed that nitroglycerin, sodium nitrosprusside, and related agents increased cGMP levels in, and relaxed, bovine tracheal smooth muscle. In addition, elevated tissue cGMP levels accompanied relaxation of ductus deferens (Bohme *et al.*, 1978), mesenteric artery (Axelsson *et al.*, 1979), taenia coli (Janis and Diamond, 1979), and coronary artery (Gruetter *et al.*, 1981a; Ignarro *et al.*, 1981a) elicited by nitrogen oxide-containing smooth muscle relaxants. Phosphodiesterase inhibitors elevated cyclic nucleotide levels in pig coronary artery and caused relaxation as well (Kramer and Wells, 1979).

Prior to the gradual accumulation of evidence relating cGMP to smooth muscle relaxation, however, cGMP was implicated in contraction. Muscarinic receptor agonists, autacoids, and related agents contracted smooth muscle and elevated cGMP levels (Lee *et al.*, 1972; Schultz *et al.*, 1973; Dunham *et al.*, 1974; Andersson *et al.*, 1975; Clyman *et al.*, 1975). Both cellular events were calcium dependent, but contraction preceded the increase in tissue cGMP levels. Spies *et al.* (1980) suggested that cGMP accumulation in contracting smooth muscle could be the result of indirect effects of intracellular calcium on guanylate cyclase. Calcium-mediated increases in smooth muscle levels of cGMP could conceivably lead to accelerated removal of calcium from contractile proteins (Schultz *et al.*, 1973) and decreased tension. Indeed, Kukovetz *et al.* (1981) demonstrated that acetylcholine-elicited accumulation of coronary arterial cGMP was inhibited by methylene blue, which concomitantly enhanced contraction. Moreover, inhibition of cGMP phosphodiesterase activity enhanced cGMP accumulation and reduced the contractile response to acetylcholine (Kukovetz *et al.*, 1981). These observations are consistent with the hypothesis that cGMP may be associated with vascular smooth muscle relaxation.

The objective of this chapter is to provide a brief account of our experimental observations that address the physiological and pharmacological roles of cGMP in vasodilatation.

2. *Vasodilator Actions of Nitric Oxide and Nitrosoamines*

Studies from our laboratory first demonstrated the potent vascular smooth muscle relaxant properties of nitric oxide and nitrosoguanidines. The principal objective of these initial studies was to ascertain whether chemical agents known to activate soluble guanylate cyclase also relax vascular smooth muscle. The rationale for this objective was that if sodium nitroprusside, which releases nitric oxide, activates guanylate cyclase, then nitric oxide should elicit relaxation. Moreover, nitrosoguanidines, which are unstable and release nitric oxide, should also relax vascular smooth muscle because they activate guanylate cyclase.

2.1. *Nitric Oxide*

The lipophilic and unstable gas nitric oxide is a potent relaxant of bovine coronary artery (Gruetter *et al.*, 1979) and intrapulmonary artery and vein (unpublished observations). Figure 1 illustrates the transient relaxant effect of nitric oxide on bovine coronary artery. In contrast, relaxant responses to sodium nitroprusside and nitroglycerin are of much longer duration (Gruetter *et al.*, 1979, 1981a). Since hemoproteins had been shown to inhibit guanylate cyclase activation by nitric oxide and related agents (Miki *et al.*, 1977; Murad *et al.*, 1978; Gruetter *et al.*, 1979), three hemoproteins were tested for their capacity to antagonize the relaxant response to nitric oxide (Fig. 1). Hemoproteins have a very high affinity for nitric oxide and react with the latter to form relatively stable nitrosyl-hemoprotein complexes. Thus, nitric oxide becomes unavailable to interact with the smooth muscle, and the relaxant response is lost.

Oxidizing agents such as ferricyanide and methylene blue also inhibit activation of guanylate cyclase by nitric oxide and nitroso compounds (Katsuki *et al.*, 1977; Arnold *et al.*, 1977a; Gruetter *et al.*, 1979). Meth-

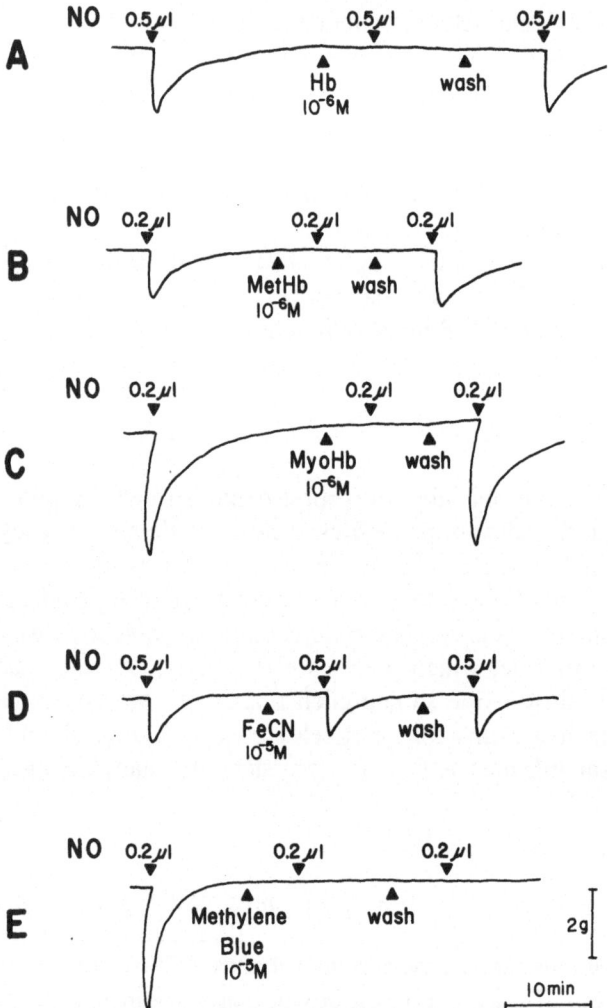

Figure 1. Effects of hemoglobin (Hb, panel A), methemoglobin (MetHb, panel B), myoglobin (MyoHb, panel C), potassium ferricyanide (FeCN, panel D), and methylene blue (panel E) on relaxation of KCl-precontracted strips of bovine coronary artery elicited by nitric oxide (NO). All concentrations are expressed as final bath concentrations. (Reproduced with permission from Gruetter *et al.*, 1979.)

ylene blue irreversibly antagonized relaxation by nitric oxide, although ferricyanide was ineffective (Fig. 1). A major difference between these two oxidants is that whereas methylene blue crosses cell membranes (vital biological stain), ferricyanide (highly charged) does not. Therefore, methylene blue likely elicits its antagonizing action in the intracellular com-

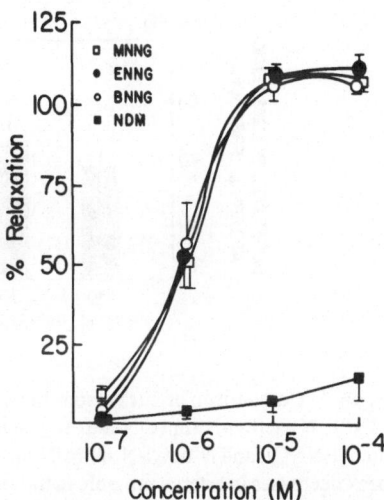

Figure 2. Concentration–response curves for relaxation of KCl-precontracted strips of bovine coronary artery elicited by N-methyl-N'-nitro-N-nitrosoguanidine (MNNG), N-ethyl-N'-nitro-N-nitrosoguanidine (ENNG), N-butyl-N'-nitro-N-nitrosoguanidine (BNNG), and N-nitrosodimethylamine (NDM). Relaxation is expressed as percentage decrease of induced tone. (Reproduced with permission from Lippton *et al.*, 1982.)

partment, to which ferricyanide is inaccessible. This interpretation supposes that nitric oxide must enter smooth muscle cells in order to elicit relaxation.

2.2. Nitrosoamines

Carcinogenic nitrosoamines such as N-methyl-N'-nitro-N-nitrosoguanidine (MNNG) are unstable, particularly in the presence of free sulfhydryls, and release nitric oxide and other reactive species (Schoental and Rive, 1965; McCalla *et al.*, 1968; Schulz and McCalla, 1969; Lawley and Thatcher, 1970; Kawachi *et al.*, 1979; Wheeler and Bowdon, 1972; Ignarro *et al.*, 1980a,b). We reported (Gruetter *et al.*, 1979) that MNNG relaxes coronary arteries and that that relaxation is antagonized by methylene blue. Similarly, the N-ethyl and N-butyl derivatives of N'-nitro-N-nitrosoguanidine caused relaxation (Fig. 2) and activated coronary arterial guanylate cyclase (Lippton *et al.*, 1982). The more stable N-nitrosodimethylamine, however, was much less active. Cigarette smoke, which contains considerable quantities of nitric oxide (Neurath *et al.*, 1976), activated guanylate cyclase and elevated tissue levels of cGMP (Arnold *et al.*, 1977b). We confirmed these observations and showed that cigarette smoke markedly relaxes bovine coronary artery (Gruetter *et al.*, 1980). Moreover, the tobacco-specific nitrosamide N'-nitrosonornicotine also caused relaxation and guanylate cyclase activation. Both effects of cigarette smoke and N'-nitrosonornicotine were inhibited by methylene blue (Gruetter *et al.*, 1980).

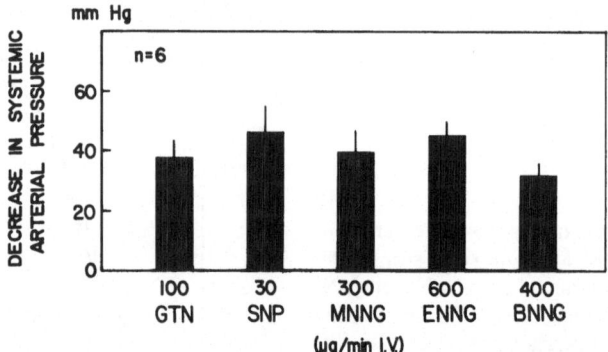

Figure 3. Comparison of intravenous infusions of nitroglycerin (GTN), sodium nitroprusside (SNP), N-methyl-N'-nitro-N-nitrosoguanidine (MNNG), N-ethyl-N'-nitro-N-nitrosoguanidine (ENNG), and N-butyl-N'-nitro-N-nitrosoguanidine (BNNG) at rates that elicited similar peak decreases in arterial pressure in the anesthetized cat during a 5-min intravenous infusion period. Results are expressed as mean ± SE; *n* = number of animals studied. (Reproduced with permission from Lippton *et al.*, 1982.)

Intravenous injections of nitrosoguanidines caused a dose-dependent decrease in systemic arterial pressure in the anesthetized cat (Fig. 3). Intravenous infusions of the nitrosoguanidines, as well as nitroglycerin and sodium nitroprusside, produced no effect on cardiac output at peak decreases in aortic pressure, indicating that a reduction in systemic vascular resistance had occurred (Lippton *et al.*, 1982). Moreover, intraarterial injections of nitrosoguanidines elicited dose-dependent decreases in perfusion pressure in the feline mesenteric vascular bed perfused at constant flow (Lippton *et al.*, 1982).

2.3. Conclusions

Collectively, these studies illustrate the vascular smooth muscle relaxant properties of nitric oxide, N-nitrosoamines, and N-nitrosamides. The latter compounds likely elicit relaxation by releasing nitric oxide (see next section). An excellent correlation was consistently found between the capacity of these compounds to relax vascular smooth muscle and to activate soluble guanylate cyclase. In addition, methylene blue antagonized both relaxation and enzyme activation by these chemical agents.

3. Nitric Oxide as an Intermediate of the Nitrogen-Oxide-Containing Vasodilators

Previous studies on guanylate cyclase activation by nitroso compounds, nitrites, azide, and hydroxylamine led to the development of the hypothesis that nitric oxide is responsible for enzyme activation by the former agents (Kimura *et al.*, 1975a,b; DeRubertis and Craven, 1976; Arnold *et al.*, 1977a; Katsuki *et al.*, 1977; Craven and DeRubertis, 1978; Murad *et al.*, 1978). Subsequent studies for this laboratory revealed the direct release of nitric oxide from various nitrogen oxide-containing substances (Ignarro *et al.*, 1980a,b). The release of nitric oxide from solutions of certain nitrosoguanidines had already been known (Schoental and Rive, 1965; McCalla *et al.*, 1968; Schulz and McCalla, 1969; Lawley and Thatcher, 1970). In view of the instability of solutions of nitrogen oxide-containing vasodilators and the knowledge that nitric oxide is a potent stimulant of cGMP formation, the hypothesis was offered that nitric oxide may mediate the vascular smooth muscle relaxant effects of this class of vasodilator drug (Gruetter *et al.*, 1979).

3.1. Nitrosoamines and Sodium Nitroprusside

These compounds release nitric oxide gas, which can be readily collected in an oxygen-free atmosphere and demonstrated to activate guanylate cyclase and relax vascular smooth muscle. Both effects are readily antagonized by hemoproteins and methylene blue. Oxidation products of nitric oxide, such as NO_2 gas, are inactive (Gruetter *et al.*, 1979). Moreover, completely decomposed solutions of nitrosoguanidines or sodium nitroprusside are inactive. These observations suggest that nitric oxide is an active intermediate of nitrosoguanidines and sodium nitroprusside in eliciting vascular smooth muscle relaxation.

3.2. Inorganic and Organic Nitrites

Nitrites readily decompose in aqueous acid to form nitrous acid (HONO) and nitric oxide (NO). $NaNO_2$ is a very weak activator of guanylate cyclase (Katsuki *et al.*, 1977) and is a week vasodilator. Studies from this laboratory demonstrated that free sulfhydryls or thiols, such as cysteine, markedly potentiate guanylate cyclase activation by $NaNO_2$ and the organic nitrite amyl nitrite (Ignarro *et al.*, 1980a,b; Ignarro and Gruetter, 1980; Gruetter *et al.*, 1980, 1981b). Thiols markedly decrease the stability of nitrites and promote the formation of nitric oxide as well as the corresponding S-nitrosothiols (Saville, 1958; Field *et al.*, 1978; Ignarro *et al.*, 1981a). S-Nitrosothiols are themselves unstable, slowly release nitric oxide, and are potent vascular smooth muscle relaxants (Ignarro *et al.*, 1981a).

3.3. Organic Nitrates

The classical example of this type of vasodilator is nitroglycerin (glyceryl trinitrate). Activation of soluble guanylate cyclase by organic nitrates specifically requires the presence of cysteine (Ignarro and Gruetter, 1980; Ignarro et al., 1981a). This requirement for cysteine is related to the reaction between organic nitrates and cysteine to form S-nitrosocysteine, which is a potent vasodilator (Ignarro et al., 1981a). The reactivity and metabolism of organic nitrates have been studied (see Needleman, 1976). Nitroglycerin does not spontaneously release nitric oxide. Denitration, however, readily occurs in the presence of certain thiols at alkaline pH to form NO_2^- (Heppel and Hilmoe, 1950). Upon acidification, NO_2^- forms HONO and NO. If the thiol employed is cysteine, the NO released reacts with the former to yield S-nitrosocysteine (Ignarro et al., 1981a).

3.4. Hydroxylamine and Sodium Azide

Both of these compounds have long been recognized as vasodilators. Activation of guanylate cyclase by hydroxylamine (NH_2OH) and sodium azide (NaN_3) was shown to require the presence of catalase (Mittal et al., 1975, 1977). The basis of this requirement is their reactivity with catalase to form NO-catalase, which is responsible for the activation of guanylate cyclase (Craven et al., 1979). As is the case with nitric oxide, guanylate cyclase activation by NO-catalase can be inhibited by methylene blue or hemoproteins (Edwards et al., 1981). Whether or not nitric oxide is involved in the vascular smooth muscle relaxant effects of NH_2OH or NaN_3 is presently unknown, but relaxation is antagonized by methylene blue or cyanide (unpublished observations). Cyanide reacts with the heme iron of NO-catalase to destroy the nitrosyl complex with the formation of NO_2.

3.5. Conclusions

The nitrogen oxide-containing vasodilators have in common that each is capable of releasing or forming nitric oxide. The characteristics of relaxation by each compound are very similar to those of relaxation by nitric oxide. Vascular smooth muscle relaxation elicited by such agents is antagonized by methylene blue but not by propranolol, indomethacine, or atropine. Likewise, activation of guanylate cyclase is inhibited by methylene blue and hemoproteins. Moreover, each drug elicits a marked but transient decrease in systemic arterial pressure while producing little or no change in cardiac output when injected intravenously. Therefore, all of these vasodilators produce a marked decrease in systemic vascular resistance. These observations strongly support the view that nitric oxide represents at least one active intermediate of the nitrogen oxide-containing vasodilators.

4. Relationship between Cyclic GMP Formation and Vascular Smooth Muscle Relaxation

The most significant early studies suggesting that cGMP might be associated with the vasodilatory action of certain compounds were discussed earlier. This view was cautiously expressed and seemingly noncommittal because earlier studies had suggested that cGMP might be involved in the contractile response to acetylcholine, bradykinin, and other agents. Some of these earlier studies, however, were likely conducted with endothelium-damaged vascular strips, which contract rather than relax to the same agents.

4.1. Cyclic GMP as a Relaxant

One of the problems with the earlier view that cGMP is involved in smooth muscle contraction is that contractile agents failed to activate guanylate cyclase. Moreover, the addition of cGMP analogues to isolated muscle strips failed to cause contraction. In contrast, 8-Br-cGMP elicited relaxation of bovine coronary artery (Napoli *et al.*, 1980), rat and rabbit aorta (Schultz *et al.*, 1979), and rat ductus deferens (Schultz *et al.*, 1979). Inclusion of phosphodiesterase inhibitors enhanced this relaxation.

4.2. Activation of Guanylate Cyclase

If cGMP is involved in mediating smooth muscle relaxation by vasodilators, the latter should be expected to stimulate the formation of cGMP provided the mechanism is unrelated to inhibition of cyclic nucleotide hydrolysis. As discussed previously, all vasodilators of this class activate soluble guanylate cyclase. Soluble enzyme from bovine coronary artery (Gruetter *et al.*, 1979, 1980, 1981b; Ignarro *et al.*, 1981a; Lippton *et al.*, 1982) and intrapulmonary artery and vein (unpublished observations) behaves similarly to enzyme from other tissue sources.

More recent studies with purified soluble guanylate cyclase have clarified the mechanism of enzyme activation by the nitrogen oxide-containing vasodilators. Earlier studies with partially purified enzyme suggested (Craven and DeRubertis, 1978; Craven *et al.*, 1979; Ignarro *et al.*,

1981b,c), and subsequent studies with purified enzyme demonstrated (Ignarro *et al.*, 1982a; Ohlstein *et al.*, 1982), that heme is required for guanylate cyclase activation by sodium nitroprusside, nitroso compounds, nitric oxide, and related agents. Nitric oxide, which is formed or released from the parent compounds, readily reacts with heme to form nitrosylheme, a highly reactive paramagnetic species that binds to (Ignarro *et al.*, 1981c) and activates guanylate cyclase (Craven and DeRubertis, 1978; Craven *et al.*, 1979; Ignarro *et al.*, 1981b,c, 1982a,b; Wolen *et al.*, 1982; Ohlstein *et al.*, 1982). Guanylate cyclase can be purified in a form that either contains stoichiometric amounts of heme (Gerzer *et al.*, 1981a,b; Ignarro *et al.*, 1982a,b; Wolin *et al.*, 1982) or is deficient in heme (Ignarro *et al.*, 1982a; Ohlstein *et al.*, 1982). The heme-enriched enzyme is markedly activated (50- to 100-fold) by nitric oxide or nitroso compounds, whereas the heme-deficient enzyme is activated only slightly (twofold) or not at all. Addition of heme or hemoproteins back to enzyme reaction mixtures, however, completely restores the activation of heme-deficient guanylate cyclase (Ignarro *et al.*, 1982a; Ohlstein *et al.*, 1982).

The structural configuration of nitrosyl-heme closely resembles that of protoporphyrin IX, and activation of guanylate cyclase by the former may be attributed to a protoporphyrin IX binding interaction (Wolin *et al.*, 1982). Protoporphyrin IX has a high binding affinity for, and markedly activates, purified guanylate cyclase in a heme-independent manner (Ignarro *et al.*, 1982b; Wolin *et al.*, 1982; Ohlstein *et al.*, 1982). Heme is, in fact, a competitive inhibitor of protoporphyrin IX. Guanylate cyclase activation by nitric oxide, nitroso compounds, or nitrosyl-heme is remarkably similar, if not identical, to activation by protoporphyrin IX with respect to several kinetic parameters (Wolin *et al.*, 1982). Thus, it appears that a common form of activated guanylate cyclase is generated by each of these enzyme activators. Protoporphyrin IX may be an important endogenous activator of guanylate cyclase. Preliminary data indicate that porphyrinogenic agents, which elevate hepatic levels of protoporphyrin IX in mice, elicit a concomitant accumulation of hepatic cGMP and an engorgement of the liver with blood. In addition, protoporhyrin IX elicits vascular smooth muscle relaxation.

4.3. Inhibition of Cyclic GMP Phosphodiesterase

Chemical agents that elevate tissue cGMP levels by inhibiting its hydrolysis to 5'-GMP also relax vascular smooth muscle. Likewise, inhibitors of cAMP hydrolysis cause relaxation. Many of these agents are nonspecific in that both cyclic nucleotide phosphodiesterases are inhibited and thus cause increased tissue levels of both cyclic nucleotides. Specific

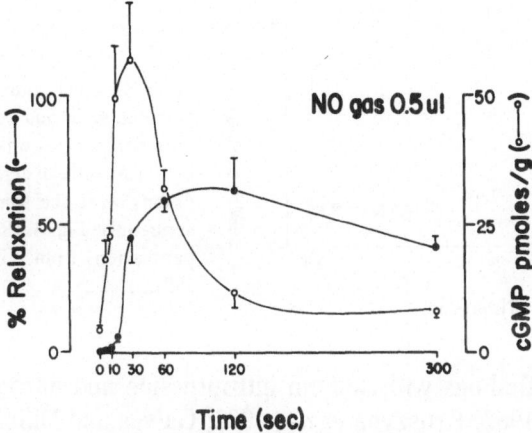

Time (sec)

Figure 4. Time course of cGMP accumulation in and relaxation of bovine coronary arterial strips elicited by 0.5 μl of nitric oxide (NO) gas. Contraction was induced with 30 mM KCl, and relaxation is expressed as percentage decrease of induced tone. One control value (zero time) and one value at each time interval after addition of NO were obtained using arterial strips from the same animal. Each point represents the mean of values from strips from four different animals. Relaxation and cGMP levels were determined in the same strips. (Reproduced with permission from Gruetter *et al.*, 1981a.)

inhibitors of either hydrolytic enzyme, however, have been synthesized and found to elicit vascular smooth muscle relaxation (Kramer and Wells, 1979). In the presence of phosphodiesterase inhibitors, relaxation by nitrogen oxide vasodilators or by cGMP itself is potentiated (Kramer and Wells, 1979; Kukovetz *et al.*, 1979c; Napoli *et al.*, 1980).

4.4. Vascular Cyclic GMP Accumulation

Vasodilators that form or release nitric oxide elevate vascular levels of cGMP (Diamond and Blisard, 1976; Bohme *et al.*, 1978; Axelsson *et al.*, 1979; Janis and Diamond, 1979; Kukovetz *et al.*, 1979c). A good association was found between relaxation and cGMP accumulation. We have recently examined time intervals as short as 5 sec after addition of several vasodilators including nitric oxide (Gruetter *et al.*, 1981b; Ignarro *et al.*, 1981a; Edwards *et al.*, 1984). Each vasodilator caused a rapid and marked accumulation of vascular cGMP that clearly preceded onset of relaxation. Two examples are illustrated in Fig. 4 (nitric oxide) and Fig. 5 (nitroglycerin). Similar observations were made for other related vasodilators (Gruetter *et al.*, 1981b; Ignarro *et al.*, 1981a; Edwards *et al.*, 1984; unpublished observations). More recent studies have confirmed cer-

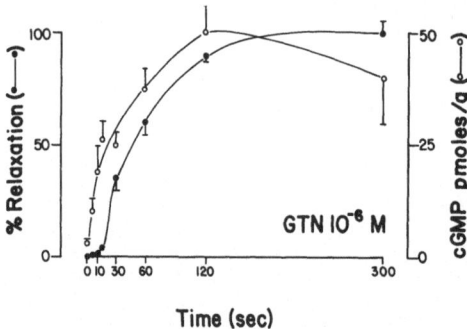

Figure 5. Time course of cGMP accumulation in and relaxation of bovine coronary arterial strips elicited by 1 μM nitroglycerin (GTN). Conditions were the same as those described for Fig. 4. (Reproduced with permission from Gruetter et al., 1981a.)

tain of these findings with sodium nitroprusside and nitroglycerin (Axelsson et al., 1982; Kruszyna et al., 1982; Galvas and DiSalvo, 1983).

Methylene blue inhibited cGMP accumulation provoked by the same vasodilators (Gruetter et al., 1981a; Ignarro et al., 1981a; Keith et al., 1982; Edwards et al. 1984). Moreover, hemoproteins prevented both relaxation (Gruetter et al., 1979) and cGMP accumulation elicited by nitric oxide (Gruetter et al., 1981a).

Nitroprusside and nitroglycerin are potent pulmonary vasodilators that act on pulmonary veins and upstream segments in the closed-chest dog (Kadowitz et al., 1981). Isolated pulmonary vein was more sensitive than intrapulmonary artery to relaxation by nitrogen oxide vasodilators (Edwards et al., 1984). Figures 6 and 7 illustrate these observations with nitroglycerin and S-nitroso-N-acetylpenicillamine. The greater sensitivity of intrapulmonary vein to relaxation by sodium nitroprusside or nitroglycerin is consistent with earlier reports both in vivo (Pagani et al., 1978; Robinson et al., 1979) and in vitro (Mackenzie and Parratt, 1977; Armstrong et al., 1980). Intrapulmonary vein was also more sensitive than intrapulmonary artery to tissue accumulation of cGMP (Figs. 8 and 9). Moreover, the onset of vascular cGMP accumulation preceded the onset of relaxation in each case, and methylene blue antagonized both pharmacological responses (Edwards et al., 1984). Preliminary experiments with unpurified soluble guanylate cyclase from bovine intrapulmonary vessels indicate clearly that enzyme from venous tissue is more markedly activated than is enzyme from arterial tissue by the same vasodilators.

4.5. Cyclic GMP as Second Messenger

The four principal criteria proposed by Sutherland and co-workers to establish a second messenger role for cAMP in a given cellular function have been satisfied for cGMP in vascular smooth muscle relaxation

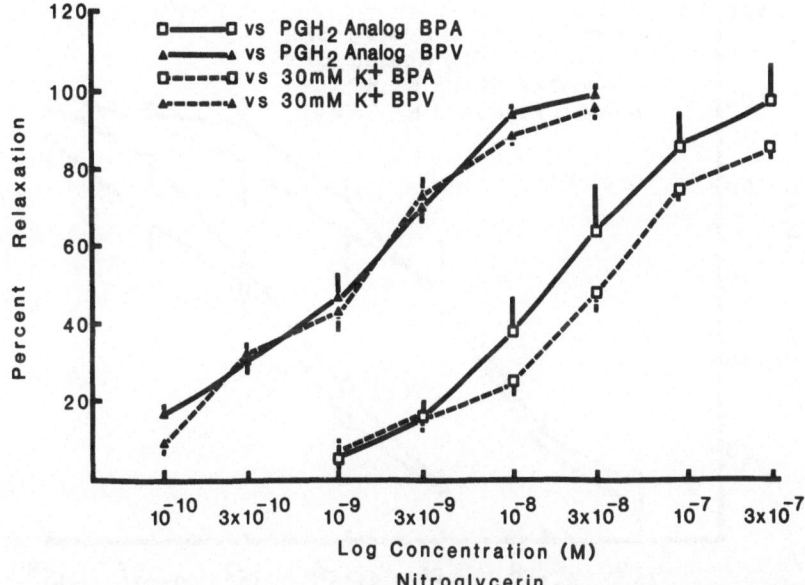

Figure 6. Concentration–relaxation curves for nitroglycerin in bovine intrapulmonary artery (BPA) and vein (BPV). Tone was induced with either 30 mM KCl (K^+) or 10^{-8} M [15S]hydroxy-11α,9α[epoxymethano]prosta-5Z,13E-dienoic acid (PGH$_2$ analogue) as indicated. Relaxation is expressed as percentage decrease of induced tone. Each point represents the mean ± S.E. from seven to ten strips. (Reproduced with permission from Edwards *et al.*, 1983.)

caused by pharmacological intervention. First, the vasodilators under consideration elicit vascular cGMP accumulation, which temporally precedes onset of relaxation. Second, each of the vasodilators markedly activates soluble guanylate cyclase. Third, inhibitors of cGMP phosphodiesterase enhance or potentiate relaxation as well as cGMP accumulation elicited by the vasodilators. Fourth, the direct addition of cGMP or 8-bromo-cGMP to precontracted muscle strips elicits relaxation. In addition to these criteria, we propose a corollary to the first. Agents that inhibit the activation or activity of guanylate cyclase should inhibit both tissue cGMp accumulation and relaxation elicited by the vasodilators. The inhibitory effects on the intact vessel would require that the inhibitor reach its site of action, which appears to be intracellular for the nitrogen oxide-containing vasodilators (Gruetter *et al.*, 1979; Ignarro *et al.*, 1981a). Methylene blue satisfies all of these requirements (Gruetter *et al.*, 1979, 1980, 1981a,b; Ignarro *et al.*, 1981a).

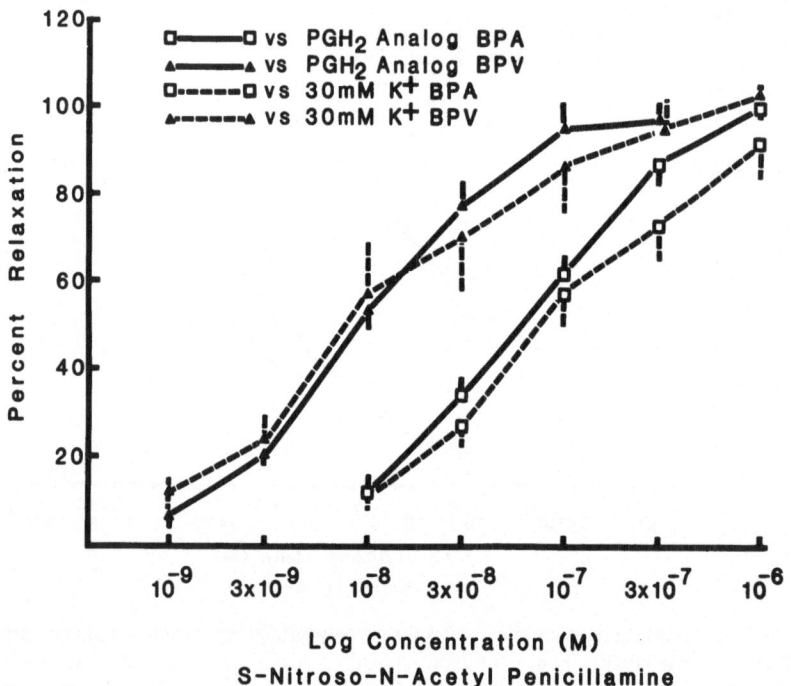

Figure 7. Concentration–relaxation curves for S-nitroso-N-acetylpenicillamine in bovine intrapulmonary artery (BPA) and vein (BPV). Tone was induced as described for Fig. 6. Relaxation is expressed as percentage decrease of induced tone. Each point represents the mean ± S.E. from seven to ten strips. (Reproduced with permission from Edwards *et al.*, 1984.)

5. Antagonism by Methylene Blue of Relaxation by Nitrogen-Oxide-Containing Vasodilators

Until recently, no antagonist of nitroglycerin or sodium nitroprusside had been known. As discussed earlier, methylene blue was found to inhibit guanylate cyclase activation and vascular smooth muscle relaxation caused by these vasodilators. Many of these observations were subsequently confirmed (Kukovetz *et al.*, 1981; Keith *et al.*, 1982).

5.1. Specificity and Mechanism of Antagonism

Several important concepts evolved from the above observations and related experiments. Most importantly, methylene blue was apparently quite specific as an antagonist of the nitrogen oxide-containing vasodilators. Relaxation by catecholamines, prostacyclin, or calcium antago-

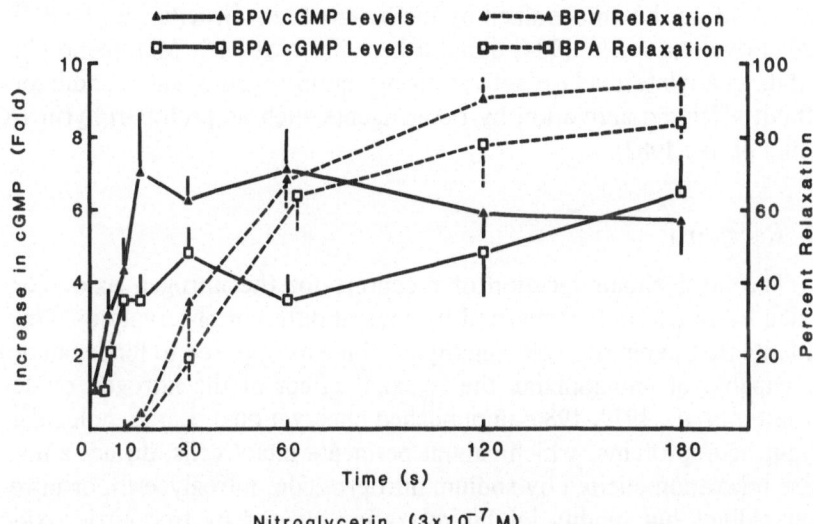

Figure 8. Time course relationships for relaxation and cGMP accumulation elicited by nitroglycerin. Tone was induced in strips of bovine intrapulmonary artery (BPA) and vein (BPV) with 30 mM KCl. Basal cGMP levels were 6.7 ± 0.8 pmole/g tissue in BPV and 9.4 ± 0.5 pmole/g tissue in BPA. Each point represents the mean $\pm$ S.E. from four strips. (Reproduced with permission from Edwards *et al.*, 1984.)

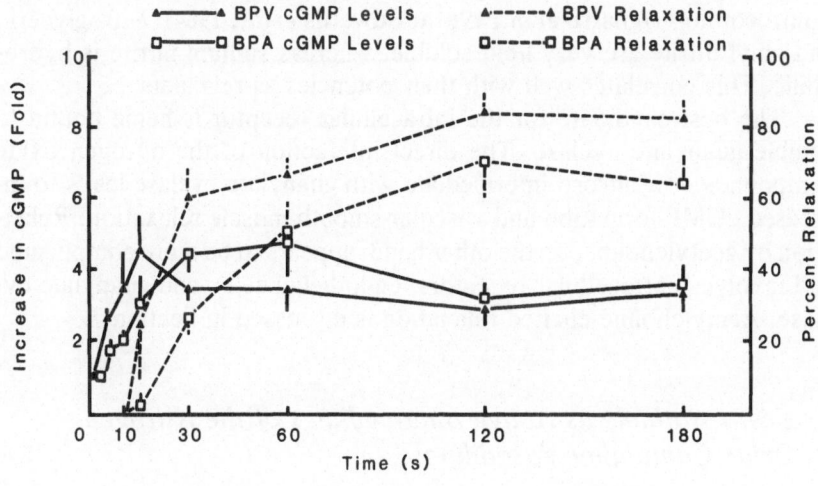

Figure 9. Time course relationships for relaxation and cGMP accumulation elicited by S-nitroso-N-acetylpenicillamine. Procedures for inducing tone and basal cGMP levels were described in Fig. 8. Each point represents the mean $\pm$ S.E. from four strips. (Reproduced with permission from Edwards *et al.*, 1984.)

nists could not be antagonized by methylene blue (Gruetter et al., 1979, 1980; Edwards et al., 1984; unpublished observations). Methylene blue inhibits guanylate cyclase activation by the nitrogen oxide vasodilators without affecting activation by other agents such as protoporphyrin IX (Wolin et al., 1982).

5.2. Receptors

The intracellular location of receptors for the nitrogen oxide-containing vasodilators is supported by several different observations. Only oxidants that penetrate cells (methylene blue as opposed to ferricyanide) are capable of antagonizing the relaxant effect of the nitrogen oxides (Gruetter et al., 1979, 1980; unpublished observations). Large-molecular-weight hemoproteins, which cannot permeate intact cells, do not antagonize relaxation elicited by sodium nitroprusside, nitroglycerin, or nitrosoguanidines but readily inhibit relaxation elicited by free nitric oxide (Gruetter et al., 1979, 1980). The nitrogen oxide vasodilators penetrate the cell membrane, and the nitric oxide released or formed within the cell escapes the sequestering effect of the hemoproteins added to the extracellular bathing medium. In addition, the potency of relaxation appears to be dependent on the lipophilic nature of the relaxant. Nitric oxide is extremely lipophilic and elicits a marked but transient relaxation at small concentrations (Gruetter et al., 1979, 1981a). The same is true for certain S-nitrosothiols (Ignarro et al., 1981a; Edwards et al., 1984). Nitroglycerin and amyl nitrite are very lipid soluble, whereas sodium nitrite is hydrophilic. This correlates well with their potencies as relaxants.

The best candidate for the intracellular receptor is heme bound to soluble guanylate cyclase. The direct interaction of the nitrogen oxide compounds or a nitroso intermediate with guanylate cyclase leads to increased cGMP formation and vascular smooth muscle relaxation. Relaxation by acetylcholine, on the other hand, appears to be more complicated and involves extracellular receptors, endothelial cells, and guanylate cyclase. Acetylcholine-elicited relaxation is discussed in Section 7.

6. S-Nitrosothiols as Active Intermediates of the Nitrogen-Oxide-Containing Vasodilators

Almost 2 years of experiments were conducted in this laboratory before the concept that S-nitrosothiols may mediate relaxation by the nitrogen oxides was appreciated. At first we believed that nitric oxide was responsible for the ultimate relaxant effect of these compounds.

6.1. Thiol Enhancement of Guanylate Cyclase Activation

Thiols enhance activation of vascular soluble guanylate cyclase by nitrogen oxide agents (Gruetter *et al.*, 1980, 1981b; Ignarro and Gruetter, 1980; Ignarro *et al.*, 1981a; unpublished observations). Nitrosoguanidines react with thiols in aqueous solution to liberate nitric oxide (Ignarro *et al.*, 1980a). Thus, we felt initially that enhanced formation of nitric oxide could explain the thiol-enhanced activation of guanylate cyclase by nitrosoguanidine. Thiol enhancement of enzyme activation by sodium nitroprusside, however, could not be similarly explained because no enhancement of nitric oxide release was observed. In fact, thiols appeared to trap the nitric oxide gas that is liberated spontaneously from neutral aqueous solutions of sodium nitroprusside (Ignarro *et al.*, 1980a). The latter observation suggested that nitric oxide reacted with thiols to form a third compound. This interpretation was supported by reports that thiols react with nitric oxide, nitrous acid, or acidic solutions of sodium nitrite to form S-nitrosothiols (Saville, 1958; Schulz and McCalla, 1969; Field *et al.*, 1978).

6.2. Cysteine Requirement for Guanylate Cyclase Activation by Organic Nitrates

A very consistent finding has been the absolute requirement of cysteine for activation of soluble guanylate cyclase by nitroglycerin, isosorbide dinitrate, and pentaerythritol tetranitrate (Ignarro and Gruetter, 1980; Ignarro *et al.*, 1981a). Other thiols including N-acetylcysteine or even homocysteine could not substitute for cysteine. The L and D isomers of cysteine produce equivalent effects. Sodium nitrite requires thiol addition to activate guanylate cyclase, but thiols other than cysteine are as effective.

6.3. S-Nitrosothiol Formation from Nitrogen-Oxide-Containing Vasodilators

Several S-nitrosothiols were synthesized and found to markedly activate soluble preparations of guanylate cyclase (Ignarro and Gruetter, 1980; Ignarro *et al.*, 1980a,b, 1981a,b,c, 1982a,b; Ohlstein *et al.*, 1982; Wolin *et al.*, 1982). Unlike the findings with the nitrogen oxide-containing vasodilators, guanylate cyclase activation by S-nitrosothiols was not enhanced by further thiol addition. Enzyme activation was inhibited, however, by methylene blue or ferricyanide. Additional experiments revealed that sodium nitroprusside, nitroglycerin, nitrosoguanidines, and amyl nitrite could react with cysteine to form S-nitrosocysteine (Ignarro *et al.*,

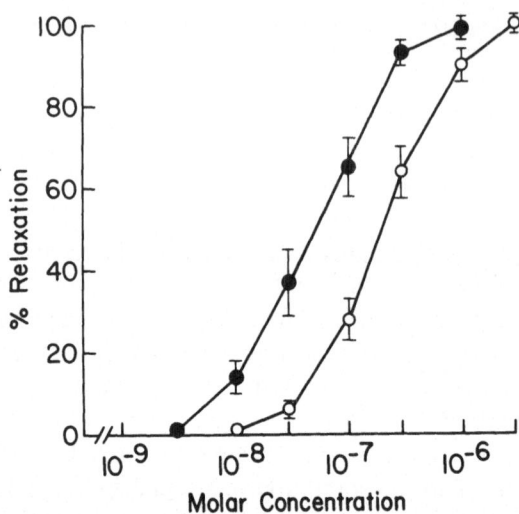

Figure 10. Relaxation of bovine coronary artery elicited by S-nitrosocysteine and S-nitroso-N-acetylpenicillamine. Relaxation of 30 mM KCl-precontracted strips by single increasing concentrations of S-nitrosocysteine (●) and cumulatively increasing concentrations of S-nitroso-N-acetylpenicillamine (○) were determined. Relaxation is expressed as percentage decrease of induced tone. Other conditions were the same as those described for Fig. 4. (Reproduced with permission from Ignarro *et al.*, 1981a.)

1981a; unpublished observations). The reaction involving nitroglycerin occurred only with cysteine. These observations were strikingly consistent with those that only cysteine enabled organic nitrates to activate guanylate cyclase.

6.4. Potent Vasodilator Action of S-Nitrosothiols

The S-nitroso derivatives of cysteine, N-acetylpenicillamine, 2-mercaptoethylamine, and 3-mercaptopropionic acid potently relaxed bovine coronary artery (Ignarro *et al.*, 1981a). The relaxant effects of S-nitrosocysteine and S-nitroso-N-acetylpenicillamine are shown in Fig. 10. S-Nitrosothiols also relaxed strips of bovine intrapulmonary artery and vein (Edwards *et al.*, 1984). The relaxant effect of S-nitroso-N-acetylpenicillamine is illustrated in Fig. 7. Intravenous injections of a wide range of doses of S-nitrosothiols in the anesthetized cat caused a decrease in systemic arterial pressure (Fig. 11). Little or no change in cardiac output accompanied the drop in systemic arterial pressure, indicating that a marked decrease in systemic vascular resistance had occurred. S-Nitrosocysteine was more potent than the other S-nitrosothiols, sodium nitro-

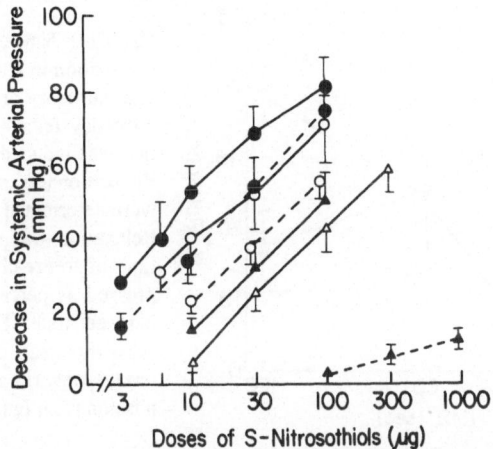

Figure 11. Effects of S-nitrosothiols, sodium nitroprusside, nitroglycerin, and NaNO₂ on systemic arterial pressure in the anesthetized cat. Symbols: ●——●, S-nitrosocysteine; ○——○, S-nitroso-N-acetylpenicillamine; ▲——▲, S-nitroso-2-mercaptoethylamine; △——△, S-nitroso-3-mercaptopropionic acid; ●–––●, sodium nitroprusside; ○–––○, nitroglycerin; ▲–––▲, NaNO₂. Each value represents the mean ± S.E. for six cats. (Reproduced with permission from Ignarro *et al.*, 1981a.)

prusside, and nitroglycerin in dilating the systemic vascular bed. The latter two vasodilators resembled the S-nitrosothiols in both onset (immediate) and duration (1–3 min) of the hypotensive response. Propranolol at doses that blocked vasodilator responses to isoproterenol did not significantly alter the decrease in systemic arterial pressure elicited by S-nitrosothiols, sodium nitroprusside, or nitroglycerin.

6.5. S-Nitrosothiols Stimulate Vascular Cyclic GMP Formation

S-Nitrosothiols markedly stimulated the accumulation of cGMP in bovine coronary artery (Ignarro *et al.*, 1981a) and bovine intrapulmonary artery and vein (Edwards *et al.*, 1984). Figure 12 illustrates the effect of S-nitrosocysteine in bovine coronary artery. Cyclic GMP accumulation temporally preceded onset of relaxation. S-Nitroso-N-acetylpenicillamine was a more potent relaxant of intrapulmonary veins than arteries (Fig. 7). Similarly, S-nitroso-N-acetylpenicillamine was more potent as a stimulator of cGMP formation in vein than in artery (Fig. 9). Again, cGMP accumulation preceded onset of relaxation. These effects of S-nitroso-N-acetylpenicillamine were remarkably similar to those of nitroglycerin (Figs. 6 and 7) and sodium nitroprusside (Edwards *et al.*, 1984).

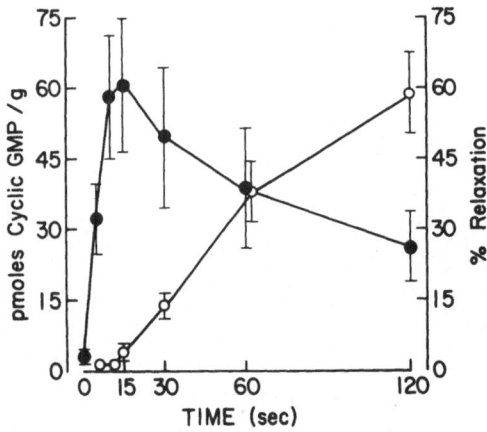

Figure 12. Time course of cGMP accumulation in and relaxation of bovine coronary artery elicited by S-nitrosocysteine (50 nM). Contraction was induced with 30 mM KCl. Relaxation (○) and cGMP levels (●) were determined in the same strips. Relaxation was recorded until the time of freeze-clamping and is expressed as percentage decrease of induced tone. Each value represents the mean ± S.E. for four arterial strips. (Reproduced with permission from Ignarro *et al.*, 1981a.)

6.6. Conclusions

Several observations support the view (Ignarro *et al.*, 1981a) that S-nitrosothiols are active intermediates in expressing vascular smooth muscle relaxation elicited by organic nitrates, nitrites, nitrosoguanidines, and sodium nitroprusside. First, thiols either enhanced or were obligatory for guanylate cyclase activation by these vasodilators. Second, the latter reacted with thiols at neutral pH to form the corresponding S-nitrosothiols. Third, S-nitrosothiols markedly activated guanylate cyclase in the absence of added thiols and elicited a marked increase in vascular cGMP levels, both of which were inhibited by methylene blue. Fourth, S-nitrosothiols were potent relaxants, and this was antagonized by methylene blue. Fifth, S-nitrosothiols were potent vasodilators, and their hemodynamic responses were strikingly similar to those of nitroglycerin and sodium nitrosprusside. Sixth, S-nitrosothiols are unstable, and this could account in part for their transient hypotensive effects as well as those of the parent vasodilator drugs (Ignarro *et al.*, 1981a). Nitric oxide, however, cannot be ruled out as an active intermediate, because the decomposition of S-nitrosothiols results in the liberation of nitric oxide. Nitric oxide is itself a potent relaxant and activates guanylate cyclase in the absence of added thiols. Since the activation of guanylate cyclase by nitric oxide or S-nitrosothiols requires the formation of nitrosyl-heme, it is conceivable that the formed S-nitrosothiol(s) serve(s) as a readily available source of nitric oxide, which subsequently causes enzyme activation. Therefore, both S-nitrosothiols and nitric oxide could be considered as active intermediates in expressing the relaxant effect of the nitrogen oxide-containing vasodilators.

7. Mechanism of the Vasodilator Action of Acetylcholine

As discussed earlier, previous studies showed an apparent correlation between acetylcholine-elicited contraction of smooth muscle and the accumulation of cGMP. Both cellular events were dependent on calcium, and contraction preceded the increase in tissue cGMP levels. Kukovetz *et al.* (1981) reported that acetylcholine-elicited accumulation of coronary arterial cGMP was inhibited by methylene blue, which concomitantly enhanced the contractile response to acetylcholine. Recent unpublished observations from our laboratory indicate that methylene blue enhances muscarinic receptor-mediated contraction of intrapulmonary artery and vein. Thus, methylene blue is not a muscarinic receptor antagonist. Methylene blue also enhances the contractile response to phenylephrine, an α-adrenergic receptor agonist.

Muscarinic receptor activation elevates vascular cGMP levels, and this effect is prevented by methylene blue. Methylene blue itself lowers basal or resting cGMP levels and elicits a concentration-dependent contraction. The above studies indicate clearly that cGMP does not mediate vascular smooth muscle contraction by muscarinic or α-adrenergic receptor agonists.

7.1. Role of Vascular Endothelial Cells

Acetylcholine dilates the systemic and pulmonary vascular beds (Nandiwada *et al.*, 1983) but elicits a marked contraction of isolated strips of most arteries and veins. This enigma was partially resolved recently by the interesting studies of Furchgott and Zawadzki (1980). Arterial strips that were carefully dissected, cut, and mounted in both chambers so that the single layer of squamous epithelia cells (endothelium) remained intact relaxed in response to muscarinic receptor agonists. Relaxation was antagonized by atropine or quinacrine. Furchgott and co-workers suggested that acetylcholine interacts with muscarinic receptors on endothelial cells to stimulate the latter to release a substance(s) that in turn interacts with smooth muscle cells to elicit relaxation. Formation of this substance(s) apparently requires oxygen and is inhibited by ETYA, a lipoxygenase inhibitor, and quinacrine, a phospholipase A_2 inhibitor (see Furchgott *et al.*, 1981).

7.2. Antagonism by Atropine, Quinacrine, and Methylene Blue

Relaxation of endothelium-intact, precontracted arterial strips by acetylcholine can be attenuated by either atropine or quinacrine (Furchgott *et al.*, 1981). Phenylephrine-precontracted strips of endothelium-intact bovine intrapulmonary artery relax to acetylcholine or carbamycholine (unpublished observations). This relaxation is inhibited not only by atropine and quinacrine but also by methylene blue. Unlike atropine, methylene blue is not a muscarinic receptor antagonist. We find that methylene blue also inhibits endothelium-dependent relaxation by arachidonic acid and bradykinin. Methylene blue is a guanylate cyclase inhibitor and may inhibit the activation of guanylate cyclase by whatever putative mediator is released from endothelial cells by muscarinic agonists.

7.3. Elevation of Cyclic GMP Levels

As discussed above, contraction of vascular smooth muscle (most likely endothelium deficient) by acetylcholine or carbamylcholine is accompanied by small increases in vascular cGMP levels. Similarly, relaxation of endothelial-intact intrapulmonary artery is accompanied by cGMP accumulation (unpublished observations). Atropine inhibits cGMP accumulation, relaxation, and contraction elicited by muscarinic receptor agonists. Methylene blue inhibits cGMP accumulation and relaxation but enchances contraction. Quinacrine is a nonselective phospholipase A_2 inhibitor that also depresses phenylephrine-elicited contraction. At concentrations that do not inhibit contraction, quinacrine partially inhibits acetylcholine-elicited relaxation without affecting vascular cGMP levels. Therefore, quinacrine may inhibit acetylcholine-elicited relaxation by a nonspecific mechanism.

7.4. Conclusions

Although more studies are necessary in order to draw more meaningful conclusions, our preliminary data suggest that intrapulmonary arterial smooth muscle relaxation elicited by muscarinic receptor agonists is at least associated with the accumulation of cGMP. One key study to be conducted entails identification of the endothelial cell substance(s) that is (are) formed during relaxation elicited by muscarinic agonists and to determine whether or not the substance(s) can activate guanylate cyclase.

8. Molecular Mechanisms of Cyclic GMP Accumulation and Vasodilatation

Our current view of the mechanism of vascular smooth muscle relaxation by nitrogen oxide-containing vasodilators is illustrated schemat-

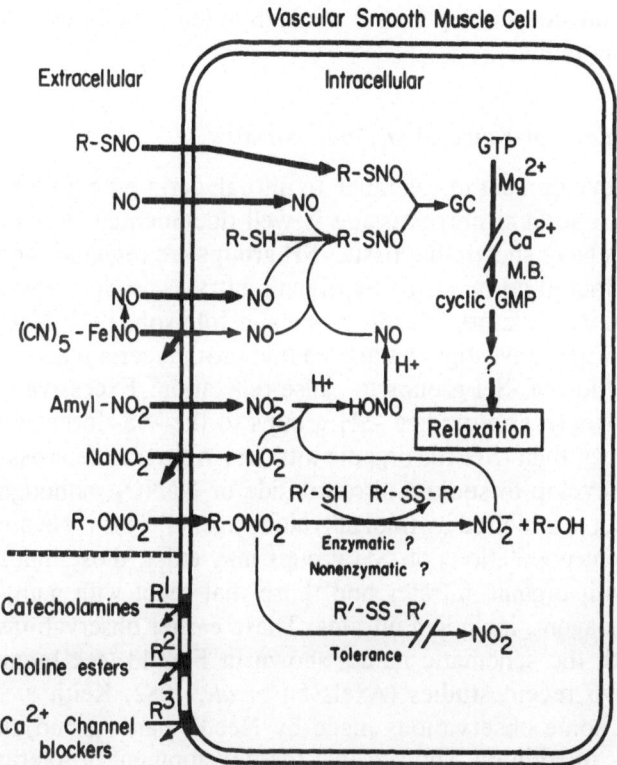

Figure 13. Schematic diagram of proposed mechanisms by which nitrogen oxide-containing vasodilators relax vascular smooth muscle. Abbreviations: R-SNO, S-nitrosothiol; NO, nitric oxide; HONO, nitrous acid; $(CN)_5$-FeNO, nitroprusside; $R-ONO_2$, organic nitrate, R-OH, denitrated organic nitrate; R-SH, low- or high-molecular-weight thiol; R'-SH, thiol that is distinct froM R-SH; GC, guanylate cyclase; M.B., methylene blue; R^1, R^2, R^3, extracellular specific receptors. (Reproduced with permission from Ignarro *et al.*, 1981a.)

ically in Fig. 13. The vasodilators (except for $NaNO_2$) are lipophilic and penetrate smooth muscle cells. Nitric oxide is either released or formed from NO_2^- as illustrated. Nitroglycerin, and probably other organic nitrates, are denitrated with the formation of NO_2^-. Nitric oxide reacts with intracellular thiols to form S-nitrosothiols. S-Nitrosothiols, either directly or by releasing nitric oxide, activate the hemoprotein guanylate cyclase and thereby stimulate cGMP formation. Cyclic GMP, in turn, causes relaxation, perhaps by rapidly lowering the intracellular concentration of calcium ion. One striking corollary of this concept is that NO_2^- is an active intermediate of nitroglycerin and related organic nitrates. Sodium nitrite is not lipophilic, and only a very small amount would be expected to penetrate cells. This may be the reason for the low potency of sodium nitrite as compared to the high potency of amyl nitrite, which is highly lipophilic.

8.1. Vascular Tolerance to Organic Nitrates

The development of tolerance to nitroglycerin with little or no cross tolerance to sodium nitroprusside is well documented. Needleman and co-workers have shown that tissue -SH groups are required for relaxation of precontracted aortic strips by organic nitrates, sodium nitroprusside, and related vasodilators (Needlem and and Johnson, 1973; Needleman et al., 1973). These investigators argued that nitroglycerin reacts with a special population of -SH groups to cause relaxation. Excessive concentrations of nitroglycerin oxidize -SH groups to the -SS- form, which has a lower affinity than -SH for organic nitrates. Appreciable cross tolerance does not develop to sodium nitroprusside or $NaNO_2$, although their relaxant effect is inhibited by thiol alkylating agents. This is because at least two different populations of -SH groups may exist: those that react specifically with organic nitrates and those that react with many types of vasodilator agent, including nitrates. These earlier observations are consistent with the schematic model shown in Fig. 13 (see Ignarro et al., 1981a). Two recent studies (Axelsson et al., 1982; Keith et al., 1982) confirmed some observations made by Needleman's group and by our group and, in addition, showed that the development of tolerance to relaxation by nitroglycerin was accompanied by a concomitant development of tolerance to the cGMP-accumulating effect of nitroglycerin. Vascular tolerance to nitroglycerin was not associated with appreciable cross tolerance to sodium nitroprusside or 8-bromo-cGMP (Keith et al., 1982).

8.2. Physiological Role of Cyclic GMP in the Control of Vascular Tone

A model is presented that attempts to associate muscarinic receptor activation, cGMP accumulation, vasodilatation, and the control of vascular smooth muscle tone (Fig. 14). Clearly, isolated arterial strips possessing an intact endothelium undergo relaxation, whereas endothelium-free strips contract in response to muscarinic receptor agonists. Both cellular events require calcium, are associated with increased tissue levels of cGMP, and are antagonized by atropine. Methylene blue, an inhibitor of guanylate cyclase activation, inhibits cGMP accumulation and relaxation but enhances contraction. At concentrations (10 μM) that inhibit relaxation, quinacrine does not inhibit the rise in cGMP levels caused by acetylcholine. Higher concentrations (100 μM) of quinacrine markedly depress contractions by phenylephrine, relaxations by acetylcholine, and

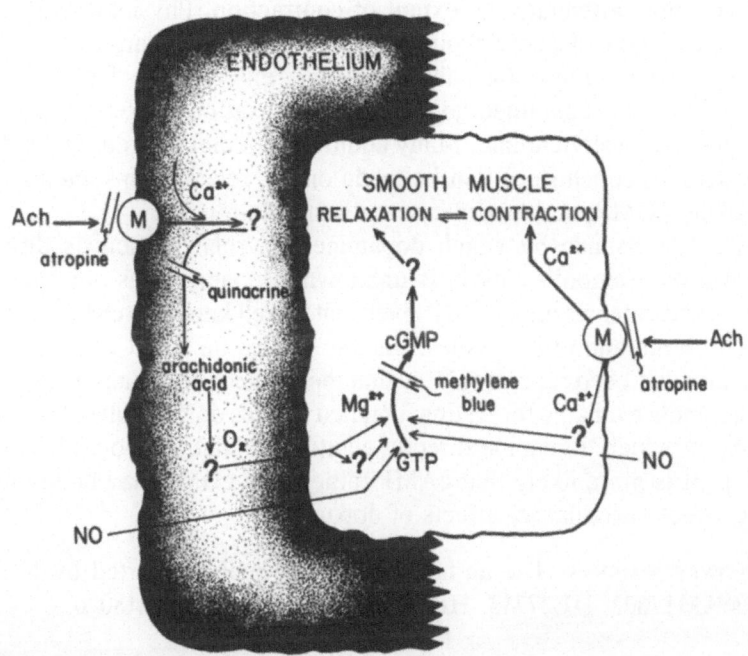

Figure 14. Schematic diagram of possible relationships among acetylcholine, cGMP, and vascular smooth muscle tone. The left side of the diagram depicts interactions involving an intact endothelium, whereas the right side describes interactions directly with smooth muscle in the absence of an intact endothelium. Abbreviations: Ach, acetylcholine; M, muscarinic receptor; NO, nitric oxide; GTP, guanosine 5'-triphosphate. Question marks signify uncertain or unknown reactions or interactions.

elevated cGMP levels caused by acetylcholine. However, these effects of quinacrine are probably nonselective and must be interpreted with caution.

Acetylcholine causes endothelial cells to form a substance(s) capable of interacting with smooth muscle cells and resulting in cGMP formation and relaxation. In the absence of endothelial cells, acetylcholine interacts directly with smooth muscle cells to cause contraction and stimulate cGMP formation. The mechanism by which acetylcholine stimulates cGMP formation in the presence and absence of endothelium may or may not be similar. Regardless of mechanism, cGMP accumulation occurs whether relaxation or contraction predominates. Assuming that cGMP mediates relaxation by acetylcholine, the accumulation of cGMP that occurs during contraction may not be of sufficient magnitude to prevent contraction or to cause relaxation. This increase in arterial cGMP levels, however, may attenuate the extent of contraction. Physiologically, any important action of acetylcholine on endothelium-free arteries may be unrealistic. Pathophysiologically, however, endothelium-damaged vessels could conceivably undergo diminished relaxation or even contraction in response to acetylcholine. Many additional studies are required before more definite conclusions can be made on the relationships among acetylcholine, cGMP, and vascular smooth muscle tone.

The mechanism by which dopamine and related agonists directly relax vascular smooth muscle is unknown. Dopamine has not been reported to elevate vascular cGMP levels but is well known to elevate cAMP levels in brain and other tissues. Similar studies on blood vessels, however, have not been reported. Now that more selective dopamine agonists are becoming available for testing, detailed studies on the molecular mechanisms by which dopamine directly elicits vasodilation should be forthcoming. It is more likely that cAMP rather than cGMP may be involved in the direct vasodilatory effects of dopamine.

ACKNOWLEDGMENTS. The authors' work has been supported by N.I.H. grants AM17692, HL27713, HL11802, HL15580, and HL18070.

References

Andersson, R., Nilsson, K., Wikberg, J., Johansson, S., Mohme-Lundholm, E., and Lundholm, L., 1975, Cyclic nucleotides and the contraction of smooth muscle, *Adv. Cyclic Nucleotide Res.* **5**:491–518.

Armstrong, J. A., Marks, G. S., and Armstrong, P. W., 1980, Absence of metabolite formation during nitroglycerin-induced relaxation of isolated blood vessels, *Mol. Pharmacol.* **18**:112–116.

Arnold, W. P., Mittal, C. K., Katsuki, S., and Murad, F., 1977a, Nitric oxide activates guanylate cyclase and increases guanosine 3',5'-cyclic monophosphate levels in various tissue preparations, *Proc. Natl. Acad. Sci. U.S.A.* **74**:3203–3207.

Arnold, W. P., Aldred, R., and Murad, F., 1977b, Cigarette smoke activates guanylate cyclase and increases guanosine 3',5'-monophosphate in tissues, *Science* **198**:934–936.

Axelsson, K. L., Wikberg, J. E. S., and Andersson, R. G. G., 1979, Relationship between nitroglycerin, cyclic GMP and relaxation of vascular smooth muscle, *Life Sci.* **24**:1779–1786.

Axelsson, K. L., Andersson, R. G. G., and Wikberg, J. E. S., 1982, Vascular smooth muscle relaxation by nitro compounds: Reduced relaxation and cyclic GMP elevation in tolerant vessels and reversal of tolerance by dithiothreitol, *Acta Pharmacol. Toxicol.* **50**:350–357.

Böhme, E., Graf, H., and Schultz, G., 1978, Effects of sodium nitroprusside and other smooth muscle relaxants on cyclic GMP formation in smooth muscle and platelets, *Adv. Cyclic Nucleotide Res.* **9**:131–143.

Clyman, R. I., Sandler, J. A., Manganiello, V. C., and Vaughan, M., 1975, Guanosine 3',5'-monophosphate and adenosine 3',5'-monophosphate content of human umbilical artery, *J. Clin. Invest.* **55**:1020–1025.

Craven, P. A., and DeRubertis, F. R., 1978, Restoration and the responsiveness of purified guanylate cyclase to nitrosoguanidine, nitric oxide, and related activators by heme and heme proteins: Evidence for the involvement of the paramagnetic nitrosyl-heme complex in enzyme activation, *J. Biol. Chem.* **253:**8433–8443.

Craven, P. A., DeRubertis, F. R., and Pratt, D. W., 1979, Electron spin resonance study of the role of NO-catalase in the activation of guanylate cyclase by NaN_3 and NH_2OH: Modulation of enzyme responses by heme protein and their nitrosyl derivatives, *J. Biol. Chem.* **254:**8213–8222.

DeRubertis, F. R., and Craven, P. A., 1976, Calcium-independent modulation of cyclic GMP and activation of guanylate cyclase by nitrosoamines, *Science* **193:**897–899.

Diamond, J., and Blisard, K. S., 1976, Effects of stimulant and relaxant drugs on tension and cyclic nucleotide levels in canine femoral artery, *Mol. Pharmacol.* **12:**688–692.

Diamond, J., and Holmes, T. G., 1975, Effects of potassium chloride and smooth muscle relaxants on tension and cyclic nucleotide levels in rat myometrium, *Can. J. Physiol. Pharmacol.* **53:**1099–1107.

Dunham, E. W., Haddox, M. K., and Goldberg, N. D., 1974, Alteration of vein cyclic 3′,5′-nucleotide concentrations during changes in contractility, *Proc. Natl. Acad. Sci. U.S.A.* **71:**815–819.

Edwards, J. C., Barry, B. K., Gruetter, D. Y., Ohlstein, E. H., Baricos, W. H., and Ignarro, L. J., 1981, Activation of hepatic guanylate cyclase by nitrosyl-heme complexes: Comparison of unpurified and partially purified enzyme, *Biochem. Pharmacol.* **30:**2531–2538.

Edwards, J. C., Ignarro, L. J., Wood, K. S., Hyman, A. L., and Kadowitz, P. J., 1984, Relaxation of intrapulmonary artery and vein by nitrogen oxide-containing vasodilators and cyclic GMP, *J. Pharmacol. Exp. Ther.*, **228:**33–42.

Field, L., Dilts, R. V., Ravichandran, R., Lenhert, P. G., and Carnahan, G. E., 1978, An unusually stable thionitrite from N-acetyl-D,L-penicillamine; X-ray crystal and molecular structure of 2-(acetylamino)-2-carboxy-1,1-dimethylethyl thionitrite, *J.C.S. Chem. Commun.* 249–250.

Furchgott, R. F., and Zawadzki, J. V., 1980, The obligatory role of endothelial cells in the relaxation of arterial smooth muscle by acetylcholine, *Nature* **288:**373–376.

Furchgott, R. F., Zawadzki, J. V., and Cherry, P. D., 1981, Role of endothelium in the vasodilator response to acetylcholine, in: *Vasodilatation* (P. M. Vanhoutte and I. Leusen, eds.), Raven Press, New York, pp. 49–66.

Galvas, P. E., and DiSalvo, J., 1983, Concentration and time-dependent relationships between isosorbide dinitrate-induced relaxation and formation of cyclic GMP in coronary arterial smooth muscle, *J. Pharmacol. Exp. Ther.* **224:**373–378.

Gerzer, R., Bohme, E., Hofmann, F., and Schultz, G., 1981a, Soluble guanylate cyclase purified from bovine lung contains heme and copper, *FEBS Lett.* **132:**71–74.

Gerzer, R., Hofmann, F., and Schultz, G., 1981b, Purification of a soluble, sodium-nitroprusside-stimulated guanylate cyclase from bovine lung, *Eur. J. Biochem.* **116:**479–486.

Gruetter, C. A., Barry, B. K., McNamara, D. B., Gruetter, D. Y., Kadowitz, P. J., and Ignarro, L. J., 1979, Relaxation of bovine coronary artery and activation of coronary arterial guanylate cyclase by nitric oxide, nitroprusside and a carcinogenic nitrosoamine, *J. Cyclic Nucleotide Res.* **5:**211–224.

Gruetter, C. A., Barry, B. K., McNamara, D. B., Kadowitz, P. J., and Ignarro, L. J., 1980, Coronary arterial relaxation and guanylate cyclase activation by cigarette smoke, N′-nitrosonornicotine and nitric oxide, *J. Pharmacol. Exp. Ther.* **214:**9–15.

Gruetter, C. A., Gruetter, D. Y., Lyon, J. E., Kadowitz, P. J., and Ignarro, L. J., 1981a, Relationship between cyclic guanosine 3′,5′-monophosphate formation and relaxation of coronary arterial smooth muscle by glyceryl trinitrate, nitroprusside, nitrite and nitric oxide: Effects of methylene blue and methemoglobin, *J. Pharmacol. Exp. Ther.* **219**:181–186.

Gruetter, C. A., Kadowitz, P. J., and Ignarro, L. J., 1981b, Methylene blue inhibits coronary arterial relaxation and guanylate cyclase activation by nitroglycerin, sodium nitrite and amyl nitrite, *Can. J. Physiol. Pharmacol.* **59**:150–156.

Heppel, L. A., and Hilmoe, R. J., 1950, Metabolism of inorganic nitrite and nitrate esters. II. The enzymatic reduction of nitroglycerin and erythritol tetranitrate by glutathione, *J. Biol. Chem.* **183**:129–138.

Ignarro, L. J., and Gruetter, C. A., 1980, Requirement of thiols for activation of coronary arterial guanylate cyclase by glyceryl trinitrate and sodium nitrite: Possible involvement of S-nitrosothiols, *Biochim. Biophys. Acta* **631**:221–231.

Ignarro, L. J., Edwards, J. C., Gruetter, D. Y., Barry, B. K., and Gruetter, C. A., 1980a, Possible involvement of S-nitrosothiols in the activation of guanylate cyclase by nitroso compounds, *FEBS Lett.* **110**:275–278.

Ignarro, L. J., Barry, B. K., Gruetter, D. Y., Edwards, J. C., Ohlstein, E. H., Gruetter, C. A., and Baricos, W. H., 1980b, Guanylate cyclase activation by nitroprusside and nitrosoguanidine is related to formation of S-nitrosothiol intermediates, *Biochem. Biophys. Res. Commun.* **94**:93–100.

Ignarro, L. J., Lippton, H., Edwards, J. C., Baricos, W. H., Hyman, A. L., Kadowitz, P. J., and Gruetter, C. A., 1981a, Mechanism of vascular smooth muscle relaxation by organic nitrates, nitrites, nitroprusside and nitric oxide: Evidence for the involvement of S-nitrosothiols as active intermediates, *J. Pharmacol. Exp. Ther.* **218**:739–749.

Ignarro, L. J., Barry, B. K., Gruetter, D. Y., Ohlstein, E. H., Gruetter, C. A., Kadowitz, P. J., and Baricos, W. H., 1981b, Selective alterations in responsiveness of guanylate cyclase to activation by nitroso compounds during enzyme purification, *Biochim. Biophys. Acta* **673**:394–407.

Ignarro, L. J., Kadowitz, P. J., and Baricos, W. H., 1981c, Evidence that regulation of hepatic guanylate cyclase activity involves interactions between catalytic site -SH groups and both substrate and activator, *Arch. Biochem. Biophys.* **208**:75–86.

Ignarro, L. J., Degnan, J. N., Baricos, W. H., Kadowitz, P. J., and Wolin, M. S., 1982a, Activation of purified guanylate cyclase by nitric oxide requires heme: Comparison of heme-deficient, heme-reconstituted and heme-containing forms of soluble enzyme from bovine lung, *Biochim. Biophys. Acta* **718**:49–59.

Ignarro, L. J., Wood, K. S., and Wolin, M. S., 1982b, Activation of purified soluble guanylate cyclase by protoporphyrin IX, *Proc. Natl. Acad. Sci. U.S.A.* **79**:2870–2873.

Janis, R. A., and Diamond, J., 1979, Relationship between cyclic nucleotide levels and drug-induced relaxation of smooth muscle, *J. Pharmacol. Exp. Ther.* **211**:480–484.

Kadowitz, P. J., Nandiwada, P., Gruetter, C. A., Ignarro, L. J., and Hyman, A. L., 1981, Pulmonary vasodilator responses to nitroprusside and nitroglycerin in the dog, *J. Clin. Invest.* **67**:893–902.

Katsuki, S., and Murad, F., 1977, Regulation of adenosine cyclic 3′,5′-monophosphate and guanosine cyclic 3′,5′-monophosphate levels and contractility in bovine tracheal smooth muscle, *Mol. Pharmacol.* **13**:330–341.

Katsuki, S., Arnold, W., Mittal, C., and Murad, F., 1977, Stimulation of guanylate cyclase by sodium nitrosprusside, nitroglycerin and nitric oxide in various tissue preparations and comparison to the effects of sodium azide and hydroxylamine, *J. Cyclic Nucleotide Res.* **3**:23–35.

Kawachi, T., Kogure, K., Kamijo, Y., and Sugimura, T., 1970, The metabolism of N-methyl-N′-nitro-N-nitrosoguanidine in rats, *Biochim. Biophys. Acta* **222**:409–415.

Keith, R. A., Burkman, A. M., Sokoloski, T. D., and Fertel, R. H., 1982, Vascular tolerance to nitroglycerin and cyclic GMP generation in rat aortic smooth muscle, *J. Pharmacol. Exp. Ther.* **221**:525–531.

Kimura, H., Mittal, C. K., and Murad, F., 1975a, Increases in cyclic GMP levels in brain and liver with sodium azide an activator of guanylate cyclase, *Nature* **257**:700–702.

Kimura, H., Mittal, C. K., and Murad, F., 1975b, Activation of guanylate cyclase from rat liver and other tissues by sodium azide, *J. Biol. Chem.* **250**:8016–8022.

Kramer, G. L., and Wells, J. N., 1979, Effects of phosphodiesterase inhibitors on cyclic nucleotide levels and relaxation of pig coronary arteries, *Mol. Pharmacol.* **16**:813–822.

Kruszyna, H., Kruszyna, R., and Smith, R. P., 1982, Nitroprusside increases cyclic guanylate monophosphate concentrations during relaxation of rabbit aortic strips and both effects are antagonized by cyanide, *Anesthesiology* **57**:303–308.

Kukovetz, W. R., Poch, G., Holzmann, S., Wurm, A., and Rinner, I., 1978, Role of cyclic nucleotides in adenosine-mediated regulation of coronary flow, *Adv. Cyclic Nucleotide Res.* **9**:397–409.

Kukovetz, W. R., Poch, G., Holzmann, S., Wurm, A., and Rinner, I., 1979a, Cyclic nucleotides and coronary flow, in: *Cyclic Nucleotides and Therapeutic Perspectives* (G. Cehovic and G. A. Robison, eds.), Pergamon Press, Oxford, pp. 109–125.

Kukovetz, W. R., Holzmann, S., Wurm, A., and Poch, G., 1979b, Prostacyclin increases cyclic AMP in coronary arteries, *J. Cyclic Nucleotide Res.* **5**:469–476.

Kukovetz, W. R., Holzmann, S., Wurm, A., and Poch, G., 1979c, Evidence for cyclic GMP-mediated relaxant effects of nitro-compounds in coronary smooth muscle, *Naunyn Schmiedebergs Arch. Pharmacol.* **310**:129–138.

Kukovetz, W. R., Poch, G., and Holzmann, S., 1981, Cyclic nucleotides and relaxation of vascular smooth muscle, in: *Vasodilatation* (P. M. Vanhoutte and I. Leusen, eds.), Raven Press, New York, pp. 339–353.

Lawley, P. D., and Thatcher, C. J., 1970, Methylation of deoxyribonucleic acid in cultured mammalian cells by N-methyl-N'-nitro-N-nitrosoguanidine, *Biochem. J.* **116**:693–707.

Lee, T. P., Kuo, J. F., and Greengard, P., 1972, Role of muscarinic cholinergic receptors in regulation of guanosine 3',5'-cyclic monophosphate content in mammalian brain, heart muscle, and intestinal smooth muscle, *Proc. Natl. Acad. Sci. U.S.A.* **69**:3287–3291.

Lippton, H. L., Gruetter, C. A., Ignarro, L. J., Meyer, R. L., and Kadowitz, P. J., 1982, Vasodilator actions of several N-nitroso compounds, *Can. J. Physiol. Pharmacol.* **60**:68–75.

Mackenzie, J. E., and Parratt, J. R., 1977, Comparative effects of glyceryl trinitrate on venous and arterial smooth muscle *in vitro*; relevance to antianginal activity, *Br. J. Pharmacol.* **60**:155–160.

McCalla, D. R., Reuvers, A., and Kitai, R., 1968, Inactivation of biologically active N-methyl-N-nitroso compounds in aqueous solution: Effect of various conditions of pH and illumination, *Can. J. Biochem.* **46**:807–811.

Miki, N., Kawabe, Y., and Kuriyama, K., 1977, Activation of cerebral guanylate cyclase by nitric oxide, *Biochem. Biophys. Res. Commun.* **75**:851–856.

Mittal, C. K., Kimura, H., and Murad, F., 1975, Requirement for a macromolecular factor for sodium azide activation of guanylate cyclase, *J. Cyclic Nucleotide Res.* **1**:261–269.

Mittal, C. K., Kimura, H., and Murad, F., 1977, Purification and properties of a protein required for sodium azide activation of guanylate cyclase, *J. Biol. Chem.* **252**:4384–4390.

Murad, F., Mittal, C. K., Arnold, W. P., Katsuki, S., and Kimura, H., 1978, Guanylate cyclase: Activation by azide, nitro compounds, nitric oxide, and hydroxyl radical and inhibition by hemoglobin and myoglobin, *Adv. Cyclic Nucleotide Res.* **9**:145–158.

Nandiwada, P. A., Hyman, A. L., and Kadowitz, P. J., 1983, Pulmonary vasodilator responses to vagal stimulation and acetylcholine in the cat, *Circ. Res.*, **53**:86–95.

Napoli, S. A., Gruetter, C. A., Ignarro, L. J., and Kadowitz, P. J., 1980, Relaxation of bovine coronary arterial smooth muscle by cyclic GMP, cyclic AMP and analogs, *J. Pharmacol. Exp. Ther.* **212**:469–473.

Needleman, P., 1976, Organic nitrate metabolism, *Annu. Rev. Pharmacol.* **16**:81–93.

Needleman, P., and Johnson, E. M., Jr., 1973, Mechanism of tolerance development to organic nitrates, *J. Pharmacol. Exp. Ther.* **184**:709–715.

Needleman, P., Jakschik, B., and Johnson, E. M., 1973, Sulfhydryl requirement for relaxation of vascular smooth muscle, *J. Pharmacol. Exp. Ther.* **187**:324–331.

Neurath, G. B., Dunger, M., and Pein, F. G., 1976, Interaction of nitrogen oxides, oxygen and amines in gaseous mixtures, *IARC Sci. Publ.* **14**:215–225.

Ohlstein, E. H., Wood, K. S., and Ignarro, L. J., 1982, Purification and properties of heme-deficient hepatic soluble guanylate cyclase: Effects of heme and other factors on enzyme activation by NO, NO-heme, and protoporphyrin IX, *Arch. Biochem. Biophys.* **218**:187–198.

Pagani, M., Vatner, S. F., and Braunwald, E., 1978, Hemodynamic effects of intravenous sodium nitroprusside in the conscious dog, *Circulation* **57**:144–151.

Robinson, B. F., Collier, J. G., and Dobbs, R. J., 1979, Comparative dilator effects of verapamil and sodium nitroprusside in forearm arterial bed and dorsal hand veins in man: Functional differences between vascular smooth muscle in arterioles and veins, *Cardiovasc. Res.* **13**:16–21.

Robison, G. A., Butcher, R. W., and Sutherland, E. W., 1968, The role of cyclic AMP in adipose tissue and smooth muscle, *Pharmacologist* **10**:145–146.

Saville, B., 1958, A scheme for the colorimetric determination of microgram amounts of thiols, *Analyst* **83**:670–672.

Schoental, R., and Rive, D. J., 1965, Interaction of N-alkyl-N-nitrosourethanes with thiols, *Biochem. J.* **97**:466–474.

Schultz, G., Hardman, J. G., and Sutherland, E. W., 1973, Cyclic nucleotides and smooth muscle function, in: *Asthma, Physiology, Immunopharmacology, and Treatment* (K. F. Austen and L. M. Lichtenstein, eds.), Academic Press, New York, pp. 123–138.

Schultz, K. D., Schultz, K., and Schultz, G., 1977, Sodium nitrosprusside and other smooth muscle-relaxants increase cyclic GMP levels in rat ductus deferens, *Nature* **265**:750–751.

Schultz, K. D., Bohme, E., Kreye, V. A. W., and Schultz, G., 1979, Relaxation of hormonally stimulated smooth muscular tissues by the 8-bromo derivative of cyclic GMP, *Naunyn Schmiedebergs Arch. Pharmacol.* **306**:1–9.

Schultz, U., and McCalla, D. R., 1969, Reactions of cysteine with N-methyl-N-nitroso-p-toluenesulfonamide and N-methyl-N'-nitro-N-nitrosoguanidine, *Can. J. Chem.* **47**:2021–2027.

Spies, C., Schultz, K. D., and Schultz, G., 1980, Inhibitory effects of mepacrine and eicosatetraynoic acid on cyclic GMP elevations caused by calcium and hormonal factors in rat ductus deferens, *Naunyn Schmiedebergs Arch. Pharmacol.* **311**:71–77.

Wheeler, G. P., and Bowdon, B. J., 1972, Comparison of the effects of cysteine upon decomposition of nitrosoureas and of 1-methyl-3-nitro-1-nitrosoguanidine, *Biochem. Pharmacol.* **21**:265–267.

Wolin, M. S., Wood, K. S., and Ignarro, L. J., 1982, Guanylate cyclase from bovine lung: A kinetic analysis of the regulation of the purified soluble enzyme by protoporphyrin IX, heme and nitrosyl-heme, *J. Biol. Chem.* **257**:13312–13320.

CLINICAL APPLICATIONS

The Relationship of Receptor Actions of Dopamine Agonists to Their Clinical Effects

LEON I. GOLDBERG

1. Introduction

We have subdivided dopamine (DA) receptors by differences in activity and potency of agonists and by demonstration of specific antagonism. The responses we have utilized can be measured in the human. Accordingly, if the subdivision is valid, the data should be useful for clinical studies.

In our classification DA receptors are divided into two subtypes: DA_1 and DA_2. Methods and results leading to this classification have been described in detail (Goldberg and Kohli, 1979, 1981, 1982). Most of the data are based on studies in the intact dog. We are not aware of significant differences in the action of DA agonists on canine and human receptors.

The principal question posed by this chapter is as follows: Can classification of DA receptors into DA_1 and DA_2 subtypes be used to help explain the effects of DA agonists in the human? Therefore, only agonists that have been administered to normal human subjects and patients are discussed.

DA_1 receptors subserve smooth muscle relaxation, which in the cardiovascular system is manifested as vasodilation (Goldberg, 1972; Goldberg *et al.*, 1978). Vasodilation is more pronounced in the renal, mesenteric, cerebral, and coronary vascular beds. DA_1 receptors are also located in other vascular beds but appear to be reduced in number. DA_2

LEON I. GOLDBERG • Committee on Clinical Pharmacology, Departments of Pharmacological and Physiological Sciences and Medicine, The University of Chicago, Chicago, Illinois 60637.

Table I. Peripheral Receptors Subserving Cardiovascular Actions

DA_1	Vasodilation (primarily in renal, mesenteric, cerebral, and coronary vascular beds)
DA_2	Inhibition of the activity of the postganglionic sympathetic nerve
β_1	Increased cardiac contractility, heart rate, and A–V conduction
β_2	Vasodilation (primarily in the skeletal muscle and mesenteric vascular beds)
α_1	Vasoconstriction
α_2	Vasoconstriction and inhibition of activity of the postganglionic sympathetic nerve

receptors subserve inhibition of the sympathetic nervous system. Activation of DA_2 receptors has also been associated with decreased secretion of prolactin and emesis (Fluckiger et al., 1978; Laubie and Schmitt, 1978; Buylaert et al., 1978; Dolak and Goldberg, 1981).

The potency series of agonists for DA_1 receptors is as follows: SK&F 82526 > DA = epinine > propylbutyl-DA > apomorphine. Ergot derivatives and piribedil are inactive. The potency series for activation of DA_2 receptors is as follows: apomorphine = propylbutyl DA > DA = epinine. Ergot derivates and piribedil are active. SK&F 82526 is inactive (Goldberg et al., 1978; Goldberg and Kohli, 1982; Hahn et al., 1982; Lokhandwala and Barrett, 1982; Kohli et al., 1982).

In addition to differences in relative DA_1 and DA_2 activity, DA agonists also differ with regard to their relative activity on other receptors. Table I lists other receptors DA and/or DA agonists act on and the responses elicited in the cardiovascular system. Table II lists several DA agonists studied in the human and the different receptors on which they have been shown to act. In addition, Table II indicates whether a compound is known to exhibit CNS activity. The significance and mechanisms responsible for the CNS actions of DA agonists is a controversial subject.

The following clinical conditions were chosen as examples for correlation of DA receptor activity and clinical response.

Table II. Characteristics of Dopamine Agonists

	DA_1	DA_2	β_1	β_2	α	CNS
					0	
SK&F 82526	+ + + +	0	0	0	+	0
Propylbutyl-DA	+ +	+ + + +	0	0	+	+
Apomorphine	+	+ + +	0	0	+, −	+
Ergots: Piribedil	0	+ +	0	0	+ → + + +	+
Dopamine	+ + +	+	+	0	+ +	0
Epinine	+ + +	+	+ +	+	+ + → + + + +	0

2. Shock

It is relatively easy to relate the effects of DA in the treatment of shock to its action on receptors. Numerous investigations in animals and humans have demonstrated that intravenous administration of DA produces dose-related changes in cardiac and renal function directly applicable to the therapy of shock (Horwitz *et al.*, 1962; MacCannell *et al.*, 1966; Goldberg *et al.*, 1977). With low rates of infusion (0.5–2 µg/kg per min), DA_1 and DA_2 receptors are activated, and there is a reduction in peripheral resistance without reflex tachycardia. Urine flow may increase with these low rates of infusion. When the infusion rate is increased to 2–4 µg/kg per min, β_1 receptors are activated, and cardiac output is increased. Systolic blood pressure is often increased, but there may be no change in diastolic blood pressure or heart rate. A further increase in urine flow is frequently observed. Finally, at higher infusion rates α-adrenergic receptors are activated, and both diastolic and systolic pressures are increased, often with further improvement in renal function. Since most patients in shock are hypotensive, higher rates of infusion are usually required with activation of all receptors.

3. Congestive Heart Failure

3.1. Dopamine

Congestive heart failure was the first clinical indication for DA (Goldberg, 1974; Goldberg *et al.*, 1963). Dopamine is administered at low rates of infusion to activate DA_1 and DA_2, but not α-adrenergic receptors (usual rates of infusion 0.5–4 µg/kg per min). Activation of α-adrenergic receptors would be deterimental because increased peripheral resistance is undesirable. A major advantage in the use of DA is that heart rate usually does not increase (presumably because of the DA_2 effect), and renal blood flow, glomerular filtration rate, and sodium excretion are usually markedly increased. The improvement in cardiac output that results from DA administration is probably related to the β_1-adrenergic effects; however, vasodilation resulting by direct action on DA_1 receptors and indirectly by reducing sympathetic nervous system activity may also be involved. Vasodilators such as nitroglycerin and nitroprusside are often added to DA therapy to produce further reductions in systemic resistance and to decrease venous and pulmonary pressures (Goldberg *et al.*, 1977).

3.2. Levodopa

Initial clinical studies by Whitsett and Goldberg (1972) demonstrated that oral administration of 1–1.5 g of levodopa to patients with Parkinson's disease caused β_1-adrenergic-induced myocardial stimulation to an extent similar to that produced by intravenous infusion of DA at an infusion rate of 4 μg/kg per min. Finlay *et al.* (1971) reported that a similar oral dose of levodopa in a patient with Parkinson's disease and mild congestive heart failure caused increments in renal blood flow, glomerular filtration rate, and sodium excretion. These effects were similar to the DA_1-induced effects produced by intravenous infusions of DA.

More recently, Rajfer *et al.* (1983) administered levodopa in a dose of 1.5–2 g to ten patients with severe (class III and class IV) congestive heart failure. Average cardiac index increased from 1.8–2.4 liters/min per m², and this effect persisted for approximately 4–6 hr. Heart rate, mean arterial pressure, and left ventricular filling pressure did not change significantly, but there was a statistically significant reduction in systemic vascular resistance. These responses appear to result from activation of β_1-adrenergic, DA_1, and DA_2 receptors. Interestingly, no α-adrenergic vasoconstriction was observed, apparently because the rate of production of DA by decarboxylation of levodopa did not result in a sufficiently high plasma level of DA to affect the α-adrenergic receptors. Levodopa dosage was gradually increased to avoid the known emetic effects of this drug (DA_2).

3.3. Ibopamine

Ibopamine is the diisobutyric ester of N-methyl-DA (epinine). When ibopamine is administered orally, epinine is released into the circulation. Epinine had previously been shown to be an active DA_1 and DA_2 agonist and differs from DA in exhibiting β_2 activity and greater α-adrenergic activity (Goldberg, 1972). When ibopamine is administered orally, however, the hemodynamic and renal effects appear to result from activation of β_1, DA_1, and DA_2 receptors. Extensive investigations of ibopamine in Italy and other European countries have been conducted in patients with severe congestive heart failure of different etiologies (Dei Cas *et al.*, 1983). Results of these studies demonstrated that ibopamine increased cardiac output and reduced systemic vascular resistance in most of these patients. Heart rate usually did not increase. In addition to the beneficial hemodynamic effects, ibopamine also produced a prolonged diuretic effect, apparently the result of increase in renal blood flow (DA_1). Ibopamine, unlike levodopa, has not been reported to produce emesis, presumably because it does not cross the blood–brain barrier to the same extent.

3.4. Propylbutyldopamine

Studies in our laboratory demonstrated that propylbutyl DA differed from DA in that it exhibited more pronounced DA_2 activity and was 1/30 as potent as DA on DA_1 receptors (Kohli *et al.*, 1978, 1980; Fennell *et al.*, 1980). In addition, propylbutyl DA does not act on β_1 receptors and has weaker α-adrenergic receptor activity than DA. Because of this difference in spectrum of receptor activity, Fennell *et al.* (1983) administered propylbutyl DA to 11 patients with severe congestive heart failure at infusion rates of 5, 10, and 20 μg/kg per min. In most patients, mean arterial pressure, left ventricular filling pressures, and pulmonary and systemic vascular resistances decreased, and cardiac index increased without change in either stroke work index or heart rate. These effects appear to result from DA_2-receptor-mediated inhibition of the sympathetic nervous system. The contribution of the relatively weak DA_1 receptor activity of this compound could not be assessed. Emesis, a common adverse effect of DA_2 agonists, did not occur with infusion rates up to 20 μg/kg per min, indicating that it is possible to separate emesis from inhibition of the sympathetic nervous system. However, one of three patients who received 40 μg/kg per min experienced emesis. As in experimental animals, the onset of propylbutyl DA action was rapid and became apparent within 2–4 min of the start of infusion.

3.5. Bromocriptine

Francis *et al.* (1983) administered bromocriptine in a single oral dose of 2.5 mg to ten patients with severe congestive heart failure. Cardiac index did not change significantly, but there was a significant increase in stroke volume index, and heart rate decreased from 87 to 78 beats/min. Left ventricular filling pressure and systemic vascular resistance were significantly reduced. In addition, plasma norepinephrine levels were lowered from the elevated values of 481 pg/ml to 366 pg/ml with no significant change in plasma renin activity. The onset of action was generally observed within 1–2 hr, and the peak response occurred at an average of 3.6 hr following the oral dose.

These hemodynamic effects can be explained by an action of bromocriptine on DA_2 receptors. Bromocriptine does not act on β_1-adrenergic or DA_1 receptors. However, evidence has been presented to suggest that bromocriptine may also inhibit sympathetic activity by action in the brain (Sowers *et al.*, 1980; Judy *et al.*, 1978; Agid *et al.*, 1979). Therefore, the hemodynamic effects of this drug may not be totally attributed to the DA_2 effect on the peripheral sympathetic nervous system.

4. Hypertension

The first hemodynamic investigations of DA demonstrated that DA differed from norepinephrine in that it reduced rather than increased systemic vascular resistance (Horwitz et al., 1962). The reduction in systemic resistance appears to result from activation of DA_1 and DA_2 receptors. In most normal subjects DA does not cause a significant reduction in blood pressure primarily because of activation of α- and β-adrenergic receptors (McDonald et al., 1964). However, the results of several investigations suggest that hypertensive patients may be more sensitive to the hypotensive effects of DA. Recently, Kikuchi et al. (1982) reported that intravenous infusions of DA at a rate of 3 μg/kg per min decreased the mean blood pressure of 44 patients with essential hypertension but did not affect the blood pressure of ten normotensive subjects. In addition, greater increments in urine volume, urinary sodium excretion, and creatinine clearance occurred in the hypertensive patients. Earlier, McNay and Goldberg (1966) reported that intravenous infusions of only 1 μg/kg per min of DA caused a pronounced reduction in the blood pressure (measured in the supine position) of four patients with severe hypertension who had previously been administered the α-adrenergic blocking agent phenoxybenzamine in an intravenous dose of 1 mg/kg. Without phenoxybenzamine, the same infusion of DA elevated blood pressure. Since α-adrenergic block prevents manifestation of DA_2 activity on blood vessels, the hypotension had to be caused by direct vasodilation produced by action on DA_1 receptors. Further evidence that action on DA_1 receptors can lower blood pressure has been demonstrated in preliminary studies of the selective DA_1 agonist SK&F 82526. Oral administration of SK&F 82526 decreased blood pressure and increased sodium excretion of several hypertensive patients (Carey et al., 1983; Ventura et al., 1983). In contrast, reduction in blood pressure did not occur in earlier studies of several normal subjects (Stote et al., 1983). Further investigations are necessary to determine whether the differences in response reflect increased receptor sensitivity in the hypertensive patients.

In contrast to the relatively limited data concerning DA_1 agonists, considerable data have accumulated demonstrating hypotensive effects of DA_2 agonists. Indeed, most investigations of the use of DA_2 agonists in the treatment of Parkinson's disease report orthostatic hypotension as a common adverse effect. Orthostatic hypotension would be expected as a result of DA_2 inhibition of sympathetic nervous system activity (Lokhandwala and Barrett, 1982). As stated above, however, a CNS mechanism could also be involved.

Several studies have reported that bromocriptine is effective in the treatment of hypertension (Stumpe et al., 1977). Again, suggestions have been made that the compound is more effective in hypertensive than in normotensive subjects (Sowers et al., 1982). In this regard, intravenous infusions of propylbutyl DA also have been shown to cause a marked reduction in blood pressure in hypertensive patients but not in normal subjects (Taylor *et al.*, 1982, 1983).

These studies suggest that both DA_1 and DA_2 agonists may offer a new approach to the treatment of hypertension. The question that must be answered is whether tolerance will occur. Tolerance to the orthostatic hypotensive effects of levodopa and the ergot derivatives appears to occur in patients with Parkinson's disease. In contrast, renal blood flow was found to increase following oral administration of levodopa despite 3 months of continuing therapy with this drug (Finlay *et al.*, 1971). These data suggest that there may be tolerance to the DA_2 or central effects of these compounds but not to the DA_1 effects.

5. Renal Failure

Several investigators have reported that intravenous infusions of DA at rates that activate only DA_1 and DA_2 receptors may be useful in the treatment of acute renal failure (Henderson *et al.*, 1980). These studies demonstrated that DA, administered alone or with furosemide, caused diuresis in previously oliguric patients. These effects appear to be caused by the increase in renal blood flow produced by an action of DA on DA_1 receptors. An action on DA_2 receptors could also cause diuresis in a patient with excessive adrenergic renal vasoconstriction. A direct tubular effect may also be involved (Bello-Reuss *et al.*, 1982).

Dopamine has also been reported to improve renal function in patients with chronic renal failure. More recently, Stefoni *et al.* (1982) reported that oral administration of ibopamine in a dose of 100 mg/day increased creatinine clearance in 21 patients by 31% after 6 months of administration. Mean creatinine clearance of the patients prior to therapy was 29 ml/min. Since continual deterioration of renal function would be expected in these patients, the finding that ibopamine can improve renal function is of considerable clinical interest. Additional studies are required to confirm this finding.

6. Endocrine Responses

A large and diverse number of endocrine functions have been reported to be affected by DA and DA agonists (Goldberg and Weder, 1980). It is difficult to prove that action on a specific DA receptor is responsible for most of these phenomena. It is clear that inhibition of prolactin release results from action on DA_2 receptors. First, both centrally and peripherally active DA_2 agonists are effective in decreasing prolactin excretion, both *in vivo* and *in vitro* (LeBlanc *et al.*, 1976; MacLeod *et al.*, 1976; Fluckiger *et al.*, 1978). Second, the selective DA_1 agonist SK&F 82526 does not inhibit the release of prolactin (Hahn *et al.*, 1982). In contrast, the effects of DA and DA agonists on the secretion of renin is much more complex (Goldberg and Weder, 1980). Both increases and reductions in renin secretion have been reported. These changes could have reflected the effects of the agonists on DA receptors and on other receptors. For example, the effect of an agonist on a DA_1 receptor would cause renal vasodilation and would tend to reduce renin activity, as would the effect of DA on DA_2 receptors to reduce sympathetic activity. On the other hand, DA acts on β_1-adrenergic receptors, which increases renin activity by direct action on cells of the juxtaglomerular apparatus.

7. Summary

This review suggests that it should be possible to begin to determine whether specific DA receptors are responsible for the actions of DA agonists in humans. This analysis is possible because of the difference in action of relatively selective DA agonists. It is important to emphasize, however, that additional studies will be required to prove the concept. First, it is possible that DA agonists may act on more than two receptors. Although we have assigned emesis, inhibition of the sympathetic nervous system, and inhibition of prolactin release to action on the same DA_2 receptor, these phenomena may be separable. Second, as stated several times in this chapter, some of the effects of DA agonists appear to be the result of a CNS effect. The unanswered question is whether this central action occurs through activation of a DA_2 receptor. Third, this chapter has been concerned almost entirely with agonists. Appropriate use of antagonists has not been possible thus far because currently available DA antagonists act on other receptors in addition to DA receptors. Preliminary studies suggest that some of the more recently synthesized antagonists are more selective and may be suitable for clinical investigations of DA actions (Kohli, *et al.*, 1983; Goldberg, *et al.*, 1984).

ACKNOWLEDGMENTS. I would like to thank Ms. Patricia Gomben for secretarial assistance. This work was supported by NIH grant GM-22220.

References

Agid, Y., Pollak, P., Bonnet, A. M., Signoret, J. L., and Lhermitte, F., 1979, Bromocriptine associated with a peripheral dopamine blocking agent in treatment of Parkinson's disease, *Lancet* 1:570–572.

Bello-Reuss, E., Higashi, Y., and Kaneda, Y., 1982, Dopamine decreases fluid reabsorption in straight portions of rabbit proximal tubule, *Am. J. Physiol.* **242**:F634–F640.

Buylaert, W. A., Willems, J. L., and Bogaert, M. G., 1978, The receptor mediating the apomorphine vasodilatation in the hindleg of the dog, *J. Pharm. Pharmacol.* **30**:113–115.

Carey, R. M., Townsend, L. H., Rose, C. E., Jr., Kaiser, D. L., Lindsay, C. C., and Ragsdale, N. V., 1983, The specific dopamine agonist, SK&F 82526-J, increases renal blood flow and lowers blood pressure in essential hypertension, *Clin. Res.* **31**:487A.

Dei Cas, L., Bolognesi, R., Cucchini, F., Fappani, A., Riva, S., and Visioli, O., 1983, Hemodynamic effects of ibopamine in patients with idiopathic congestive cardiomyopathy, *J. Cardiovasc. Pharmacol.* **5**:249–253.

Dolak, T. M., and Goldberg, L. I., 1981, Renal blood flow and dopaminergic agonists, *Annu. Rep. Med. Chem.* **16**:103–111.

Fennell, W. H., Kohli, J. D., and Goldberg, L. I., 1980, Hypotensive effects of N-N-di-*n*-propyl dopamine in the anesthetized dog: Comparison with sodium nitroprusside, *J. Cardiovasc. Pharmacol.* **2**:247–255.

Fennell, W. H., Taylor, A. A., Young, J. B., Brandon, T. A., Ginos, J. Z., Goldberg, L. I., and Mitchell, J. R., 1983, Propylbutyldopamine: Hemodynamic effects in conscious dogs, normal human volunteers, and patients with heart failure, *Circulation* **67**:829–836.

Finlay, G. D., Whitsett, T. L., Cucinell, E. A., and Goldberg, L. I., 1971, Augmentation of sodium and potassium excretion, glomerular filtration rate and renal plasma flow by levodopa, *N. Engl. J. Med.* **284**:865–870.

Fluckiger, E., Vigouret, J. M., and Wagner, H. R., 1978, Ergot compounds and prolactin secretion, in: *Progress in Prolactin Physiology and Pathology* (C. Robyn and M. Harter, eds.), Elsevier/North-Holland Biomedical Press, Amsterdam, pp. 383–396.

Francis, G. S., Parks, R., and Cohn, J. N., 1983, The effects of bromocriptine in patients with congestive heart failure, *Amer. Heart J.* **106**:100–106.

Glock, D., Kohli, J. D., and Goldberg, L. I., 1982, Domperidone: A potent and highly selective DA$_2$ peripheral dopamine receptor antagonist, *Fed. Proc.* **41**:1651.

Goldberg, L. I., 1972, Cardiovascular and renal actions of dopamine: Potential clinical applications, *Pharmacol. Rev.* **24**:1–29.

Goldberg, L. I., 1974, Dopamine: Clinical uses of an endogenous catecholamine, *N. Engl. J. Med.* **291**:707–710.

Goldberg, L. I., and Kohli, J. D., 1979, Peripheral pre- and post-synaptic dopamine receptors: Are they different from dopamine receptors in the central nervous system?, *Commun. Psychopharmacol.* **3**:447–456.

Goldberg, L. I., and Kohli, J. D., 1981, Agonists and antagonists of peripheral pre- and post-synaptic dopamine receptors: Clinical implications, in: *Apomorphine and other Dopaminomimetics*, Volume 1, *Basic Pharmacology* (G. L. Gessa and G. U. Corsini, eds.), Raven Press, New York, pp. 273–284.

Goldberg, L. I., and Kohli, J. D., 1982, Peripheral post-synaptic dopamine (DA$_1$) receptors, in: *Advances in the Biosciences*, Volume 37 *Advances in Dopamine Research* (M. Kohsaka, T. Shohmori, Y. Tsukada, G. N. Woodruff, eds.), Pergamon Press, Oxford, pp. 41–49.

Goldberg, L. I., and Weder, A. B., 1980, Connections between endogenous dopamine, dopamine receptors, and sodium excretion: Evidences and hypotheses, in: *Recent Advances in Clinical Pharmacology* (P. Turner and D. G. Shand, eds.), Churchill Livingstone, Edinburgh, pp. 149–166.

Goldberg, L. I., McDonald, R. H., Jr., and Zimmerman, A. M., 1963, Sodium diuresis produced by dopamine in patients with congestive heart failure, *N. Engl. J. Med.* **269**:1060–1064.

Goldberg, L. I., Hsieh, Y. Y., and Resnekov, L., 1977, Newer catecholamines for treatment of heart failure and shock. An update on dopamine and a first look at dobutamine, *Prog. Cardiovasc. Dis.* **4**:327–340.

Goldberg, L. I., Volkman, P. H., and Kohli, J. D., 1978, A comparison of the vascular dopamine receptor with other dopamine receptors, *Annu. Rev. Pharmacol. Toxicol.* **18**:57–79.

Goldberg, L. I., Glock, D., Kohli, J. D., and Barnett, A., 1984, Separation of peripheral dopamine receptors by a selective DA₁ antagonist, *SCH 23390. Hypertension,* (in press).

Hahn, R. A., Wardell, J. R., Jr., Sarau, H. M., and Ridley, P. T., 1982, Characterization of the peripheral and central effects of SK&F 82526, a novel dopamine receptor agonist, *J. Pharmacol. Exp. Ther.* **223**:305–313.

Henderson, I. S., Beattie, T. J., and Kennedy, A. C., 1980, Dopamine hydrochloride in oliguric states, *Lancet* **2**:827–829.

Horwitz, D., Fox, S. M., and Goldberg, L. I., 1962, Effects of dopamine in man, *Circ. Res.* **10**:237–243.

Judy, W. V., Watanabe, A. M., Henry, D. P., Besch, H. R., Jr., and Aprison, B., 1978, Effect of L-dopa on sympathetic nerve activity and blood pressure in the spontaneously hypertensive rat, *Circ. Res.* **43**:24–28.

Kikuchi, K., Miyama, A., Nakao, T., Takigami, Y., Kondo, A., Mito, T., Ura, N., Tsuzuki, M., and Iimura, O., 1982, Hemodynamic and natriuretic responses to intravenous infusion of dopamine in patients with essential hypertension, *Jpn. Circ. J.* **46**:486–493.

Kohli, J. D., Glock, D., and Goldberg, L. I., 1982, Differential antagonism of postsynaptic (DA₁) and presynaptic (DA₂) peripheral dopamine receptors by substituted benzamides, in: *The Benzamides: Pharmacology, Neurobiology, and Clinical Aspects* (J. Rotrosen and M. Stanley, eds.), Raven Press, New York, pp. 97–108.

Kohli, J. D., Glock, D., and Goldberg, L. I., 1983, Selective DA₂ versus DA₁ antagonist activity of domperidone in the periphery, *Eur. J. Pharmacol.* **89**:137–141.

Kohli, J. D., Goldberg, L. I., Volkman, P. H., and Cannon, J. G., 1978, N,N-Di-*n*-propyl dopamine: A qualitatively different dopamine vascular agonist, *J. Pharmacol. Exp. Ther.* **207**:16–22.

Kohli, J. D., Weder, A. B., Goldberg, L. I., and Ginos, J. Z., 1980, Structure activity relationships of N-substituted dopamine derivatives as agonists of the dopamine vascular and other cardiovascular receptors, *J. Pharmacol. Exp. Ther.* **213**:370–374.

Laubie, M., and Schmitt, H., 1978, Inhibitory effects of piribedil on adrenergic neurotransmission, *Eur. J. Pharmacol.* **52**:99–107.

LeBlanc, H., Lachelin, G. C. L., Abu-Fadil, S., and Yen, S. S. C., 1976, Effects of dopamine infusion on pituitary hormone secretion in humans, *J. Clin. Endocrinol. Metab.* **43**:668–674.

Lokhandwala, M. F., and Barrett, R. J., 1982, Cardiovascular dopamine receptors: Physiological, pharmacological and therapeutic implications, *J. Autonom. Pharmacol.* **3**:189–215.

MacCannell, K. L., McNay, J. L., Meyer, M. B., and Goldberg, L. I., 1966, The use of dopamine in the treatment of hypotension and shock, *N. Engl. J. Med.* **275**:1389–1398.

MacLeod, R. M., Kumura, H., and Login, I., 1976, Inhibition of prolactin secretion by dopamine and piribedil (ET-495), in: *Growth Hormones and Related Peptides* (A. Pecile and E. E. Muller, eds.), Excerpta Medica, Amsterdam, pp. 443–453.

McDonald, R. H., Jr., Goldberg, L. I., McNay, J. L., and Tuttle, E. P., Jr., 1964, Effects of dopamine in man: Augmentation of sodium excretion, glomerular filtration rate, and renal plasma flow, *J. Clin. Invest.* **43:**1116–1124.

McNay, J. L., MacCannell, K. L., Meyer, M. B., and Goldberg, L. I., 1966, Hypotensive effects of dopamine in dogs and hypertensive patients after phenoxybenzamine, *J. Clin. Invest.* **45:**1045–1046.

Rajfer, S. I., Anton, A. H., Rowland, J., and Goldberg, L. I., 1983, Beneficial hemodynamic effects of oral levodopa in heart failure: Relationship to the generation of dopamine, *Clin. Res.* **31:**526A.

Sowers, J. R., Sollars, E. G., Tuck, M. L., and Asp, N. D., 1980, Dopaminergic modulation of renin activity and aldosterone and prolactin secretion in the spontaneously hypertensive rat (40923), *Proc. Soc. Exp. Biol. Med.* **164:**598–603.

Sowers, J. R., Nyby, M., and Jasberg, K., 1982, Dopaminergic control of prolactin and blood pressure: Altered control in essential hypertension, *Hypertension* **4:**431–437.

Stefoni, S., Docci, D., Mosconi, G., Coli, L., and Prandini, R., 1982, Longterm treatment of chronic renal insufficiency by ibopamine (SB 7505), a new orally active dopamine-related drug, *Clin. Nephrol.* **18:**168–173.

Stote, R. M., Dubb, J. W., Familiar, R. G., Erb, B. B., and Alexander, F., 1983, A new oral renal vasodilator, fenoldopam, *Clin. Pharmacol. & Therap.* **34:**309–315.

Stumpe, K. O., Kolloch, R., Higuchi, M., Kurck, F., and Vetter, H., 1977, Hyperprolactinemia and antihypertensive effect of bromocriptine in essential hypertension, *Lancet,* **2:**211–214.

Taylor, A. A., Fennell, W. H., and Mitchell, J. R., 1982, Propylbutyldopamine increases renal blood flow and decreases blood pressure in man by activation of DA$_1$ and DA$_2$ dopamine receptors, *Clin. Res.* **30:**259A.

Taylor, A. A., Fennell, W. H., Feldman, M. B., Brandon, T. A., Ginos, J. Z., and Mitchell, J. R., 1983, Activation of peripheral dopamine presynaptic receptors lowers blood pressure and heart rate in dogs, *Hypertension* **5:**226–234.

Ventura, H. O., Messerli, F. H., Oigman, W., Dunn, F. G., Kobrin, I., and Frohlich, E. D., 1983, Immediate hemodynamic effects of SK&F 82526J—A dopamine agonist—in hypertension, *Circulation* **68:**III-46, #181.

Whitsett, T. L., and Goldberg, L. I., 1972, Effects of levodopa on systolic preejection period, blood pressure and heart rate during acute and chronic treatment of Parkinson's disease, *Circulation* **45:**97–106.

14

Hemodynamic Factors Involved in the Regulation of Sodium Balance

JAY H. STEIN

1. Introduction

Sodium salts constitute more than 90% of the total solute contained in extracellular fluid. Therefore, the content of the extracellular fluid volume is dependent on the regulation of sodium balance. Since sodium salts are excreted primarily by the kidney, it follows that the regulation of sodium balance will be determined by the relationship between sodium intake and the renal handling of sodium. In this chapter I briefly review the factors involved in the renal handling of sodium, emphasize how hemodynamic alterations may play a major regulatory role in the system, and, last, discuss the possible role of the dopaminergic receptor in this model.

2. Renal Handling of Sodium

Approximately 20,000 meq of sodium are filtered at the glomerulus each day. Of this amount, the urinary excretion of sodium in the steady state (which equals the dietary sodium intake) is usually around 1% of the filtered load. Thus, the vast amount of filtered sodium is reabsorbed at some point along the nephron. Approximately 50–65% of the filtered sodium load is reabsorbed along the proximal convoluted tubule (Burg, 1981). In the early proximal tubule, there is a lumen-negative potential difference created by active sodium reabsorption, which is coupled with the majority of glucose and amino acid transport. At this site there is also

JAY H. STEIN • Department of Medicine, The University of Texas Health Science Center at San Antonio, San Antonio, Texas 78284.

active hydrogen ion secretion with resultant reabsorption of sodium bicarbonate. There is a progressive decrement in luminal bicarbonate concentration and a reciprocal increment in luminal chloride concentration along the proximal convoluted tubule. With this progressive rise in chloride concentration, the luminal potential becomes positive in the late proximal tubule because of the diffusion potential caused by passive chloride reabsorption in this segment.

The proximal convoluted tubule is considered a "leaky" epithelium analogous to the well-studied mammalian gallbladder and jejunum. The leakiness of this epithelium reflects the ability of solute to migrate between cells, presumably through the morphologically well-defined lateral intercellular space. Although the exact transport process is not totally established, one view holds that sodium that enters a proximal tubular cell is actively transported into the intercellular space, increasing compartmental tonicity and thus generating an osmotic gradient, causing water to follow (Whittembury et al., 1973). This would then cause an increase in hydrostatic pressure within the space, which would act as a driving force to expel the salt and water into the interstitial compartment. Further, back leak of fluid from interstitium to lumen might occur across the tight junction located at the apical end of the channel (Fig. 1). The magnitude of this back leak would seemingly be dependent on the permeability of the tight junction and the hydraulic pressure within the interspace and renal interstitium. Recently, an alternative formulation has been proposed to explain the movement of salt and water through the intercellular channel that does not necessitate more than a small increase in osmolality in this compartment (Andreoli and Schafer, 1979). In any case, the presence of this compartment and its linkage with the postglomerular circulation will be discussed in detail subsequently.

The straight portion of the proximal tubule reabsorbs 5–10% of the filtered sodium load by an active transport process (Burg, 1981). There is presumably no sodium reabsorption in the descending limb of Henle's loop. On the other hand, a substantial amount of sodium reabsorption may occur in the thin ascending limb (Imai and Kokko, 1974). As water is being extracted along the descending limb, the sodium concentration within the tubular lumen rises, and by the time the fluid reaches the thin ascending limb, the sodium concentration within the tubular fluid exceeds that in the renal interstitium. Since the permeability of this segment is quite high for sodium, the cation will be passively reabsorbed as long as the appropriate concentration gradient is present. As will be subsequently discussed, the presence of this concentration gradient is markedly affected by alterations in blood flow in the renal medulla.

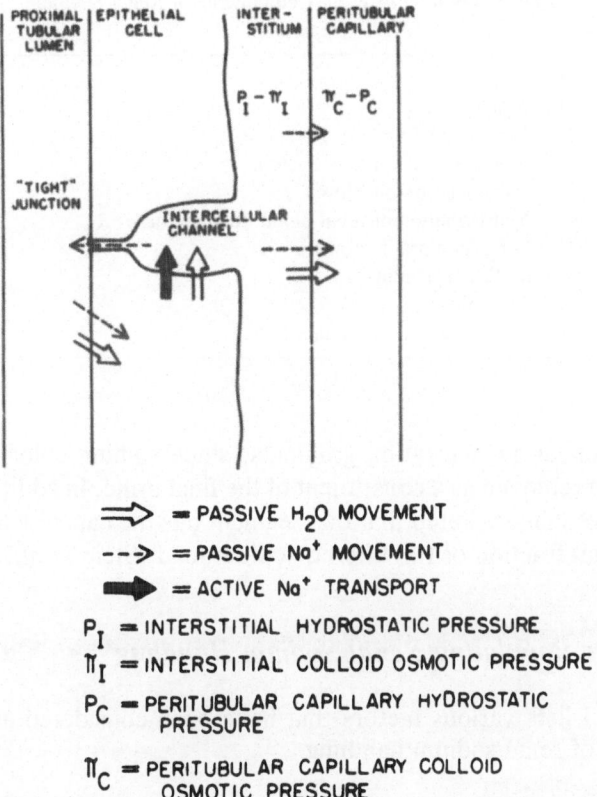

Figure 1. Schematic representation of the "pump–leak" model of proximal tubular sodium reabsorption. Filtered sodium is passively reabsorbed from the tubular lumen into the epithelial cell down a concentration gradient. It is then actively transported into the lateral intercellular channel, which communicates directly with the interstitial space. The uptake of reabsorbate from the interstitium into the peritubular capillary is determined by the Starling forces across the capillary wall. If the net force for uptake of reabsorbate into the capillary is decreased, conductive and geometric changes in the tight junction interspace complex may occur that favor increased "back leak" of reabsorbate into the tubular lumen, diminishing net absorption.

The thick ascending limb, distal convoluted tubule, and collecting duct system are all capable of active sodium chloride reabsorption (Burg, 1981). Although it had been previously thought that the chloride ion was actively transported in the thick ascending limb, this view has recently been seriously questioned (Greger, 1981). Both the thick ascending limb and distal tubule have been shown to be capable of markedly increasing absolute reabsorption when delivery to that segment is enhanced (Burg, 1981). The papillary collecting duct is capable of creating remarkable

Table I. Possible Efferent Components of Renal Sodium
Regulation

I.	GFR
II.	Aldosterone
III.	Peritubular Capillary Forces
IV.	Sympathetic Nervous System
V.	Medullary Blood Flow
VI.	Redistribution of renal blood flow and/or GFR
VII.	Other humoral factors
	a. Prostaglandins
	b. Kinins
	c. "Natriuretic hormone"?

electrochemical concentration gradients, since sodium chloride can essentially be removed as a constituent of the final urine. In addition, recent studies have demonstrated that this segment has the capacity to reabsorb a substantial fraction of the filtered sodium load (Stein *et al.*, 1976).

3. Factors Regulating Renal Sodium Handling

Table I lists various factors that have been considered as potential regulators of renal sodium handling.

3.1. Glomerular Filtration Rate

It is apparent that small increases in the glomerular filtration rate (GFR) without a concomitant rise in tubular reabsorption would lead to a marked natriuresis. Because of the technical difficulties in determining small changes in GFR (as measured by inulin clearance), it is difficult to disprove that a given natriuretic state is caused by an alteration in GFR even though no measurable change might be noted. Yet, a number of investigations starting with the work of deWarderner and associates (1961) have clearly demonstrated that a natriuresis may occur during expansion of the extracellular fluid volume in spite of a decrease in GFR. Further, a large number of studies have demonstrated the presence of glomerular tubular balance, i.e., a coupling between filtered sodium load and renal tubular sodium reabsorption. The mechanisms involved in this phenomenon are still not clear. There are data that factors extrinsic to the proximal tubule are responsible, i.e., hydrostatic and oncotic pressure in the peritubular capillary circulation (Brenner *et al.*, 1973). There is, however, continuing evidence that a change in tubular load will cause a directionally similar alteration in proximal tubular sodium reabsorption independent of these hemodynamic factors (Haberle *et al.*, 1981).

3.2. Hormonal Factors

Table I lists the various hormonal factors that have been suggested to play a role in regulating sodium balance.

The renin–angiotensin–aldosterone system is clearly altered during changes in extracellular volume. With a decrease in effective arterial volume, the system is activated in an attempt to restore homeostatic balance. This may have various effects on renal sodium balance as well. Angiotensin II has been proposed to have a direct effect on sodium transport (Harris and Young, 1977). In addition, the release of intrarenal angiotensin II may preferentially increase proximal tubular reabsorption by an effect on efferent arteriolar tone (see below). Aldosterone enhances sodium reabsorption in the collecting duct (Gross *et al.*, 1975). Yet, it is clear that aldosterone is not the final determinant of urinary sodium excretion. Sodium balance can be well regulated in adrenalectomized man on a small fixed dose of mineralocorticoids (Rosenbaum *et al.*, 1959). As is also well known, the chronic administration of mineralocorticoid causes only a transient period of salt retention, after which sodium balance is restored (the "DOCA escape" phenomenon). This would seem to indicate that the magnitude of salt delivery to the aldosterone-dependent collecting duct site is a major determinant of sodium balance and can overide the effect of aldosterone.

Prostaglandins of various types have been studied extensively in regard to their possible role in the regulation of sodium balance. Although there is *in vitro* evidence indicative of a direct inhibitory action of PGE_2 on thick ascending limb and cortical collecting tubule salt transport (Stokes and Kokko, 1977; Stokes, 1979), these findings have not been universally confirmed (Fine and Trizna, 1977). It is also possible that prostaglandins may have an effect on sodium balance that is hemodynamically mediated. Brenner and his group have suggested a vasodilatory effect of prostaglandins on the postglomerular circulation, which could decrease proximal tubular sodium reabsorption (Ichikawa and Brenner, 1980). In addition, a prostaglandin-mediated change in medullary blood flow could alter sodium excretion.

The kallikrein–kinin system has also been extensively studied in the past decade. Kinins are also potent vasodilators, a phenomenon that is partially prostaglandin dependent. The direct role of the kinin system on sodium excretion is not presently clear.

Aside from these well-defined humoral agents, there continues to be a search for additional humoral substances that decrease sodium transport when extracellular fluid volume is expanded. Although a number of potentially exciting physiological results have been reported, there has not been, to date, the biochemical characterization of such a putative substance.

3.3. Sympathetic Activity

Altered adrenergic nervous activity can modify urinary sodium excretion by influencing Starling's forces in the peripheral capillary bed, by affecting the central blood volume, or by changing renal hemodynamics. A more direct effect of autonomic nerve activity on renal sodium handling has also been demonstrated. Numerous studies have demonstrated that alterations in sympathetic activity may affect renal sodium handling without any discernible change in renal hemodynamics. Low-level renal nerve stimulation without measurable alterations in GFR or renal blood flow can decrease sodium excretion (Zambraski and DiBona, 1976). Renal denervation in the rat depresses proximal tubular sodium reabsorption and increases sodium excretion without a change in GFR (Bello-Reuss et al., 1975). These findings have a possible histological correlate, since sympathetic fibers have been found in close proximity to tubular epithelium (Barajas, 1978). In addition, L-norepinephrine (10^{-6} M) reversibly increases fluid reabsorption in the isolated rabbit proximal convoluted tubule (Bello-Reuss, 1980). This effect is blocked by propranolol but not by phentolamine and can be reproduced with isoproterenol and phentolamine.

The overall importance of adrenergic activity to the regulation of sodium balance must be questioned, however, since a totally denervated kidney (i.e., transplant recipient) maintains sodium balance normally.

4. Hemodynamic Factors

Ludwig initially proposed that tubular reabsorption was totally a passive phenomenon related to a fall in hydrostatic pressure in the postglomerular capillaries coupled with the concentration of nonfilterable solutes in the capillary circulation (Ludwig, 1844). This view was quite intuitive, since Starling's classic description of the forces affecting solute and water movement across the capillary was not to be published until more than 60 years later (Starling, 1908). Yet, tubular transport cannot be explained on the basis of the Ludwig hypothesis alone. First, active transport of sodium has been demonstrated in virtually every portion of the nephron (Burg, 1981). Second, the passive reabsorption thesis is not compatible with the ability of the mammalian kidney to both concentrate and dilute the final urine. These two points in particular dissuaded a number of investigators from seriously considering the role of the capillary circulation in the regulation of salt and water balance. Although there is clearly active transport of sodium and/or chloride along the nephron, changes in hydrostatic and/or oncotic pressure in the peritubular capillary circulation may in some manner modify the net reabsorption of electrolytes. In fact, Green *et al.* (1974) showed that an effect of oncotic pressure on proximal tubular sodium reabsorption could only be demonstrated in the presence of an intact active transport system. Thus, the active transport of sodium and other electrolytes in no way obviates a role for these passive forces in altering the composition of the final urine.

In order to more clearly explain the role of these so-called "physical factors," a few basic comments are warranted. Along the glomerular capillary, net ultrafiltration is favored in at least a portion of the glomerulus because of the greater transcapillary hydrostatic pressure gradient (ΔP). As filtration occurs, the transcapillary colloid osmotic pressure difference ($\Delta\pi$) rises until it equals ΔP. The reverse forces are operative in the peritubular capillary. Because of the marked pressure drop from the glomerulus to the peritubular capillary, $\Delta\pi$ exceeds ΔP, and absorption of reabsorbate into the capillary occurs. ΔP is equal to $P_C - P_I$, where P_C and P_I are the capillary and interstitial hydrostatic pressure, and $\Delta\pi$ is equal to $\pi_C - \pi_I$, where π_C and π_I are the capillary and interstitial colloid osmotic pressures, respectively. Thus, the fluid exchanges across the capillary wall at any point can be expressed by:

$$J_v = K\left[(\pi_C - \pi_I) - (P_C - P_I)\right] \tag{1}$$

where J_v is the net transcapillary fluid flux, and K is the effective hydraulic permeability of the capillary wall.

Although it has recently become popular to consider these passive forces totally as a function of the mass balances shown in equation 1, it must be remembered that the primary regulatory events that alter either ΔP or $\Delta\pi$ are hemodynamic. For example, increases in renal blood flow caused by various stimuli (i.e., vasodilator agents, extracellular volume expansion, etc.) are usually associated with a fall in filtration fraction (FF). As originally derived by Bresler (1956):

$$C_E = C_A\, 1/(1 - FF) \tag{2}$$

where C_E and C_A are efferent and afferent arteriolar protein concentrations, respectively. Rearranging,

$$FF = 1 - C_E/C_A \qquad (3)$$

From this equation, it is clear that at any given C_A, a fall in FF will decrease C_E. In addition, vasodilatation will increase P_C because of the fall in resistance at the efferent arteriole. Thus, renal vasodilatation will decrease C_E and increase P_C, both alterations that would tend to decrease capillary uptake.

Even with this basic understanding of the relationship between capillary uptake and the Starling forces acting across the peritubular capillary, a rather complex mechanism is required to explain how alterations in these parameters may modify urinary sodium excretion.

The linkage between peritubular capillary dynamics and proximal tubular reabsorption primarily involves the lateral intercellular channel (Section 2). As previously discussed, fluid moves from the intercellular channel into the interstitium by a hydrostatic pressure gradient generated in the channel. The reabsorbate entering the interstitium is then removed at a rate determined by the Starling forces acting across the peritubular capillary. If, in a given setting, the rate of reabsorption exceeds the rate of capillary uptake, interstitial volume will increase. For example, a decrease in capillary oncotic pressure and/or a rise in capillary hydrostatic pressure would decrease the rate of uptake out of the renal interstitium. This alteration in interstitial volume may then lead to a change in the conductance and/or the geometry of the tight junction–intercellular channel complex with a resultant increase in the flux of sodium back into the lumen of the proximal tubule (back leak). The net effect of this particular alteration would be a decrease in net sodium transport in the proximal tubule even though active transport was unchanged (Fig. 1). Although a number of the specific aspects of this model are still controversial, the general description would seem to be a reasonable working hypothesis. In any case, from this model, one can see how alterations in Starling's forces in the peritubular capillary circulation may modify net sodium transport in the proximal convoluted tubule.

Thus, the natriuretic action of various vasodilators such as dopamine may be mediated through such a mechanism. It should be noted, however, that not all renal vasodilators cause an increase in sodium excretion (see below).

Finally, it should be emphasized that the control of peritubular capillary forces may be mediated by vasoactive agents. Ichikawa and Brenner (1980) have, in fact, suggested that efferent arteriolar tone is regulated by the balance between vasodilatory prostaglandins and vasoconstrictor substances such as angiotensin II.

5. Medullary Blood Flow

Although the blood flow in the inner medulla is only a small fraction of that in the renal cortex, the regulation of medullary blood flow may be critical to the regulation of both salt and water balance. To exemplify this proposal, recent studies from our laboratory have compared the vasodilators bradykinin, acetylcholine, and secretin (Fadem *et al.*, 1982). All three compounds caused a comparable rise in total renal blood flow, but only bradykinin and acetylcholine were natriuretic. Of interest, both natriuretic vasodilators increased medullary blood flow, but secretin did not (Fig. 2). Thus, it would seem that an increase in medullary blood flow was critical for a natriuresis in this setting.

Several suggestions have been made to explain this relationship between medullary blood flow and sodium excretion. Earley and Friedler (1964), in considering both drug-induced vasodilatation and volume expansion, first suggested that a washout of the medullary interstitium may be natriuretic. Their theory is as follows: states associated with an increase in medullary blood flow will "wash out" the hypertonic medullary interstitium. This will decrease the abstraction of water out of the descending limb of Henle's loop, which normally occurs because of the high medullary osmolality. Thus, an increased volume of fluid with the same total sodium content will be delivered to the water-impermeable ascending limb. If there is a lower limit to the sodium concentration that can be generated along the ascending limb, then more sodium will be delivered to the distal portion of the nephron.

More recently, studies from our laboratory have suggested another mechanism for the relationship between medullary blood flow and urinary sodium excretion (Osgood *et al.*, 1978). Ringer loading, a model that presumably increases medullary blood flow, was shown to abolish the sodium concentration gradient between the thin ascending limb and the medullary interstitium (Fig. 3). This consequence of medullary washout would abolish any sodium transport in this segment, which presumably only transports sodium passively, and cause a marked increase in delivery of sodium to more distal nephron sites.

One possible contradiction to this proposal is the fact that a natriuresis is not seen during water diuresis, a model in which medullary washout occurs. To investigate this question, Reineck and Parma (1982) performed micropuncture studies in the rat comparing water diuresis and

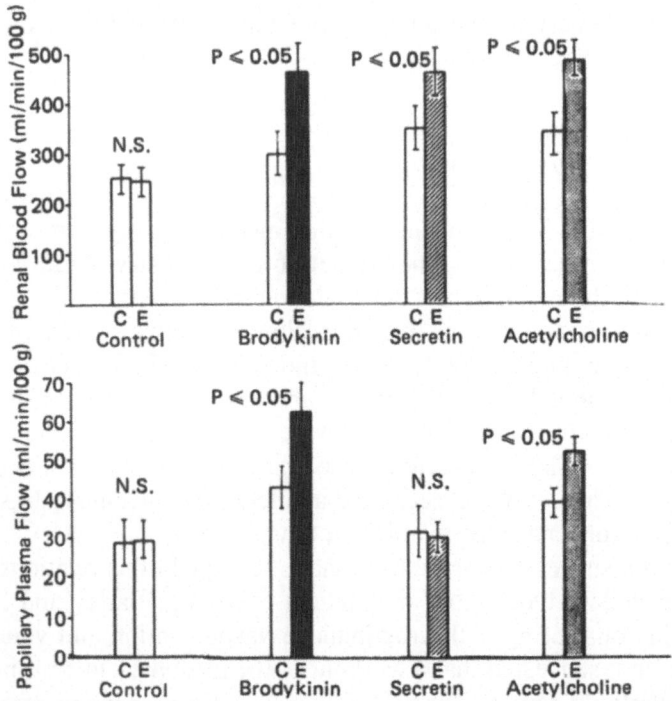

Figure 2. Summary of total renal blood flow and papillary plasma flow (PPF). Adjacent bars represent values from the two kidneys in each animal. Although bradykinin, secretin, and acetylcholine all increased total renal blood, only bradykinin and acetylcholine increased PPF (Reproduced with permission from Fadem *et al.*, 1982).

mild extracellular volume expansion. Water diuresis *per se* did not alter sodium delivery out of the proximal tubule or urinary sodium excretion. On the other hand, the superimposition of a salt load that normally caused only a trivial natriuresis with water diuresis caused a marked increase in sodium excretion. It was concluded that the natriuretic effect of medullary washout required a setting in which there was a concomitant increase in sodium delivery out of the proximal tubule (i.e., saline loading).

6. Redistribution of Blood Flow and/or Filtrate

Alterations in the distribution of renal blood flow have also been suggested to affect urinary sodium excretion. According to this original theory, deep nephrons may have a greater sodium reabsorption capacity than more superficial nephrons, and thus the redistribution of flow to deep nephrons would result in sodium retention (Goodyer and Jaeger, 1955).

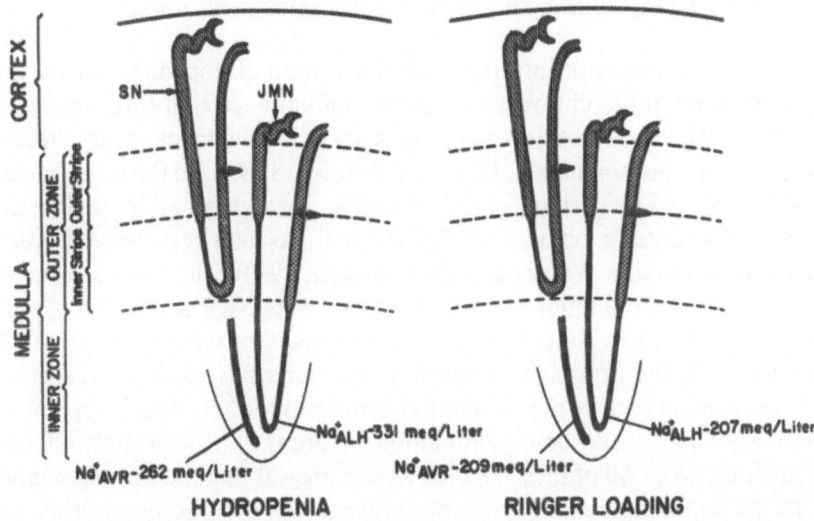

Figure 3. Proposed model to explain heterogeneity of Na$^+$ transport during Ringer loading. Arrows denote active salt transport in thick ascending limb of both superficial (SN) and juxtamedullary nephrons (JMN). In hydropenia (left panel), a sodium concentration gradient exists between thin ascending limb (ALH) and ascending vasa recta (AVR), 331 *vs.* 262 meq/liter. During Ringer loading, however, this gradient is abolished. Thus, sodium transport would be markedly decreased in the thin ascending limb of JMN because transport in this segment presumably occurs totally by passive means (Reproduced with permission from Osgood *et al.*, 1978).

Utilizing an inert gas washout technique, Thornburn *et al.* (1963) presented data to support this hypothesis. In a recent review, however, Lameire *et al.* (1977) summarized the current status of this controversial field. Compiling data from a large number of studies employing the radiolabeled microsphere method, they found no correlation between the changes in distribution and urinary sodium excretion. From these studies, it was concluded that there was no clear-cut evidence that redistribution of cortical blood flow *per se* was a major determinant of urinary sodium excretion.

A redistribution of renal blood flow does not necessarily indicate a redistribution of glomerular filtrate. Many laboratories have utilized micropuncture methods as well as a technique that determines the nephron uptake of [^{14}C]-ferrocyanide (Hanssen technique) to determine the distribution of nephron GFR. As recently summarized, the results are somewhat conflicting (Lameire *et al.*, 1977). Yet, it would seem fair to say that there is generally no evidence to suggest that a redistribution of glomerular filtrate is consistently noted in a given experimental setting.

7. Effect of Dopamine on Urinary Sodium Excretion

The intravenous or intrarenal administration of dopamine causes an increase in renal blood flow and urinary sodium excretion (McDonald *et al.*, 1964). The action of dopamine on renal hemodynamics is not altered by α-adrenoceptor blockade (Hahn and Wardell, 1980). On the other hand, agents such as haloperidol, chlorpromazine, metoclopramide, and ergometrine attenuate or obviate the fall in renal vascular resistance usually seen with dopamine (Yeh *et al.*, 1969; Brotzu, 1970). The renal effects of dopamine may be mimicked by agonists such as SKF 38393 (Lang and Woodman, 1982). Although dopamine decreases resistance in the renal vascular bed, the drug administered at the same dose may be vasoconstrictor in areas such as the hindlimb (Hahn and Wardell, 1980). Dopamine also vasodilates the coronary circulation, whereas SKF 38393 only affects renal blood flow. All of these studies would suggest that the hemodynamic effect of dopamine results from the presence of specific renal vascular receptors. Further, the renal receptor seems to differ from that in other vascular beds.

Although it might be assumed that the natriuretic effect of dopamine is hemodynamically mediated, recent studies by Bello-Reuss *et al.* (1982) suggest an alternative possibility. Dopamine (10^{-6} M) markedly inhibited sodium transport in the straight portion of the isolated rabbit proximal tubule. There was no effect in the proximal convoluted tubule. Haloperidol, lisuride, and metoclopramide abolished this inhibitory effect. Since this inhibitory effect of dopamine was obviously not related to any change in hemodynamics in this study, the agent must have a more direct effect on sodium transport. The relevance of these findings to *in vivo* sodium balance is not clear, since the total sodium transport by the pars recta is relatively small. In addition, there are no adequate anatomic data concerning the proximity of dopaminergic nerve endings to renal tubular cells.

ACKNOWLEDGMENTS. Portions of this work were supported by National Institutes of Health grant AM 17387.

References

Andreoli, T. E., and Schafer, J. A., 1979, External solution driving forces for isotonic fluid absorption in proximal tubules, *Fed. Proc.* **38**:154–160.

Barajas, L., 1978, Innervation of the renal cortex, *Fed. Proc.* **37**:1192–1201.

Bello-Reuss, E., 1980, Effect of catecholemines on fluid reabsorption by the isolated proximal convoluted tubule, *Am. J. Physiol.* **238**:F347–F352.

Bello-Reuss, E., Colindres, R. E., Pastoriza-Munoz, E., Mueller, R. A., and Gottschalk, C. W., 1975, Effects of acute unilateral renal denervation in the rat, *J. Clin. Invest.* 56:208–217.

Bello-Reuss, E., Higashi, Y., and Kaneda, Y., 1982, Dopamine decreases fluid reabsorption in straight portions of rabbit proximal tubule, *Am. J. Physiol.* 242:F634–F640.

Brenner, B. M., Troy, J. L., Daugharty, T. M., and MacInnes, R. M., 1973, Quantitative importance of changes in postglomerular colloid osmotic pressure in mediating glomerulotubular balance in the rat, *J. Clin. Invest.* 52:190–197.

Bresler, E. H., 1956. Problem of volume component of body fluid homeostasis, *Am. J. Med. Sci.* 232:93–104.

Brotzu, G., 1970, Inhibition by chlorpromazine of the effects of dopamine on the dog kidney, *J. Pharm. Pharmacol.* 22:664–667.

Burg, M. B., 1981, The renal handling of sodium chloride, water, amino acids, and glucose, in: *The Kidney*, 2nd ed. (B. M. Brenner and F. C. Rector, eds.), W. B. Saunders, Philadelphia, pp. 328–370.

Earley, L. E., and Friedler, R. M., 1965, Changes in renal blood flow and possibly intrarenal distribution of blood during the natriuresis accompanying saline loading in the dog, *J. Clin. Invest.* 44:929–941.

Fadem, S. Z., Hernandez-Llamas, G., Patak, R. V., Rosenblatt, S. G., Lifschitz, M. D., and Stein, J. H., 1982. Studies on the mechanism of sodium excretion during drug-induced vasodilatation in the dog, *J. Clin. Invest.* 69:604–610.

Fine, L. G., and Trizna, W., 1977, Influence of prostaglandins on sodium transport of isolated medullary nephron segments, *Am. J. Physiol.* 232:F383–F390.

Goodyer, A. V. N., and Jaeger, C. A., 1955, Renal response to non-shocking hemorrhage: Role of the autonomic nervous system and of the renal circulation, *Am. J. Physiol.* 180:69–74.

Green, R., Windhager, E. E., and Giebisch, G., 1974, Protein oncotic pressure effects on proximal tubular movement in the rat, *Am. J. Physiol.* 226:265–276.

Greger, R., 1981, Chloride reabsorption in the rabbit cortical thick ascending limb of Henle's loop of rabbit kidney, *Pfluegers Arch* 392:92–94.

Gross, J. B., Imai, M., and Kokko, J. P., 1975, A functional comparison of the cortical collecting tubule and the distal convoluted tubule, *J. Clin. Invest.* 55:1284–1294.

Haberle, D. A., Shiigai, T. T., Maier, G., Schiffl, H., and Davis, J. M., 1981, Dependency of proximal tubular fluid transport on the load of glomerular filtrate, *Kidney Int.* 20:18–28.

Hahn, R. A., and Wardell, J. R., Jr., 1980, Antagonism of the renal vasodilator activity of dopamine by metoclopramide, *Arch. Pharmacol.* 314:177–182.

Harris, P. I., and Young, J. A., 1977, Dose-dependent stimulation and inhibition of proximal tubular sodium reabsorption by angiotensin II in the rat kidney, *Pfluegers Arch.* 367:295–297.

Ichikawa, I., and Brenner, B. M., 1980, Importance of efferent arteriolar vascular tone in regulation of proximal tubule fluid reabsorption and glomerulotubular balance in the rat, *J. Clin. Invest.* 65:1192–1201.

Imai, M., and Kokko, J., 1974, Sodium chloride, urea, and water transport in the thin ascending limb of Henle: Generation of osmotic gradients by passive diffusion of solutes, *J. Clin. Invest.* 53:393–402.

Lameire, N. H., Lifschitz, M. D., and Stein, J. H., 1977, Heterogeneity of nephron function, *Annu. Rev. Physiol.* 39:159–184.

Lang, W. J., and Woodman. O. L., 1982, Comparison of the vasodilator action of dopamine and dopamine agonists in the renal and coronary beds of the dog, *Br. J. Pharmacol.* 77:023–028.

Ludwig, C., 1844, Nieren und Harnbereitung, in: *Handworterbuch der Physiologie*, Volume 2 (Wanger, ed.), Vieweg & Sohn, Braunschweig, p. 628.

McDonald, R. H., Jr., Goldberg, L. I., McNay, J. L., and Tuttle, E. P., Jr., 1964, Effects of dopamine in man: Augmentation of sodium excretion, glomerular filtration rate, and renal plasma flow, *J. Clin. Invest.* **43**:1116–1124.

Osgood, R. W., Reineck, H. J., and Stein, J. H., 1978, Further studies on segmental sodium transport in the rat kidney during expansion of the extracellular fluid volume, *J. Clin. Invest.* **64**:311–320.

Reineck, H. J., and Parma, R., 1982, Effect of medullary tonicity on urinary sodium excretion in the rat, *J. Clin. Invest.* **69**:971–978.

Rosenbaum, J. D., Papper, S., and Ashley, M. M., 1959, Variations on renal excretion of sodium independent of change in adrenocortical hormone dosage in patients with Addison's disease, *J. Clin. Endocrinol. Metab.* **15**:1459–1474.

Starling, E. H., 1908, in: *The Fluids of the Body* (Keener, ed.), Chicago.

Stein, J. H., Osgood, R. W., and Kunau, R. T., Jr., 1976, Direct measurement of papillary collecting duct sodium transport in the rat, *J. Clin. Invest.* **58**:767–773.

Stokes, J. B., 1979, Effect of prostaglandin E_2 on chloride transport across the rabbit thick ascending limb of Henle, *J. Clin. Invest.* **64**:495–502.

Stokes, J. B., and Kokko, J. P., 1977, Inhibition of sodium transport by prostaglandin E_2 across the isolated, perfused rabbit collecting tubule, *J. Clin. Invest.* **59**:1099–1104.

Thorburn, G. D., Kopald, H. H., Herd, J. A., Hollenberg, M., O'Morchoe, C. C. C., and Barger, A. C., 1963, Intrarenal distribution of nutrient blood flow determined with krypton[85] in the unanesthetized dog, *Circ. Res.* **13**:290–307.

Wardener, H. E. de, Mills, I. H., Clapham, W. F., and Hayter, C. J., 1961, Studies on the efferent mechanism of the sodium diuresis which follows the administration of intravenous saline in the dog, *Clin. Sci.* **21**:249–264.

Whittembury, G. F., Rawlins, F. A., and Boulpaep, E. L., 1973, Paracellular pathway in kidney tubules: Electrophysiological and morphological evidence, in: *Transport Mechanisms in Epithelia* (H. H. Ussing and N. A. Thorn, eds.), Academic Press, New York, pp. 577–595.

Yeh, B. K., McNay, J. L., and Goldberg, L. I., 1969, Attenuation of dopamine renal and mesenteric vasodilatation by haloperidol: Evidence for a specific dopamine receptor, *J. Pharmacol. Exp. Ther.* **168**:303–309.

Zambraski, E. J., and DiBona, G. F., 1976, Angiotensin II in antinatriuresis of low-level renal nerve stimulation, *Am. J. Physiol.* **231**:1105–1110.

15

Dopaminergic Mechanisms in the Control of Aldosterone Secretion
A Critical Appraisal

ROBERT M. CAREY

1. Introduction

Dopamine, a precursor of the sympathetic neurotransmitter norepinephrine, is itself a neurotransmitter in the central nervous system (Hornykiewicz, 1966). Dopamine also may serve as a neurotransmitter in the periphery, as it inhibits prolactin secretion directly at the pituitary lactotroph and dilates the renal and mesenteric vascular beds (MacLeod, 1976; Goldberg, 1975).

Studies during the past 5 years have suggested that aldosterone secretion may be inhibited by dopaminergic mechanisms (Carey et al., 1979, 1980). Administration of the dopamine antagonist metoclopramide to normal man increases aldosterone secretion independent of known regulating factors (Norbiato et al., 1977; Carey et al., 1979). Additional support for the concept that dopamine inhibits aldosterone secretion has been provided by in vitro studies demonstrating that angiotensin II-induced aldosterone secretion is inhibited by dopamine (McKenna et al., 1979). The observations that metoclopramide increases aldosterone secretion and that the dopamine agonists, dopamine and bromocriptine, do not decrease basal aldosterone secretion have led to the hypothesis that aldosterone secretion is under maximum tonic dopaminergic inhibition (Carey et al., 1979, 1980; Noth et al., 1980).

ROBERT M. CAREY • Division of Endocrinology and Metabolism, Department of Internal Medicine, University of Virginia Medical Center, Charlottesville, Virginia 22908.

2. Dopamine Antagonists

2.1. Metoclopramide

The vast majority of the evidence that dopaminergic mechanisms regulate aldosterone secretion derives from *in vivo* studies with metoclopramide in man and experimental animals.

Metoclopramide (N-diethylaminoethyl-2-methoxy-4-amino-5-chlorobenzamide) is a procainamide derivative with well-established dopamine antagonist properties (Jenner and Marsden, 1979). Metoclopramide is a competitive antagonist of dopamine in the central nervous system, gastrointestinal tract, and cardiovascular system (Dolphin *et al.*, 1975; Jenner *et al.*, 1975, 1978; Peringer *et al.*, 1976; Valenzuela, 1976; Day and Blower, 1975). Metoclopramide stimulates prolactin secretion from the pituitary gland *in vivo* in experimental animals and man and antagonizes the inhibitory action of dopamine on prolactin secretion *in vitro* (Delitala *et al.*, 1975; McCallum *et al.*, 1976; Sowers *et al.*, 1976, 1977; Carlson *et al.*, 1977; Healy and Burger, 1978; Aona *et al.*, 1978; Yeo *et al.*, 1978).

Although some of the biological effects metoclopramide may be related to nondopamine mechanisms, metoclopramide appears to be the most specific dopamine antagonist available for human investigation in the United States (Goldberg 1978; Goldberg and Weder, 1980). Under certain circumstances, metoclopramide may act as a serotonin antagonist (Pinder *et al.*, 1976; Fozard and Mobarok, 1978; Niemegeers and Jamssen, 1979). However, since serotonin stimulates aldosterone secretion *in vivo* and *in vitro*, metoclopramide could not stimulate aldosterone secretion by means of serotonin mechanisms (Haning *et al.*, 1970; Mantero *et al.*, 1980). Metoclopramide also increases gastroesophageal tone and motility by dopamine-dependent and -independent mechanisms (Hay, 1975; Valenzuela, 1976; Goldberg, 1978).

Kebabian and Calne (1979) recently emphasized the diversity of dopamine receptors in various tissues. At least two different classes of dopamine receptors can be identified on the basis of biochemical criteria. The so-called D-1 receptor is linked to adenylate cyclase; stimulation of this receptor results in intracellular accumulation of cyclic AMP. Postsynaptic nigrostriatal and renal vascular dopamine receptors are D-1 receptors. D-2 receptors are not adenylate cyclase linked; pituitary lactotrophs contain D-2 receptors, and metoclopramide has been proposed as a specific D-2 antagonist.

With the exception of the initial study of Ogihara *et al.* (1979), all studies from many different groups have reported an increase in plasma aldosterone secretion as a result of metoclopramide administration in man (Norbiato *et al.*, 1977; Carey *et al.*, 1979, 1980; Carpenter *et al.*, 1979; Noth *et al.*, 1980; Sowers *et al.*, 1980). An intravenous bolus dose of 10 mg of metoclopramide produces an increase in plasma aldosterone concentration within 5 min with a peak two- to threefold increase at 10–15 min and a return to baseline over 1–3 hr. In the rat, whether or not metoclopramide stimulates aldosterone secretion is controversial (Sowers *et al.*, 1980c; Campbell *et al.*, 1981), and metoclopramide does not stimulate aldosterone secretion in the rabbit, dog, or cat (Sowers *et al.*, 1981b). However, metoclopramide increases aldosterone secretion in the monkey, and this response is similar in onset, magnitude, and duration to that in man (Brown *et al.*, 1982; Sowers *et al.*, 1982b). Also, metoclopramide increases plasma aldosterone concentration in the sheep, although the response is not as marked and is more variable than in man (Coghlan *et al.*, 1980; Wilson *et al.*, 1983a). The increase in plasma aldosterone concentration evoked by metoclopramide in man is associated with an increase in urinary aldosterone excretion and no change in aldosterone metabolic clearance (Carey *et al.*, 1979; Carpenter *et al.*, 1979). Thus, a true increase in aldosterone secretion occurs.

In the studies with metoclopramide, none of the known stimuli for aldosterone secretion was altered. Thus, metoclopramide-induced increases in plasma aldosterone concentration were not associated with any changes in blood pressure, heart rate, plasma renin activity, or plasma concentrations of sodium, potassium, or cortisol (Norbiato *et al.*, 1977; Carey *et al.*, 1979, 1980; Carpenter *et al.*, 1979; Noth *et al.*, 1980; Sowers *et al.*, 1980a,b; Coghlan *et al.*, 1980). Further, metoclopramide-induced aldosterone secretion is not influenced by bilateral nephrectomy (absence of renin secretion), angiotensin blockers (saralasin or captopril), or dexamethasone (ACTH suppression) (Sowers *et al.*, 1980a–c, 1981a). Taken together, these results strongly suggest that metoclopramide stimulates aldosterone secretion independent of known aldosterone-regulating mechanisms.

Metoclopramide-induced aldosterone secretion is probably not related to pituitary factors, since metoclopramide increases aldosterone in hypopituitary patients in whom no detectable rise in serum prolactin concentration can be demonstrated (Pratt *et al.*, 1979).

McKenna *et al.* (1980) reported (in abstract form) that the catecholamine norepinephrine stimulates aldosterone secretion in bovine adrenal cells *in vitro*. This observation raised the issue that metoclopramide-induced aldosterone secretion might be related to sympathetic nervous system stimulation. In fact, ganglionic blockade with trimethaphan increased basal plasma aldosterone concentration and prevented metoclopramide from increasing aldosterone secretion in conscious sheep (Wilson *et al.*, 1983a). However, in man, trimethaphan in doses causing postural hypotension and lowering plasma norepinephrine by 75% failed to alter metclopramide-induced aldosterone secretion (Wilson *et al.*, 1983b). Further, metoclopramide administration did not influence circulating norepinephrine or epinephrine levels in these experiments. Thus, metoclopramide increases aldosterone secretion in man independent of the sympathetic nervous system (Wilson *et al.*, 1983b).

Previous studies have suggested that prolactin may increase aldosterone secretion (McCaa *et al.*, 1974; Solyom, 1974; Lichtenstein *et al.*, 1976; Carroll *et al.*, 1980). Since metoclopramide increases prolactin secretion, it was possible that prolactin secondarily increased aldosterone secretion. However, an overwhelming amount of evidence mitigates against this possibility. Ovine prolactin does not increase aldosterone secretion in man (Carey *et al.*, 1977). Administration of thyrotropin-releasing hormone, which acutely raises circulating prolactin, has no effect on aldosterone secretion (Bauman and Loriaux, 1976). Glucocorticoid administration depresses prolactin responses to metoclopramide without altering metoclopramide-induced aldosterone secretion (Sowers *et al.*, 1981a). Patients with markedly increased serum prolactin concentrations secondary to prolactin-secreting pituitary adenomas do not have increased aldosterone levels, and reduction of prolactin to undetectable levels with dopamine agonists (dopamine or bromocriptine) does not alter aldosterone secretion (R. M. Carey, unpublished observations). Thus, prolactin is highly unlikely to affect aldosterone secretion.

2.2. Sulpiride

Sulpiride is a substituted benzamide structurally related to metoclopramide. Sulpiride is the most specific antagonist of dopamine receptors thus far studied and has many biological effects similar to those of metoclopramide.

Mori *et al.* (1980) have reported that 50 mg sulpiride injected intramuscularly failed to increase plasma aldosterone concentration in man. However, recently Costa *et al.* (1980) demonstrated that sulpiride stimulates aldosterone production by superfused bovine adrenal cortical cells. Since the aldosterone response to metoclopramide is dependent on dose and route of administration, it is important that higher doses of sulpiride be administered intravenously to determine the effects of sulpiride on aldosterone secretion *in vivo*.

2.3. Chlorpromazine

Chlorpromazine is a phenothiazine with a relatively narrow range of specificity for dopamine receptors compared with sulpiride or metoclopramide (Goldberg *et al.*, 1978). Chlorpromazine is a central and peripheral dopamine antagonist and also has α-adrenoceptor-blocking activity (Brotzu, 1970; Caron *et al.*, 1978). Chlorpromazine increases plasma aldosterone concentration when given intravenously to schizophrenic patients (Szalay, 1973). However, chlorpromazine does not increase aldosterone secretion in rat adrenal cells *in vitro* (Szalay, 1973).

2.4. Domperidone

Domperidone is a benzimidazole derivative that possesses specific dopamine antagonist effects in the central nervous system and at the pituitary gland. However, in contrast to the aforementioned dopamine antagonists, domperidone does not cross the blood–brain barrier in appreciable quantities. Administration of domperidone into the peripheral circulation does not stimulate aldosterone secretion in man or the sheep (R. M. Carey, unpublished observations; Wilson *et al.*, 1983a; Sowers *et al.*, 1983b). These results may be interpreted as indicating either that dopaminergic control of aldosterone secretion is mediated by way of the central nervous system or, alternatively, that domperidone does not interact with the dopamine receptor involved in aldosterone regulation.

3. Dopamine Agonists

3.1. Dopamine

Dopamine interacts with specific receptors in the central nervous system and in peripheral tissues. In the periphery, dopamine interacts with specific presynaptic neuronal receptors at sympathetic ganglia and at postganglionic nerve terminals to inhibit norepinephrine release (Goldberg and Weder, 1980). In various vascular beds, dopamine stimulates postsynaptic dopaminergic receptors to produce vasodilation. In addition to its agonist activity at dopamine receptors, dopamine also stimulates α- and β_1-adrenergic receptors (Goldberg, 1972a). However, combined α- and β_1-adrenergic blockade does not block dopaminergic inhibition of prolactin secretion by 1.5 μg/kg per min of dopamine in man, indicating that dopamine acts preferentially at its own receptor to suppress prolactin secretion (Lorenzi *et al.*, 1979).

We have demonstrated that intravenous infusion of dopamine in man at doses (2 and 4 µg/kg per min) that suppress basal serum prolactin to a nondetectable level does not alter basal plasma aldosterone concentration (Carey et al., 1980). However, intravenous dopamine infusion blocks metoclopramide-induced increases in circulating aldosterone in a dose-dependent manner (Carey et al., 1980). Although this effect could be related to a nonspecific effect of dopamine, this possibility seems unlikely. None of the known mediators of aldosterone secretion (renin, ACTH, sodium, or potassium) changed as a result of metoclopramide or dopamine alone or in combination. Although there was a slight increase of pulse pressure with administration of dopamine, it is unlikely that α-adrenergic receptors were stimulated significantly at the doses of dopamine employed (Lorenzi et al., 1979). Further, as discussed above, metoclopramide-induced aldosterone secretion is not related to the sympathetic nervous system. These results thus indicate that the aldosterone response to metoclopramide is mediated by an antagonist activity at dopamine receptors.

The observation that dopamine inhibits metoclopramide-induced aldosterone secretion without influencing basal aldosterone secretion in man has been confirmed by several other groups (Noth et al., 1980; Sowers et al., 1981a). In addition, pretreatment with dopamine or L-dopa inhibits the increase in aldosterone secretion induced by metoclopramide in the monkey and rat, respectively (Sowers et al., 1980a, 1982b). Thus, the evidence to date is consistent with the concept that the aldosterone response to metoclopramide is related to dopamine antagonism.

In the studies demonstrating that dopamine inhibits metoclopramide-induced aldosterone secretion, it is possible that dopamine increased the metabolic clearance of aldosterone by increasing hepatic blood flow (Innes and Nickerson, 1975). However, the failure of dopamine to alter circulating cortisol, also metabolized by the liver, argues strongly against this possibility.

Dopamine is an agonist at both D-1 and D-2 receptors (Kebabian and Calne, 1979). Relatively large quantities (micromolar concentrations) of dopamine are required for D-1 receptor stimulation. Relatively smaller quantities (nanomolar concentrations) are required for stimulation of D-2 receptors. Inhibition of metoclopramide-induced aldosterone secretion by dopamine does not demonstrate conclusively which class of dopamine receptors is involved. Nevertheless, on the basis of the dose-related inhibitory effect of dopamine to suppress prolactin secretion, we have postulated that we were dealing with nanomolar quantities of dopamine. We gave almost enough dopamine to suppress prolactin secretion maximally and thus for stimulation of D-2 receptors. This quantity of dopamine would be insufficient to stimulate D-1 receptors.

It is obvious that the dopamine receptors modulating aldosterone secretion cannot be characterized exclusively as D-1 or D-2. The possibility that another type of dopamine receptor may inhibit aldosterone secretion will have to await studies of a wide range of dopamine agonists and antagonists as well as of the intracellular mechanism mediating the biological response.

3.2. Bromocriptine

Bromocriptine (2-brom-α-ergocriptine) acts as a dopamine agonist in the central nervous system, at the pituitary gland to inhibit prolactin release *in vivo* and *in vitro*, and at peripheral vascular receptors to produce vasodilation (Fluckiger and Wagner, 1968; Corrodi *et al.*, 1973; Besser *et al.*, 1972; Fluckiger *et al.*, 1976; Yeo *et al.*, 1979; Clarke *et al.*, 1978). In addition to its agonist activity at dopamine receptors, bromocriptine stimulates central α-adrenergic and serotoninergic receptors, but its order of potency is much greater for dopamine receptors (Fuxe *et al.*, 1974; Lew *et al.*, 1977). Actions of bromocriptine at central or peripheral presynaptic dopamine receptors may decrease peripheral sympathetic nervous system activity (DiChiara *et al.*, 1977; Judy *et al.*, 1978; Hertting *et al.*, 1979; Van Loon *et al.*, 1979; Carey *et al.*, 1983). These effects may at least partially account for the hypotensive action of the compound (Judy *et al.*, 1978).

Recent investigations have documented almost uniformly that bromocriptine is without effect on aldosterone secretion. Administration of bromocriptine in man does not alter basal aldosterone secretion (del Pozo *et al.*, 1977; Carey *et al.*, 1979, 1980; Birkhauser *et al.*, 1979) the circadian rhythm of plasma aldosterone concentration (Uberti *et al.*, 1979), the urinary excretion of aldosterone (Birkhauser *et al.*, 1979), or the aldosterone response to upright posture (del Pozo *et al.*, 1977; Birkhauser *et al.*, 1979) or dietary sodium depletion (Semple and Mason, 1978; Carey and Van Loon, 1982). Even more convincingly, we showed that bromocriptine, at doses that completely suppress the prolactin response to metoclopramide, does not inhibit the aldosterone response to that dopamine antagonist (Carey *et al.*, 1980). Further, bromocriptine does not affect the increase in aldosterone secretion engendered by cumulative administration of angiotensin II (Carey *et al.*, 1982a). Since bromocriptine is classified as a D-2 receptor agonist, these findings indicate that receptors mediating the adrenal response to dopamine are not exclusively D-2.

3.3. SKF 82526-J

SKF 82526-J (6-chloro-7,8-dihydroxy-1-(4-hydroxyphenyl)-2,3,4,5-tetrahydro-1H-3-benzazepine), a benzazepine derivative, is a dopamine agonist that appears specific for dopamine receptors (Ackerman *et al.*, 1982). No cross activity with α- or β-adrenergic receptors has been demonstrated. SKF 82526-J acts at dopamine receptors in the central nervous system. In the periphery, the compound appears selective for renal vascular receptors, producing vasodilation with an increase in renal blood flow. In this respect, SKF 82526-J has approximately fourfold the potency of dopamine. In man and experimental animals, SKF 82526-J reproducibly increases renal blood flow and produces natriuresis without altering glomerular filtration rate. SKF 82526-J binds poorly to dopamine receptors on pituitary lactotrophs and does not inhibit prolactin secretion.

In experimental animals, SKF 82526-J increases plasma aldosterone concentration as a result of its marked stimulation of plasma renin activity. In man, acute administration of a single oral dose of SKF 82526-J increases plasma renin activity in association with a marked decrease in renal vascular resistance (Carey *et al.*, 1984). Plasma aldosterone concentration rise slightly in association with this vasodilatory stimulation of renin release. SKF 82526-J has been shown not to inhibit metoclopramide-induced increases of circulating aldosterone in normal human subjects (R. M. Carey and R. Stote, unpublished observations).

4. Site of Dopaminergic Inhibition of Aldosterone Secretion

If aldosterone secretion is modulated by a dopaminergic inhibitory mechanism, it is important to clarify the site of this mechanism. At present, the majority of evidence would seem to indicate a direct adrenal cortical site of dopamine action, although a central nervous system mechanism also is possible.

Regarding an adrenal site for this mechanism, recent studies from our laboratories have indicated that the adrenal cortex contains a high concentration of dopamine (R. McCarty and R. M. Carey, unpublished observations). Adrenal medullectomy in rats is associated with a 60% decrease in dopamine. These results are in agreement with those of Kvetnansky *et al.* (1979). The 40% of adrenal dopamine remaining after medullectomy is located in the cortex, but the origin of adrenocortical dopamine is unknown. Possibilities include uptake from the medulla with subsequent storage in the cortex, primary adrenocortical dopamine synthesis, or secretion by dopaminergic neurons. A further source of adrenocortical dopamine would be via the subarcuate arteries of the kidney, where large quantities of dopamine are formed. Since circulating quantities of dopamine are low (Carey *et al.*, 1981), and orders of magnitude higher concentrations of circulating dopamine are required to inhibit metoclopramide-induced aldosterone secretion, it is unlikely that plasma dopamine contributes to aldosterone regulation.

Several *in vitro* studies of adrenocortical tissue have been performed in different species, including man, with conflicting results. Initial studies by McKenna *et al.* (1979) determined the effects of dopamine on aldosterone secretion in bovine adrenal glomerulosa cells in suspension. Dopamine did not alter basal aldosterone secretion but significantly inhibited angiotensin II-induced aldosterone secretion, probably by inhibiting late steps (deoxycorticosterone to aldosterone) in the biosynthetic pathway. Inhibition of 50% was observed at 10 μM dopamine, and 20% at 10 nM dopamine. Brown and colleagues (1981) have demonstrated stimulation of aldosterone secretion by metoclopramide in human adrenal adenoma cells *in vitro*. Metoclopramide, 10^{-8} M, was required for significant aldosterone stimulation. Rat adrenal zona glomerulosa cells on a Bio-gel® column have been shown to respond to metoclopramide with an increase in aldosterone secretion, which was inhibited by dopamine (Edwards *et al.*, 1980). However, no dose–response curve was described. In recent studies, we found no direct effect of metoclopramide or dopamine on aldosterone secretion from sheep adrenal zona glomerulosa cells *in vitro* (Wilson *et al.*, 1983a).

Recently, dopamine receptors have been identified in rat and calf adrenal zona glomerulosa cells *in vitro* (Dunn and Bosmann, 1981; Norbiato *et al.*, 1982). These dopamine receptors were characterized as D-1 on the basis of preliminary pharmacological studies.

From the above discussion, it is apparent that the weight of the evidence would favor a direct adrenal site of action of dopamine in the regulation of aldosterone secretion. Other evidence favoring this hypothesis includes the *in vivo* finding that metoclopramide seems to increase the immediate aldosterone precursor, 18-hydroxycorticosterone, in parallel with aldosterone in man and the monkey (Sowers and Stern, 1982). Thus, a specific site of stimulation late in the aldosterone biosynthetic pathway would argue for a direct site of dopamine action. Additionally, since peripheral administration of dopamine blocks metoclopramide-induced aldosterone secretion, and since dopamine crosses the blood–brain barrier poorly, the current data favor a peripheral site of action for dopamine in the adrenal cortex.

5. Physiological Significance of Dopamine in the Control of Aldosterone Secretion

We have studied *in vivo* responses of plasma aldosterone concentration to angiotensin II and ACTH in the presence and absence of dopamine in man during normal sodium intake (150 meq/day) (Carey, 1982). Aldosterone responses to graded doses of angiotensin II (2, 4, and 6 pmole/kg per min) were not altered by dopamine, 4 μg/kg per min intravenously. This dose of dopamine resulted in approximately 70% attenuation of the aldosterone response to metoclopramide. In addition, this dose of dopamine failed to inhibit ACTH-induced aldosterone secretion. These observations are consistent with our earlier observations that metoclopramide does not modify the aldosterone response to angiotensin II in sodium-repleted normal man.

In contrast to the above observations, recent studies from our laboratory (Williams *et al.*, 1984) have indicated that dopaminergic mechanisms may regulate the aldosterone response to sodium depletion. A single oral dose (500 mg) of L-dopa, which does not affect plasma aldosterone concentration in sodium-replete subjects, decreases basal plasma aldosterone concentrations in sodium-depleted subjects in balance at 10 meq/day sodium intake. Again, no changes in the known factors that regulate aldosterone secretion were observed with L-dopa.

Although dopamine does not inhibit angiotensin-induced aldosterone secretion in subjects on normal sodium intake, a quite different response is observed in sodium-deprived subjects (Drake *et al.*, 1984). Dopamine, 4 μg/kg per min, significantly inhibited the aldosterone response to 4 and 6 pmole/kg per min of angiotensin II. Other studies have shown enhanced aldosterone responses to metoclopramine in sodium-depleted man (Gordon *et al.*, 1983). Further, Aguilera and Catt (1984) have demonstrated in rats that simultaneous infusion of metoclopramide and angiotensin II enhanced the aldosterone secretion more than either agent alone. This enhancing effect of metoclopramide on angiotensin II-induced aldosterone secretion was blocked by dopamine, indicating a specific effect involving dopamine receptors. Thus, dopaminergic mechanisms appear to be more active in sodium-depleted than normal-sodium man and seem to block angiotensin II steroidogenic action.

Consistent with these observations, we and others have demonstrated a decrease in urinary dopamine during the course of dietary sodium depletion in normal human subjects (Carey *et al.*, 1981; Alexander *et al.*, 1974). It is possible, therefore, that the aldosterone response to sodium deprivation may be modulated via decreased dopaminergic activity. This proposed decrease in dopaminergic activity could occur by means of decreased activity of peripheral dopaminergic neurons or of nonneuronal dopamine-secreting cells, for example, in the kidney or the adrenal gland.

6. Summary and Conclusions

The evidence cited in this chapter strongly supports the concept that dopaminergic mechanisms regulate aldosterone secretion. The data indicate that in normal man, aldosterone secretion is under maximum tonic dopaminergic inhibiton.

Although the anatomic site of dopamine mechanisms operating to control aldosterone secretion is not unequivocally defined, most of the evidence suggests a direct action of dopamine at the adrenal cortex, where specific zona glomerulosa receptors for dopamine have been identified and characterized.

Dopamine mechanisms controlling aldosterone secretion appear to act predominantly in the setting of sodium depletion in man and experimental animals. In man, dopamine inhibits aldosterone responses to angiotensin II only during sodium depletion. The precise physiological role of dopamine in the regulation of aldosterone secretion in normal man and in pathological states has yet to be defined.

References

Ackerman, D. M., Weinstock, J., Wiebelhans, V. D., and Berkowitz, B., 1982, Renal vasodilators and hypertension, *Drug Dev. Res.* 2:283–297.

Aguilera, G., and Catt, K. J., 1984, Regulation of aldosterone secretion during altered sodium intake, *J. Steroid Biochem.* (in press).

Alexander, R. W., Gill, J. R., Jr., Yamabe, H., Lovenberg, W., and Kaiser, H. R., 1974, Effects of dietary sodium and of acute saline infusion on the interrelationship between dopamine excretion and adrenergic activity in man, *J. Clin. Invest.* 54:194–200.

Aona, T., Shioji, T., Kinugasa, T., Onishi, T., and Kurachi, K., 1978, Clinical and endocrinological analysis of patients with galactorrhea and menstrual disorders due to sulpiride and metoclopramide, *J. Clin. Endocrinol. Metab.* 47:675–680.

Bauman, G., and Loriaux, D. L., 1976, Failure of endogenous prolactin to alter renal salt and water excretion and adrenal function in man, *J. Clin. Endocrinol. Metab.* 43:643–649.

Besser, G. M., Parke, L., Edwards, C. R. W., Forsyth, I. A., and McNeilly, A. S., 1972, Galactorrhea: Successful treatment with reduction of plasma prolactin levels by bromergocryptine, *Br. Med. J.* 3:669–672.

Birkhauser, M., Riondel, A., and Vallotton, M. B., 1979, Bromocriptine-induced modulation of the plasma aldosterone response to acute stimulation, *Acta Endocrinol. (Kbh.)* 91:294–302.

Brotzu, G., 1970, Inhibition by chlorpromazine of the effects of dopamine on the dog kidney, *J. Pharm. Pharmacol.* 22:664–667.

Brown, R. D., Wisgerhof, M., Jiang, N. S., Kao, P., and Hagstad, R., 1981, Effect of metoclopramide on the secretion and metabolism of aldosterone in man, *J. Clin. Endocrinol. Metab.* **52**:1014–1018.

Brown, R. D., Billman, G. E., Kem, D. C., Stone, H. L., Jiang, N., Kao, P., and Hegstad, R., 1982, The effect of metoclopramide and dopamine on plasma aldosterone concentration in normal man and rhesus monkeys: A new model to study dopamine control of aldosterone secretion, *J. Clin. Endocrinol. Metab.* **55**:828–832.

Campbell, D. J., Mendelsohn, F. A. O., Adam, W. R., and Funder, J. W., 1981, Is aldosterone secretion under dopaminergic control? *Circ. Res.* **49**:1217–1227.

Carey, R. M., 1982, Acute dopaminergic inhibition of aldosterone secretion in man is independent of angiotensin II and adrenocorticotropin, *J. Clin. Endocrinol. Metab.* **54**:463–469.

Carey, R. M., and Van Loon, G. R., 1982, Bromocriptine does not inhibit the aldosterone response to sodium depletion, *J. Clin. Endocrinol. Metab.* **55**:162–165.

Carey, R. M., Johanson, A. J., and Sief, S. M., 1977, The effects of ovine prolactin on water and electrolyte excretion in man are attributable to vasopressin contamination, *J. Clin. Endocrinol. Metab.* **44**:850–858.

Carey, R. M., Thorner, M. O., and Ortt, E. M., 1979, Effects of metoclopramide and bromocriptine on the renin–angiotensin–aldosterone system in man: Dopaminergic control of aldosterone, *J. Clin. Invest.* **63**:727–735.

Carey, R. M., Thorner, M. O., and Ortt, E. M., 1980, Dopaminergic inhibition of metoclopramide-induced aldosterone secretion in man: Dissociation of responses to dopamine and bromocriptine, *J. Clin. Invest.* **66**:10–18.

Carey, R. M., Van Loon, G. R., Baines, A. D., and Ortt, E. M., 1981, Decreased plasma and urinary dopamine during dietary sodium depletion in man, *J. Clin. Endocrinol. Metab.* **52**:903–909.

Carey, R. M., Van Loon, G. R., Baines, A. D., and Kaiser, D. L., 1983, Suppression of basal and stimulated noradrenergic activity by the dopamine agonist, bromocriptine, in man, *J. Clin. Endocrinol. Metab.* **56**(3):595–602.

Carey, R. M., Townsend, L. M., Rose, C. E., Jr., Kaiser, D. L., and Ragsdale, N. V., 1984, The specific dopamine agonist, SKF 82526-J, increases renal blood flow and lowers blood pressure in essential hypertension, *Hypertension* (in press).

Carlson, H. E., Briggs, J. E., and McCallum, R. W., 1977, Stimulation of prolactin secretion by metoclopramide in the rat, *Proc. Soc. Exp. Biol. Med.* **154**:475–478.

Caron, M. G., Beaulieu, M., Raymond, V., Gagne, B., Drouin, J., Lefkowitz, R. J., and Labrie, F., 1978, Dopaminergic receptors in the anterior pituitary gland. Correlation of (^{3}H)dihydroergocryptine binding with the dopaminergic control of prolactin release, *J. Biol. Chem.* **253**:2244–2253.

Carroll, J. E., Campanile, C. P., and Goodfriend, T. L., 1980, Role of prolactin in aldosterone secretion, *Clin. Res.* **28**:772A.

Clarke, B. J., Scholtysik, G., and Fluckiger, E., 1978, Cardiovascular actions of bromocriptine, *Acta Endocrinol. (Kbh.)* **216**(Suppl. 88):75–81.

Carrodi, H., Fuxe, K., Hokfelt, T., Lidbrink, P., and Ungerstedt, U., 1973, Effect of ergot drugs on central catecholamine neurons. Evidence for stimulation of central dopamine neurons, *J. Pharm. Pharmacol.* **25**:409–411.

Costa, G., Frisina, N., and DePasquale, R., 1980, Increased aldosterone secretion by sulpiride, *Clin. Endocrinol. (Oxf.)* **13**:1–7.

Day, M. D., and Blower, P. R., 1975, Cardiovascular dopamine receptor stimulation antagonized by metoclopramide, *J. Pharm. Pharmacol.* **27**:276–278.

del Pozo, E., Darragh, A., Lancranjan, I., Ebling, D., Burmeister, P., Buhler, F., Marbach, P., and Braun, P., 1977, Effect of bromocriptine on the endocrine system and fetal development, *Clin. Endocrinol. (Suppl.)* **6**:47s–55s.

Delitala, G., Masala, A., Alagna, S., and Devilla, L., 1975, Metoclopramide and prolactin secretion in man: Effects of pretreatment with L-DOPA and 2-brom-*alpha*-ergocriptine (CB-154), *IRCS, Med. Sci. Libr. Compend.* **3**:274.

DiChiara, G., Vargiu, L., Porceddu, M. L., and Gessa, G. L., 1977, Bromocriptine: A rather specific stimulant of dopamine receptors regulating dopamine metabolism, *Adv. Biochem. Psychopharmacol.* **16**:443–446.

Dolphin, A., Jenner, P., Marsden, C. D., Pycock, C., and Tarsy, D., 1975, Pharmacological evidence for cerebral dopamine receptor blockade by metoclopramide in rodents, *Psychopharmacologia* **41**:133–138.

Drake, C. R.f, Ragsdale, N. V., Kaiser, D. L., and Carey, R. M., 1984, Dopamine inhibits aldosterone responses to angiotensin II during sodium depletion in man, *Metabolism* (in press).

Dunn, M. G., and Bosmann, H. B., 1981, Peripheral dopamine receptor identification: Properties of a specific dopamine receptor in the rat adrenal zona glomerulosa, *Biochem. Biophys. Res. Commun.* **99**:1081–1087.

Edwards, C. R. W., Al-Dujaili, E. A. S., Boscaro, M., Zuyyumi, S., Miall, P. A., and Rees, L. H., 1980, *In vivo* and *in vitro* studies on the effect of metoclopramide on aldosterone secretion, *Clin. Endocrinol. (Oxf.)* **13**:45–50.

Fluckiger, E., and Wagner, H. R., 1968, 2-Br-*alpha*-Ergocriptine. Beeinflussung von Fertilitat and Lactation bei der Ratte, *Experientia* **24**:1130.

Fluckiger, E., Marko, M., Doepfner, W., and Niederer, W., 1976, Effects of ergot alkaloids on the hypothalamopituitary axis, *Postgrad. Med. J.* **52**(Suppl. I):57–61.

Fozard, J. R., and Mobarok Aki, A. T. M., 1978, Blockade of neuronal tryptamine receptors by metoclopramide, *Eur. J. Pharmacol.* **49**:109–112.

Fuxe, K., Carrodi, H., Hokfelt, T., Lidbrink, P., and Ungerstedt, U., 1974, Ergocornine and 2-Br-*alpha*-ergocriptine. Evidence for prolonged dopamine receptor stimulation, *Med. Biol.* **52**:121–132.

Goldberg, L. I., 1972, Cardiovascular and renal actions of dopamine: Potential clinical applications, *Pharmacol. Rev.* **24**:1–29.

Goldberg, L. I., 1975, The dopamine vascular receptor, *Biochem. Pharmacol.* **24**:651–653.

Goldberg, L. I., 1978, Characteristics of the vascular dopamine receptor: Comparison with other receptors, *Fed. Proc.* **37**:2396–2402.

Goldberg, L. I., and Weder, A. B., 1980, Connections between endogenous dopamine, dopamine receptors and sodium excretion: Evidence and hypotheses, in: *Recent Advances in Clinical Pharmacology* (P. Turner and D. Shand, eds.), Churchill Livingstone, Edinburgh, pp. 149–166.

Gordon, M. B., Moore, T. J., Dluhy, R. G., and Williams, G. H., 1983, Dopaminergic modulation of aldosterone responsiveness to angiotensin II with changes in sodium intake, *J. Clin. Endocrinol. Metab.* **56**:340–345.

Haning, R., Tait, S. A. S., and Tait, J. F., 1970, In vitro effects of ACTH, angiotensins, serotonin and potassium on steroid output and conversion of corticosterone to aldosterone by isolated adrenal cells, *Endocrinology* **87**:1146–1167.

Hay, A. M., 1975, The mechanism of action of metoclopramide, *Gut* **16**:403.

Healy, D. L., and Burger, H. G., 1978, Sustained elevation of serum prolactin by metoclopramide: A clinical model of idiopathic hyperprolactinemia, *J. Clin. Endocrinol. Metab.* **46**:709–714.

Hertting, G., Reimann, W., Zumstein, A., Jackisch, R., and Starke, K., 1979, Dopaminergic feedback regulation of dopamine release in slices of caudate nucleus of the rabbit, *Adv. Biosci.* **18:**145–150.

Hornykiewicz, O., 1966, Dopamine (3-hydroxytyramine) and brain function, *Pharmacol. Rev.* **18:**925–964.

Innes, I. R., and Nickerson, M., 1975, Norepinephrine, epinephrine, and the sympathomimetic amines. In: *The Pharmacological Basis of Therapeutics* (L. S. Goodman and A. Gilman, eds.), pp. 477–513, Macmillan, New York.

Jenner, P., and Marsden, C. D., 1979, The substituted benzamides—a novel class of dopamine antagonists, *Life Sci.* **25:**479–486.

Jenner, P., Marsden, C. D., and Perringer, E., 1975, Behavioral and biochemical evidence for cerebral dopamine receptor blockade by metoclopramide in rodents, *Br. J. Pharmacol.* **54:**275P–276P.

Jenner, P., Elliott, N. C., Clow, A., Reavill, C., and Marsden, C. D., 1978, A comparison of *in vitro* and *in vivo* dopamine receptor antagonism produced by substituted benzamide drugs, *J. Pharm. Pharmacol.* **30:**46–48.

Judy, W. V., Watanabe, A. M., Henry, D., Besch, H. R., and Aprison, B., 1978, Effect of L-dopa on sympathetic nerve activity and blood pressure in the spontaneously hypertensive rat, *Circ. Res.* **43:**24–28.

Kebabian, J. W., and Calne, D. B., 1979, Multiple receptors for dopamine, *Nature* **277:**93–96.

Kvetnansky, R., Weise, V. K., Thoa, N. B., and Kopin, I. J., 1979, Effects of chronic guanethidine treatment and adrenal medullectomy on plasma levels of catecholamines and corticosterone in forcibly immobilized rats, *J. Pharmacol. Exp. Ther.* **209:**287–291.

Lew, J. Y., Hata, F., Ohashi, T., and Goldstein, M., 1977, The interactions of bromocriptine and lergotrile with dopamine and β-adrenergic receptors, *J. Neural Transm.* **41:**109–121.

Lichtenstein, L. S., Colwell, J. A., and Levine, J. H., 1976, Prolactin stimulates aldosterone biosynthesis, in: *Program and Abstracts of the Sixth International Congress of Endocrinology,* Union Offset Co., Canberra, Australia, p. 86.

Lorenzi, M., Karam, J. H., Tsalikian, E., Bohannon, N. V., Gerich, J. E., and Forsham, P., 1979, Dopamine during *alpha*- and *beta*-blockade in man, *J. Clin. Invest.* **63:**310–317.

MacLeod, R. M., 1976, Regulation of prolactin secretion, in: *Frontiers in Neuroendocrinology* (L. Martini and W. F. Ganong, eds.), Raven Press, New York, pp. 169–194.

Mantero, F., Boscaro, M., Opocher, G., Aramini, D., and Edwards, C. R. W., 1980, *In vitro* and *in vivo* effect of metergoline on aldosterone secretion, in: *Program and Abstracts of the Sixth International Congress of Endocrinology*, Union Offset Co., Canberra, Australia, p. 405.

McCaa, R. E., Young, D. B., and Guyton, A. C., 1974, Evidence of a role of an unidentified pituitary factor regulating aldosterone secretion during altered sodium balance, *Circ. Res. (Suppl. 1)*:34–35.

McCallum, R. W., Sowers, J. R., Hershman, J. M., and Sturdevant, R. A. L., 1976, Metoclopramide stimulates prolactin secretion in man, *J. Clin. Endocrinol. Metab.* **42:**1148–1152.

McKenna, T. J., Island, D. P., Nicholson, W. E., and Liddle, G. W., 1979, Dopamine inhibits angiotensin-stimulated aldosterone biosynthesis in bovine adrenal cells, *J. Clin. Invest.* **64:**287–291.

McKenna, T. J., Island, D. P., Nicholson, W. E., and Liddle, G. W., 1980, Stimulation of aldosterone prolactin by catecholamines *in vitro*, in: *Program and Abstracts, Sixth*

International Congress of Endocrinology, Melbourne, Union Offset Co., Canberra, Australia, p. 407.

Mori, M., Kobayashi, I., Ohshima, K., Maruta, S., Shomomura, Y., and Fukuda, H., 1980, Potentiation of sulpiride-induced prolactin secretion by sodium deprivation in man, *Acta Endocrinol. (Kbh.)* **94:**25–29.

Niemegeers, C. J. E., and Janssen, P. A. J., 1979, A systematic study of the pharmacological activities of the dopamine antagonists, *Life Sci.* **24:**2201–2216.

Norbiato, G., Bevilacqua, M., Raggi, U., Micossi, P., and Moroni, C., 1977, Metoclopramide increases plasma aldosterone in man, *J. Clin. Endocrinol. Metab.* **45:**1313–1316.

Norbiato, G., Bevilacqua, M., Vago, T., Reggi, U., and Malacco, E., 1982, Characterization of dopaminergic receptors by [H^3]-ADTN binding in calf adrenal glomerulosa cells, in: *Endocrinology of Hypertension* (F. Mantero, E. G. Biglieri, and C. R. W. Edwards, eds.), Proceedings of the Serono Symposia, Vol. 50, Academic Press, London, pp. 133–141.

Noth, R. H., McCallum, W., Contino, C., and Havelick, J., 1980, Tonic dopaminergic suppression of plasma aldosterone, *J. Clin. Endocrinol. Metab.* **51:**64–69.

Ogihara, T. S., Matsumara, S., Onishi, T., Miyai, K., Uozumi, T., and Kumahara, Y., 1977, Effect of metoclopramide-induced prolactin on aldosterone secretion in normal subjects, *Life Sci.* **20:**523–526.

Peringer, E., Jenner, P., Donaldson, I. M., and Marsden, C. D., 1976, Metoclopramide and dopamine receptor blockade, *Neuropharmacology* **15:**463–469.

Pinder, R. M., Brogden, R. M., Sawyer, P. R., Speight, T. M., and Avery, F. S., 1976, Metoclopramide: A review of its pharmacological properties and clinical use, *Drugs* **12:**81–131.

Pratt, J. H., Ganguly, A., and Weinberger, M. H., 1979, Metoclopramide-induced aldosterone stimulation: Independence from pituitary and renal factors, *Clin. Res.* **27:**680A.

Semple, P. F., and Mason, P. A., 1978, Bromocriptine: Lack of effect on the angiotensin II and aldosterone responses to sodium deprivation, *Clin. Endocrinol.* **9:**155–161.

Solyom, J., 1974, Anterior pituitary and aldosterone secretion, *Lancet* **2:**507.

Sowers, J. R., and Stern, N., 1982, Influence of sodium homeostasis and circadean rhythm on dopaminergic modulation of 18-hydroxycorticosterone secretion in man, *J. Clin. Endocrinol. Metab.* **55:**1046–1051.

Sowers, J. R., McCallum, R. W., Hershman, J. M., Carlson, H. E., Sturdevant, R. A. L., and Meyer, N., 1976, Comparison of metoclopramide with other dynamic tests of prolactin secretion, *J. Clin. Endocrinol. Metab.* **43:**679–681.

Sowers, J. R., Carlson, H. E., Brautbar, N., and Hershman, J. M., 1977, Effects of dexamethasone on prolactin and TSH responses to TRH and metoclopramide in man, *J. Clin. Endocrinol. Metab.* **44:**327–341.

Sowers, J. R., Sollars, E., Barrett, J. D., and Sambhi, M. P., 1980a, Effect of L-DOPA and bilateral nephrectomy on the aldosterone response to metoclopramide, *Life Sci.* **27:**497–501.

Sowers, J. R., Sollars, E., Tuck, M. L., and Asp, N., 1980b, Dopaminergic modulation of renin activity, aldosterone and prolactin secretion in the spontaneously hypertensive rat, *Proc. Soc. Exp. Biol. Med.* **164:**598–601.

Sowers, J. R., Tuck, M. L., Golub, M. S., and Sollars, E. G., 1980c, Dopaminergic control of aldosterone secretion is independent of alterations in renin secretion, *Endocrinology* **107:**937–941.

Sowers, J. R., Brickman, A. S., Sowers, D. K., and Berg, G., 1981a, Dopaminergic modulation of aldosterone secretion in man is unaffected by glucocorticoids and angiotensin blockade, *J. Clin. Endocrinol. Metab.* **52:**1078–1084.

Sowers, J. R., Sharp, B., Levin, E. R., Golub, M. S., Eggena, P., 1981b, Metoclopramide, a dopamine antagonist, stimulates aldosterone secretion in rhesus monkeys, but not in dogs or rabbits, *Life Sci.* **29:**2171.

Sowers, J. R., Sharp, B., and McCallum, R. W., 1982a, Effect of domperidone, an extracerebral inhibitor of dopamine receptors, on thyrotropin, prolactin, renin, aldosterone and 18-hydroxycorticosterone secretion in man, *J. Clin. Endocrinol. Metab.* **54:**869–871.

Sowers, J. R., Berg, G., Martin, V. S., and Mayes, D. M., 1982b, Dopaminergic modulation of aldosterone secretion in the rhesus monkey, *Endocrinology* **54:**523.

Szalay, K. S., 1973, *In vitro* aldosterone production: Effect of ethacrynic acid, chlorpromazine and veratrine, *Acta Physiol. Acad. Sci. Hung.* **43:**275–279.

Uberti, E. C., Fabbri, B. L., Margutti, A. R., Fersini, C. M., and Pansini, R., 1979, Effect of bromocriptine on the control of plasma aldosterone diurnal variation in normal supine man, *Horm. Res.* **10:**64–78.

Valenzuela, J. E., 1976, Dopamine as a possible neurotransmitter in gastric relaxation, *Gastroenterology* **71:**1019–1022.

VanLoon, G. R., Sole, M. J., Bain, J., and Ruse, J. L., 1979, Effects of bromocriptine on plasma catecholamines in normal men, *Neuroendocrinology* **28:**425–434.

Williams, F. A., Jr., Ragsdale, N. V., Kaiser, D. L., and Carey, R. M., 1984, Suppression of basal aldosterone secretion by L-DOPA in sodium deplete man, *J. Clin. Endocrinol. Metab.* (in press).

Wilson, T. A., Kaiser, D. L., Peach, M. J., and Carey, R. M., 1983a, Possible mechanism of action of metoclopramide-induced aldosterone secretion: *In vivo* and *in vitro* studies in the sheep, *Endocrinology* **113:**887–892.

Wilson, T. A., Kaiser, D. L., and Carey, R. M., 1983b, Dopaminergic inhibition of aldosterone secretion in man is independent of the autonomic nervous system, *J. Clin. Endocrinol. Metab.* **57:**200–203.

Yeo, T., Thorner, M. O., Jones, A., Lowry, P. J., and Besser, G. M., 1978, Release from continuous perfused columns of isolated rat pituitary cells, *Clin. Endocrinol.* **10:**123–130.

Yeo, T., Thorner, M. O., Jones, A., Lowry, P. J., and Besser, G. M., 1979, The effects of dopamine, bromocriptine, lergotrile and metoclopramide on prolactin release from continuous perfused columns of isolated rat pituitary cells, *Clin. Endocrinol.* **10:**123–130.

16

Dopamine Agonists/Antagonists in the Treatment of Gastrointestinal Diseases

HERBERT S. ORMSBEE III

1. Introduction

The smooth muscle relaxant effects of dopamine observed in vascular tissue also extend to the smooth muscle of the gastrointestinal tract. For example, dopamine is known to relax the lower esophageal sphincter and has been suggested as a mediator of receptive relaxation of the stomach (Valenzuela, 1976). In contrast, contraction of GI muscle to dopamine has been reported from several locations in the GI tract in at least two species (Lanfranchi *et al.*, 1978a; Anuras, 1981). Besides these smooth muscle effects, dopamine has a number of other interesting effects on GI function. Dopamine reduces pentagastrin-stimulated acid secretion in man, and it has been implicated in animal experiments to be involved in the pathogenesis of duodenal ulcer disease (Szabo, 1979). In fact, dopamine agonists may be antiulcerogenic drugs. A dopaminergic effect on electrolyte absorption has been demonstrated for the rabbit ileum. An additional effect of dopamine on GI function is its ability to increase blood flow through the arteries supplying most of the stomach and small intestine. Whether some or all of these GI effects of dopamine are physiologically relevant, especially in man, is still very much open to question. The presence of gut dopamine receptors appears to vary not only among species but among organs of the GI tract within one species. A thorough characterization of these receptors has not been performed. The evidence to date will be presented in the text of this chapter.

HERBERT S. ORMSBEE III • Department of Pharmacology, Smith Kline & French Laboratories, Philadelphia, Pennsylvania 19101.

One additional feature of dopamine agonists relating to gastrointestinal function is the ability of dopamine$_2$ receptor agonists (DA$_2$) such as apomorphine to produce emesis via stimulation of the chemoreceptor trigger zone (Goldberg and Kohli, 1983). The emetic effects of dopamine agonists can be inhibited by a number of antagonists from different chemical classes. Several of these compounds have potent effects on gastrointestinal contractility as well. The motility-enhancing effects of the dopamine antagonists have considerable therapeutic potential in gastrointestinal disorders characterized by abnormally reduced motor function. The prototype agent in this category is metoclopramide, which was originally synthesized and examined for its antiemetic properties. It is currently recognized as a GI "prokinetic" drug, one that enhances the contractility of and transit through the stomach and small intestine. Metoclopramide and other dopamine antagonists also appear to enhance the pressure of the lower esophageal sphincter. The therapeutic relevance and the pharmacological actions of the dopamine antagonists are also discussed briefly in this review. The discussion attempts to outline the available evidence for the peripheral mechanism of action of these compounds. Finally, the recognition of dopamine agonists and antagonists as therapeutic candidates for GI diseases is placed in perspective by presenting an overview of the pharmaceutical development work currently proceeding on agents of this type.

2. Actions of Dopamine on the Gastrointestinal Tract

2.1. Esophagus

Studies performed in anesthetized opossums have demonstrated that dopamine causes a dose-dependent relaxation of the lower esophageal sphincter (LES) and contraction of the distal esophageal body (Rattan and Goyal, 1976; Mukhopodhyay and Weisbrodt, 1977). *Alpha-* and β-adrenergic receptor antagonists, vagotomy, and tetrodotoxin failed to block the responses to dopamine, which were antagonized by haloperidol and bulbocapnine. These data suggest that the effect of dopamine on the esophagus and LES is via peripheral dopaminergic postsynaptic receptors. This conclusion has also been supported by work *in vitro* by DeCarle and Christensen (1976).

2.2. Stomach

2.2.1. Motility

The effects of dopamine on the motility of the stomach have been investigated in at least three species. In all cases, dopamine is an inhibitor of contractility. In man, dopamine reduced the amplitude and frequency of spontaneous gastric antral contractions, an effect blocked by the dopamine antagonist sulpiride (Lanfranchi *et al.*, 1978b). In dogs with gastric fistulas, dopamine caused a dose-related decrease in the intragastric pressure, thus suggesting that dopamine may be a mediator of receptive relaxation (Valenzuela, 1976). In this experiment as with the experiment in man, dopamine antagonists inhibited the agonist response. Dopamine also inhibits bethanechol-stimulated antral contractions in the dog (Beck and Hovendal, 1982). Several studies have appeared in the literature from the Janssen Pharmaceutica Research Laboratories reporting the results of experiments on the effects of dopamine and domperidone on the isolated guinea pig stomach preparation. Unquestionably, dopamine relaxes the preparation, thus increasing the volume of the stomach and, thereby, delaying its emptying, decreases the amplitude of phasic gastric contractions, inhibits proximal duodenal contractility, and reduces antral-to-duodenal coordination of contractions (Van Nueten *et al.*, 1978; Schuurkes and Van Nueten, 1981a,b, 1982). Unlike the opossum LES, dopamine inhibits the guinea pig stomach by a tetrodotoxin-sensitive mechanism, thus suggesting a presynaptic action for at least part of the gastric dopamine response (Van Nueten and Janssen, 1978).

2.2.2. Acid Secretion and Ulcerogenesis

The inhibitory dopamine receptors in the stomach also appear to be associated with the production of hydrogen ion secretion. In man, dopamine has been demonstrated to inhibit the acid secretion induced by pentagastrin stimulation (Valenzuela *et al.*, 1979). The dopamine effect was blocked by haloperidol without affecting basal acid secretion. In the rat, experimental acute and chronic duodenal ulcers can be produced by the administration of cysteamine hydrochloride (Szabo, 1978). Part of the pathogenesis of these ulcers appears to be attributable to an increased gastric acid secretion (Szabo *et al.*, 1977). The incidence and intensity of the ulcers are inhibited by histamine H_2-receptor antagonism, by truncal vagotomy, and by the dopamine agonists bromocriptine, lergotrile, and apomorphine (Szabo *et al.*, 1979; Szabo, 1978). These dopamine agonists inhibited acid secretion and the cysteamine-induced ulcers, whereas the administration of dopamine antagonists exacerbated the ulcers (Szabo, 1978). This evidence suggested to Szabo that a dopaminergic system may be involved in the pathogenesis of experimental ulcer disease. Interestingly, intracerebroventricular administration of dopamine (but not norepinephrine) significantly reduced the intensity of the cysteamine ulcer, thus emphasizing the potential central site of action of dopamine agonists as antiulcer agents (Horner and Szabo, 1981). Recently, Szabo and Neu-meyer (1983) identified two apomorphine derivatives, (−)-N-*n*-propyl-norapomorphine and (−)-10,11-methylenedioxy-N-*n*-propylaporphine, as potent antiulcerogens in the cysteamine ulcer model. Selective dopamine agonists may have therapeutic potential as antiulcer drugs.

2.2.3. Gastrin Secretion

Dopamine itself has not been shown to affect gastrin secretion. How-ever, apomorphine has been demonstrated to induce vomiting and in-crease the levels of peripheral circulating gastrin in the dog (Uvnas-Wal-lensten *et al.*, 1978). On the other hand, haloperidol enhanced meal-induced gastrin secretion in normal subjects (Schrumpf and Linnestad, 1982). Thus, the data at hand on the role of dopamine in gastrin secretion are equivocal and need substantiation.

2.3. Small Intestine and Colon

2.3.1. Motility

Like the smooth muscle of the lower esophagus, the longitudinal and circular muscle of the opossum duodenum contracts to dopamine (Anuras, 1981). Isolated strips of duodenal longitudinal muscle were 6.5 times more sensitive to dopamine ($ED_{50} = 2.8 \times 10^{-6}$ M) than the isolated circular muscle (Anuras, 1981). Whether these responses involve an interaction with dopamine receptors is questionable, since in only one-third of the strips were the dopamine responses reduced or blocked by dopamine antagonists.

The responses of the ileum to dopamine have been examined *in vitro* in the guinea pig. Dopamine inhibited the responses to exogenous ace-tylcholine and to electrical field stimulation (Ennis *et al.*, 1979; Gorich *et al.*, 1982). Whether or not the effects of dopamine and apomorphine, which also inhibits the response to electrical field stimulation, represent an interaction with specific dopamine receptors is controversial, as is presented in Section 4 of this chapter.

In the human sigmoid colon, the effect of dopamine is once again excitatory as in the esophagus and duodenum. Both the resting base-line pressure (tone) and phasic contractions are enhanced during an intrave-nous infusion of dopamine (Lanfranchi *et al.*, 1978a). An uncontrolled clinical study has reported the effects of haloperidol, sulpiride, and pi-mozide on distal colonic motility (Lechin and Van Der Dijs, 1979). The effects of the first two drugs appeared to be dependent on the preexisting pattern of motility at the time of administration of the drug. The effect of pimozide, which suppressed sigmoidal motility, is consistent with the previously reported excitatory effects of dopamine, but a conclusion cannot be reached concerning the effects of the other antagonists. Taken together, these two studies on distal colonic motility indicate that dopamine can modulate contractility in this organ as well.

2.3.2. Secretion

The role of dopamine as a potential mediator in the control of water and electrolyte balance across the GI mucosa is a relatively new topic. It makes sense that dopamine should have effects on the function of the small bowel because it has been found to be present in the mucosa and/ or the muscularis of the small intestine of several species including the dog, rat, and rabbit (Holzbauer and Sharman, 1972). The catecholamines epinephrine and norepinephrine stimulated active sodium ion and chloride ion absorption across the rabbit ileum (Field and McColl, 1973). Similarly, recent work by Donowitz *et al.* (1982) using the Ussing chamber voltage-clamp technique has demonstrated that dopamine also increases net absorption of sodium and chloride ions across the rabbit ileal mucosa. This pharmacological investigation suggests that dopamine may play a physiological role in the regulation of active intestinal ion absorption.

2.4. Gastrointestinal Circulation

The proper control of the gastrointestinal circulation is important to the normal multiplicity of functions within the GI tract. A large array of vasoactive substances affects both the gastric and the mesenteric blood flow (Lanciault and Jacobson, 1976; Jacobson, 1982; Kauffman, 1982). Included in this category is dopamine (Yeh *et al.*, 1969). Intravenous or intraarterial administration of dopamine to anesthetized dogs increased mesenteric arterial blood flow (Yeh *et al.*, 1969; Ackerman and Woodward, 1983). The selective dopamine agonist SK&F 82526 also increases mesenteric arterial blood flow and decreases mesenteric vascular resistance dose relatedly (Ackerman and Woodward, 1983). A species difference appears to exist with the vascular response to dopamine, since the effects of dopamine and SK&F 82526 on the mesenteric artery are not observed in the rat (D. M. Ackerman, personal communication). In the rabbit, however, dopamine increases blood flow in the left gastric artery when injected into the common hepatic artery, and this response is inhibited by dopamine antagonists (Reinsberg and Kullman, 1982).

2.5. Pancreas

Depending on the dose of dopamine administered, the isolated perfused canine pancreas exhibits a vasodilation that is inhibited by haloperidol (Bastie *et al.*, 1977). In this same preparation, dopamine significantly increases the rate of secretion and the volume of pancreatic juice. The volume of secretion but not its protein content was inhibited by haloperidol. A similar but weaker response on pancreatic secretion was also observed for apomorphine. Increases in pancreatic juice output including protein also have been demonstrated in the anesthetized and the conscious dog. These responses have been inhibited with haloperidol, sulpiride, and domperidone (Satoh *et al.*, 1980; Delcenserie *et al.*, 1982). Fragments of mouse pancreas responded to dopamine with an increase in amylase release that was abolished with domperidone (Delcenserie and Laugier, 1982). In contrast, studies in man have shown no modification of basal or stimulated bicarbonate pancreatic secretion (Caldara *et al.*, 1978; Valenzuela *et al.*, 1979) and an apparent reduction in stimulated amylase and lipase secretion (Valenzuela *et al.*, 1979). The pancreatic actions of dopamine also include an interaction with endocrine peptide secretion as well. The dopamine agonist bromocriptine has been shown to reduce the secretion of human pancreatic polypeptide, whereas the dopamine antagonist domperidone significantly increases pancreatic polypeptide secretion in man (Sowers *et al.*, 1982).

3. Evidence for Dopamine Receptors in the Gastrointestinal Tract

A number of classification systems for dopamine receptors have been proposed primarily on the basis of agonist and antagonist orders of potency, radioligand binding, and link to cyclic nucleotides (Kebabian and Calne, 1979; Goldberg *et al.*, 1978; Costall and Naylor, 1981). The binding assays and the cyclic nucleotide assays have been, for the most part, from central nervous system tissues and may not relate directly to the situation in the periphery. At present, the majority of the evidence for dopamine receptors in the GI tract comes from pharmacological studies using dopamine agonists and antagonists with the following exception. The binding properties of dopamine receptors in the GI tract have been reported in a single study in the rat by Sandrock (1981). Sandrock demonstrated saturable, low-affinity binding of [^{3}H]-dopamine to tissue membrane fractions of the mucosa and muscularis of the stomach and duodenum. The data were interpreted to suggest that these areas of the rat gut contain postsynaptic D-1 receptors, since no [³H]-haloperidol binding was observed in their preparations. In addition, the ulcerogen cysteamine (see Section 2.2.2) significantly enhanced [³H]-dopamine binding in the gut and [³H]-haloperidol binding to the cortex of the rats, thus lending further support to the speculated role for dopamine receptor involvement in the pathogenesis of experimental duodenal ulcer disease.

Pharmacological evidence supporting the presence of specific dopamine receptors in the GI tract comes from several sources. In the isolated LES preparation from the opossum, both dopamine and epinine are agonists for LES relaxation (De Carle and Christensen, 1976). This dopaminergic response is significantly inhibited by bulbocapnine and by haloperidol but not by phenoxybenzamine, propranolol, or tetrodotoxin. Therefore, the ability of dopamine to relax the LES appears to be via specific dopamine receptors located on the smooth muscle of the sphincter. As noted previously (Section 2.1), this conclusion is supported by experiments *in vivo* in the anesthetized opossum (Rattan and Goyal, 1976; Mukhopadhyay and Weisbrodt, 1977). Interestingly, the purported dopamine antagonists metoclopramide and domperidone each have been suggested to increase the resting tone of the LES in man (Schulze-Delrieu, 1981; Brogden *et al.*, 1982). No studies are available that report the order of potency of a series of dopaminergic agonists and antagonists on esophageal or LES muscle. This must be done before any final conclusions can be reached regarding the number and classification of dopamine receptor subtypes present in the esophagus, LES, and other organs within the GI tract.

Although dopamine possesses inhibitory characteristics in the smooth muscle of the stomach of several species, the best evidence for specific dopamine receptors in the mediation of this response comes from the dog. Both pimozide and metoclopramide but not phenoxybenzamine, propranolol, guanethidine, or FLA-63 (a dopamine-β-hydroxylase inhibitor) decreased the dopamine-mediated fall in intragastric pressure (Valenzuela, 1976). The precise location of the inhibitory dopamine receptors in the stomach is not known, but there is some evidence in the guinea pig stomach that the effect may be in part presynaptic (Van Nueten and Janssen, 1978). One weakness of the argument for a specific dopamine receptor in the guinea pig mediating its gastric effects is the ability of prazosin to significantly inhibit the relaxant effects of dopamine (Schuurkes and Van Nueten, 1981a). Since domperidone was capable of completely abolishing the effects of dopamine and prazosin was not, Schuurkes and Van Nueten (1981a) concede that dopamine may act through an α_1-adrenoceptor as well as a dopaminergic receptor in the stomach. Despite this finding, the weight of the evidence supports the presence of specific gastric dopaminergic receptors.

The evidence for dopamine receptors from other parts of the gut is based on the assumption that the agents that were used to antagonize the effects of dopamine were specific for peripheral dopaminergic receptors. For example, the ability of dopamine to inhibit pentagastrin-stimulated acid secretion in the human stomach or to stimulate the active net absorption of sodium and chloride in the rabbit ileum were each inhibited by haloperidol (Valenzuela *et al.*, 1979; Donowitz *et al.*, 1982). The ileal dopamine response on short-circuit current was also inhibited by yohimbine but not by 6-hydroxydopamine, prazosin, or propranolol. The dopamine-stimulated absorption of sodium and chloride in the small intestine may, therefore, be dependent on interactions with α_2-adrenoceptors as well as dopaminergic receptors. In the rabbit, a series of dopamine antagonists has been examined on the blood flow response of the left gastric artery to dopamine (Reinsberg and Kullman, 1982). The order of potency of the antagonists was flupenthixol > haloperidol > bulbocapnine > sulpiride. These data suggest that the dopamine receptor in the rabbit gastric vasculature is similar to the central nervous system dopamine receptor linked to adenylate cyclase, the D-1 receptor (Kebabian and Calne, 1979).

4. Evidence against Dopamine Receptors in the Gastrointestinal Tract

Not all the experimental evidence supports the presence of specific dopamine receptors in the GI tract. Investigators working with isolated gastrointestinal tissues from the guinea pig, in particular, have had difficulty pharmacologically demonstrating dopamine receptors. When longitudinal smooth muscle strips from the region of the guinea pig gastroesophageal (GE) junction are treated with dopamine, relaxation is observed (Cox and Ennis, 1980). Phentolamine plus propranolol abolished the response of this tissue to dopamine. The order of antagonist potency was prazosin > spiroperidol > phentolamine > domperidone > haloperidol, whereas metoclopramide and pimozide were not active as antagonists. A pA_2 value analysis for the several antagonists versus dopamine and phenylephrine provided no substantial supporting evidence for specific receptors in the guinea pig GE junction. In this preparation, dopamine appears to act via an α_1-adrenoceptor in contrast to the LES of the opossum, where dopamine appears to act via a postsynaptic dopamine receptor (cf. DeCarle and Christensen, 1976).

It is clear that species differences exist in the responses of the GI tract to dopamine and in the presence of specific dopamine receptors. Recently, Gorich *et al.* (1982) discovered a similar situation in the isolated guinea pig ileum. Dopamine, norepinephrine, and clonidine inhibited the response of the tissue to electrical field stimulation. The dopamine response was not antagonized by flupenthixol, pimozide, or domperidone. The antagonists metoclopramide, sulpiride, and tolazoline each had the same pA_2 values against the three respective agonists. Thus, it appears that in the guinea pig ileum the dopamine responses are mediated by adrenoceptors.

This is controversial, as others have suggested that the guinea pig ileum contains two populations of prejunctional receptors on cholinergic neurons, one of which is an adrenoceptor and the other a dopamine receptor (Ennis *et al.*, 1979). Evidence for adrenergically mediated dopamine responses is also available from isolated opossum duodenal longitudinal smooth muscle, where the responses were abolished by either phenoxybenzamine or phentolamine in each preparation tested (Anuras, 1981). This is to be compared with the one-third of duodenal tissues that were inhibited by the dopamine antagonists haloperidol and bulbocapnine. Thus, not only are there species differences in responses to dopamine but responses and participation of dopamine receptors in the responses may also differ within organs of the same species.

The available evidence from experiments *in vivo* in man supports the conclusion of specific dopamine receptors in the gastric musculature mediating relaxation (e.g., Lanfranchi *et al.*, 1978b). A conflicting report has been published recently from work using human gastric smooth muscle strips obtained during gastric surgery (Thompson and DeCarle, 1982). In this *in vitro* preparation, dopamine had only weak relaxant effects, which were not inhibited by haloperidol and were abolished by phenoxybenzamine plus propranolol. These data stress the need for futher systematic studies of the dopamine receptor in the GI tract using orders of potency relationships and selective agonists and antagonists for peripheral dopamine receptor subtypes. At the moment, the totality of the evidence favors specific dopamine receptors in certain specified GI locations. The characterization is far from complete.

5. Pharmacology of Dopamine Antagonists in the Gastrointestinal Tract

The use of dopamine antagonists in the treatment of GI diseases began with the recognition that drugs such as metoclopramide, which were synthesized as antiemetics, could actually enhance smooth muscle contractility in the GI tract. In this section, two dopamine antagonist drugs with utility in GI disease, metoclopramide and domperidone, are featured. In addition, several of the impending new dopamine antagonists with potential therapeutic utility in GI disease are briefly discussed so as to provide an understanding of the growing interest in these compounds within the pharmaceutical industry.

5.1. Pharmacology of Metoclopramide

Since metoclopramide has been reviewed several times within the past few years (Pinder *et al.*, 1976; Schulze-Delrieu, 1981; Kilbinger and Weihrauch, 1982), only a brief account of its experimental and clinical pharmacology is presented. Metoclopramide is a substituted benzamide that acts both centrally and peripherally to produce its profile of effects. Centrally, it alters behavior, presumably by interacting with presynaptic dopamine receptors (Alander *et al.*, 1980). Peripherally, metoclopramide appears to interact at a number of sites not all of which are dopaminergic in character. The potent antiemetic effects of metoclopramide result from an interaction with dopamine receptors in the chemoreceptor trigger zone (CTZ) on the floor of the fourth ventricle (Pinder *et al.*, 1976), an area of the brain that appears not to have a blood–brain barrier (Cheng and Long, 1974). Metoclopramide blocks the emetic effects of the dopamine agonist apomorphine on the CTZ (Thorner, 1975). Clinically, metoclopramide is a potent antiemetic that has recently found a role in the prevention of nausea and vomiting associated with chemotherapeutic agents such as *cis*-dichlorodiammineplatinum (II) (Schulze-Delrieu, 1981; Kahn *et al.*, 1978).

Not only is metoclopramide a potent antiemetic but it is also excitatory to the smooth muscle of the GI tract, expecially the upper GI tract. The motility-enhancing effects of the drug have been referred to as "gastrokinetic" or "prokinetic," indicating its ability to hasten esophageal clearance, strengthen the resting pressure of the lower esophageal sphincter, accelerate gastric emptying, and decrease the time of transit through the small intestine (Schulze-Delrieu, 1981). The gastrokinetic or emptying-enhancing effects appear to be caused by a decrease in the physiological accommodation of the stomach, since metoclopramide impairs distension and swallowing-induced gastric relaxation in the dog (Valenzuela, 1976). Metoclopramide also stimulates the contractile activity of the canine antrum and duodenum in both the interdigestive and digestive states (Ormsbee and Bass, 1976) and in anesthetized dogs (Johnson, 1971). In the digestive state, however, a much greater effect on the antral-to-duodenal gradient of activity was observed, suggesting that a second reason metoclopramide enhances gastric emptying is a greater antral pumping mechanism associated with an enhanced capability of the duodenum to receive gastric contents.

Clinically, metoclopramide has been found to be useful in disorders of GI motility characterized by impaired motor function. It is useful in gastroesophageal reflux disease not only because it elevates the resting pressure of the lower esophageal sphincter but also because it appears to enhance the clearance of the esophageal body and stimulates gastric emptying, thus removing gastric acid from the irritated esophageal mucosa (Behar and Biancani, 1976; Richter and Castell, 1982). Although metoclopramide increases LES pressure, it appears to be less effective in patients with esophageal reflux than in normals (Kilbinger and Weihrauch, 1982). Postoperative motor dysfunction in the esophagus and delayed gastric emptying also have been successfully treated with metoclopramide (Telford *et al.*, 1978). Gastric emptying and motility have been improved in patients with diabetic gastroparesis as well (Malagelada, 1982; Snape *et al.*, 1982). Metoclopramide has not been of benefit in treating postoperative ileus or intestinal pseudoobstruction, but it has accepted use in facilitating radiological examination and intubation of the small intestine (Kilbinger and Weihrauch, 1982; Schulze-Delrieu, 1981).

In the gastrointestinal tract, the mechanism of action of metoclopramide appears to be related more to its cholinergic-agonist-like effects than to its dopaminergic antagonist effects. The first evidence in support of a cholinergic action of metoclopramide is that its responses in the GI tract are blocked with atropine and with tetrodotoxin, implying that part of its action may be neurally mediated (Jacoby and Brodie, 1967; Kilbinger and Weihrauch, 1982). In the guinea pig ileum, metoclopramide potentiates the responses to ACh and to electrical field stimulation and does not affect the inhibitory response on field stimulation produced by dopamine (Fontaine and Reuse, 1979; Zar *et al.*, 1982).

The sensitization of ileal smooth muscle to ACh by metoclopramide requires the presence of calcium in the bathing medium (Fontaine and Reuse, 1978). The actual release of ACh by metoclopramide has been demonstrated in the guinea pig ileum (Kilbinger *et al.*, 1982). Acetylcholine release by metoclopramide in the guinea pig stomach has also been suggested by the reduction of response to metoclopramide in antral muscle strips following pretreatment of the tissue with hemicholinium-3 (Hay and Man, 1979). Such a mechanism of action for metoclopramide suggests that the drug will be an effective stimulator of GI motility except where ACh is absent (Johnson, 1971; Schulze-Delrieu, 1981). In addition to its actions on the dopaminergic and cholinergic systems in the gut, metoclopramide also inhibits the contractile effects of serotonin on the guinea pig ileum (Fontaine and Reuse, 1978). Metoclopramide is clearly not a selective dopamine antagonist in the periphery.

Metoclopramide exhibits variable oral bioavailability but appears to be rapidly absorbed following oral administration. Its plasma half-life is less than 4 hr. The drug is eliminated primarily in the urine; 80% of the drug is excreted unchanged. The side effects of metoclopramide appear to be related to the dopaminergic antagonist effects of the drug in the CNS and include nervousness, irritability, somnolence, dystonic reactions, and prolactin release (Pinder et al., 1976; Schulze-Delrieu, 1981).

5.2. Pharmacology of Domperidone

Although domperidone is not yet available on the United States market, several monographs and reviews of domperidone have been published recently (Hoffbrand, 1979; Towse, 1981; Brogden et al., 1982), reporting the results of studies performed mainly outside the United States. The actions of domperidone are in large measure similar to those of metoclopramide, with the major exception being that the substituted benzimidazolone structure of domperidone does not penetrate the CNS to the extent that metoclopramide does (Brogden et al., 1982; Wauquier et al., 1981). This difference appears to afford domperidone a better side effect profile but does not affect its potency as an antiemetic. Indeed, domperidone has demonstrated antiemetic efficacy against apomorphine- and radiation-induced vomiting in the dog (Niemegeers and Janssen, 1979; Dubois et al., 1981) and against pediatric vomiting or postoperative and chemotherapy-induced vomiting in man (DeLoore et al., 1979; Brogden et al., 1982). In the dog, domperidone also has been shown to inhibit reversed peristalsis preceding an episode of vomiting (Ehrlein, 1981).

The gastrokinetic and prokinetic properties of domperidone are also similar to those of metoclopramide. Experimental and clinical studies show that domperidone enhances antral–duodenal coordination (Schuurkes and Van Nueten, 1982; Eyre-Brook et al., 1982). The drug augments spontaneous contractile activity, enhancing the amplitude and the duration of gastric contractions (Van Nueten and Janssen, 1978; Kilbinger and Weihrauch, 1982; Weihrauch and Ehl, 1981). These factors appear to facilitate antral peristalsis and accelerate gastric emptying (Baeyens et al., 1979). Although Baeyens and co-workers (1979) observed that domperidone enhanced intestinal transit, they suggested that domperidone was less useful than metoclopramide in facilitating radiological examinations of the small intestine.

Following the lead set by the purported dopamine antagonist metoclopramide to increase LES pressure and alleviate the symptoms of gastroesophageal reflux disease, domperidone has been evaluated on the human LES in several studies. The studies on normal human subjects indicate that domperidone increases the resting LES pressure when given intravenously (Weihrauch *et al.*, 1979; Bron and Massih, 1980; Lux *et al.*, 1981). In patients with symptoms of gastroesophageal reflux, domperidone has been shown to have an LES effect less than that in normal subjects (Weihrauch *et al.*, 1979) or to improve symptoms with little or no measurable change in LES pressure (Pozzessere *et al.*, 1982; Valenzuela, 1981). In fact, Brogden *et al.* (1982) have stated that domperidone has not been shown to increase LES pressure in patients with esophagitis confirmed by endoscopy. Nevertheless, domperidone will probably find use as a preanesthetic medication, since its sphincter-tightening effects on the LES should reduce the incidence of postoperative reflux and counter the sphincter-relaxing effects of atropine (Brock-Utne, 1980).

In a limited number of studies, domperidone has been evaluated for relief of symptoms in functional bowel diseases of the upper and lower GI tract. Under double-blind, placebo-controlled conditions domperidone produced good or excellent improvement in symptoms in 79% of a group of patients studied with the irritable bowel syndrome (IBS) versus 34% in the placebo group (Milo, 1980). This result is controversial, since Fielding (1982) has shown that IBS patients ingesting a high-fiber diet do not differ in symptomatology from placebo controls. One controlled study in patients with upper GI functional disease has shown domperidone to be of benefit on symptoms of nausea and vomiting, pain, and early satiety (Chey *et al.*, 1982). Whether the alleviation of symptoms by domperidone in functional bowel disorders of the GI tract is a result of the antiemetic effects of the drug or of a motility effect is not known.

There is little doubt that the mechanism of action of domperidone on central structures is mediated by an interaction with dopamine receptors. In the GI tract, the mechanism of domperidone is largely unknown. Most of the studies reported argue that since domperidone antagonizes the inhibitory effects of dopamine and apomorphine on gastric emptying, it is acting via specific dopamine receptors (Brogden *et al.*, 1982; Van Nueten *et al.*, 1978). As has been noted previously, evidence is available that suggests that the effects of domperidone may be on α_1-adrenoceptors (Cox and Ennis, 1980). This is currently being debated in the literature (Schuurkes and Van Nueten, 1982). There is no evidence to date that domperidone possesses any of the cholinergiclike effects of metoclopramide.

Domperidone exhibits good parenteral but modest enteral bioavailability and is well absorbed. It binds to plasma proteins, undergoes a rapid biotransformation, and has an elimination half-life of approximately 7.5 hr. The drug is eliminated by urinary (31%) and fecal (66%) excretion. Side effects with domperidone are reportedly few, and CNS side effects are rare. Domperidone, like metoclopramide, stimulates prolactin release and may cause a transient skin rash, headache, diarrhea, and nervousness (Brogden et al., 1982; Bron and Massih, 1980; Malagelada, 1982).

5.3. Newer Dopamine Antagonists

In the last several years the promise of metoclopramide appears to have spawned the development of several new substituted benzamides from a number of pharmaceutical firms. When these new compounds (or older ones as well) have been examined for their effects on the gastrointestinal tract, their profiles have been very similar to the prototype GI compound they chemically resemble, either metoclopramide or domperidone. For example, haloperidol inhibited the effects of dopamine on the opossum LES (Rattan and Goyal, 1976). Bromopride (10 mg intravenously) significantly increased the LES pressure in man (Lux et al., 1981) and enhanced resting tension and contractions evoked by ACh in the guinea pig intestine (Kilbinger and Weihrauch, 1982). Although less potent than metoclopramide, sulpiride stimulated GI motor activity in man and dog and was also a potent antiemetic in these species (Stadaas and Aune, 1972; O'Connor and Brown, 1982). In contrast to metoclopramide, sulpiride also abolished the gastric acid response to insulin in the dog and prevented the development of experimental restraint stress ulcers (O'Connor and Brown, 1982).

Another substituted benzamide, clebopride, with a profile like that of metoclopramide, has recently been described (Masso and Roberts, 1980; Roberts, 1982). In the rat fundus, guinea pig ileum, and colon, clebopride is more potent in stimulating contractions than either metoclopramide or sulpiride. The complete clinical profile of clebopride and other new dopamine antagonists with prokinetic GI effects is not known as yet. Clinical investigation of clebopride has been ongoing in Europe for over 2 years (Roberts, 1982). Clearly, an agent is being sought with fewer CNS side effects than metoclopramide and one that is a selective dopamine antagonist for GI smooth muscle. Figure 1 shows the chemical structures of several new substituted benzamides and the pharmaceutical companies in which they are under development. This list does not include all the known compounds or all of the companies with such programs but is presented as an indication of the recognition of this chemical class in the

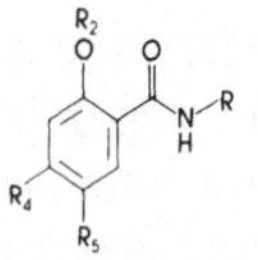

				STRUCTURE	
COMPOUND NAME	COMPANY	R	R_2	R_4	R_5
Alepride	Almirall	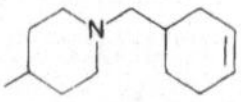	$-CH_2CH{=}CH_2$	$-NH_2$	-Cl
Alizapride	Delagrange	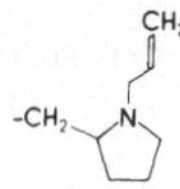	$-CH_3$	-NH-N=N-	
Bromopride	Delagrange	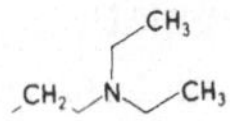	$-CH_3$	$-NH_2$	-Br
Broclepride	Almirall	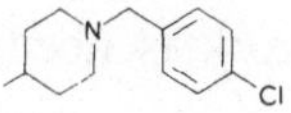	$-CH_3$	$-NH_2$	-Br
Cinitapride	Almirall	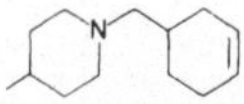	$-CH_2CH_3$	$-NH_2$	$-NO_2$
Cipropride	Synthelabo	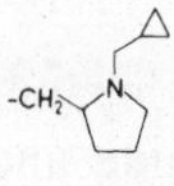	$-CH_3$	-H	$-SO_2NH_2$
Clebopride	Almirall	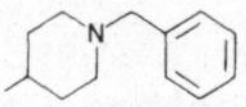	$-CH_3$	$-NH_2$	-Cl
Tinisulpiride	Pierre Fabre	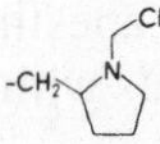	$-CH_3$	-H	$-SO_2NH\,C(CH_3)_2C{\equiv}CH$

Figure 1. Structural comparisons of several substituted benzamide derivatives currently in development in the pharmaceutical industry as dopamine antagonists. The prototype benzamide structure is shown at the top of the figure. The names of the compounds and companies developing them are listed along the left.

future treatment of GI disorders. Of the compounds shown, alizapride, bromopride, cipropride, and cleopride have been tested for their efficacy in man.

6. *Therapeutic Implications of Dopamine Agonists and Antagonists—Present and Future*

6.1. *Dopamine Agonists*

Dopamine agonists are not currently in use in the treatment of GI disorders. The data reviewed in this chapter suggest at least three potential uses of selective dopamine agonists. First, the interesting work of Szabo and his colleagues suggesting a role for dopamine in the pathogenesis of duodenal ulcer disease indicates that dopamine agonists may have a place in the treatment of this disease. It is not known what function the central actions of dopamine have in the pathogenesis and treatment of peptic ulcer disease, but this central pathway may play an important new role in considerations for therapy of this multifactorial disease. Secondly, since selective dopamine agonists such as SK&F 82526 have been shown to be effective dilators of the mesenteric circulation, such drugs may find therapeutic potential in mesenteric ischemia. The third potential use of a selective dopamine agonist in GI disease comes from the potential physiological effects of dopamine in the regulation of electrolyte absorption in the small intestine. A dopamine agonist may have a role in regulating electrolyte absorption and, therefore, have utility in diarrheal disease. Clearly, much more investigative work is needed before any of these potentialities come to pass.

6.2. Dopamine Antagonists

The therapeutic implications of the dopamine antagonists are in large measure those for which metoclopramide and domperidone are being used. These are to:

1. Increase LES pressure and esophageal clearance in patients with gastroesophageal reflux or as an anesthetic premedicant.
2. Hasten gastric emptying in patients with gastroparesis and/or duodenogastric reflux.
3. Prevent nausea and emesis from a number of causes including chemotherapy and anesthesia and surgery.
4. Facilitate diagnostic radiological examination and intubation of the gastrointestinal tract.
5. Improve the effectiveness of oral medications dependent on gastric emptying for absorption, particularly when emptying is delayed.
6. Alleviate the syndrome of unexplained nausea, vomiting, abdominal pain, and early satiety (upper GI functional bowel disease).

The key therapeutic actions or targets of the dopamine antagonists are as antiemetics, as agents for gastroesophageal reflux disease, and as prokinetic drugs. Their use in ulcer disease and the irritable bowel syndrome is unlikely and in need of further evaluation, respectively. The clinical success of metoclopramide and domperidone has generated an active area of drug development research. It can be anticipated that compounds will become available that are devoid of the deleterious CNS side effects of metoclopramide. The future development of compounds in this field will be greatly assisted by the thorough characterization of dopamine receptors in the specific target areas of the GI tract. At present, it appears that dopamine antagonists will have a solid place in the therapy of GI disorders in the years ahead.

ACKNOWLEDGMENTS. The author acknowledges valuable discussions with Dr. Dennis Ackerman and Dr. William Bondinell of Smith Kline and French Laboratories. Special thanks are extended to Dr. Bondinell for the preparation of Fig. 1, to Dr. Martin A. Wasserman for reading the manuscript, and to Ms. Tinamaria Kadelski for typing and editorial assistance.

References

Ackerman, D. M., and Woodward, P., 1983, Effect of SK&F 82526 on mesenteric blood flow (MBF) and resistance under normal and ischemic conditions in the dog, *Fed. Proc.* **42:**748.

Alander, T., Anden, N.-E., and Grabowska-Anden, M., 1980, Metoclopramide and sulpiride as selective blocking agents of pre- and postsynaptic dopamine receptors, *Naunyn Schmiedebergs Arch. Pharmacol.* **312:**145–150.

Anuras, S., 1981, Effect of dopamine on opossum duodenal smooth muscle, *Gastroenterology* **80:**51–54.

Baeyens, R., Van de Velde, E., DeSchepper, A., Wollaert, F., and Reyntjens, A., 1979, Effects of intravenous and oral domperidone on the motor function of the stomach and small intestine, *Postgrad. Med. J.* **55**(Suppl. 1):19–23.

Bastie, M. J., Vaysse, N., Brenac, B., Pascal, J. P., and Ribet, A., 1977, Effects of catecholamines and their inhibitors on the isolated canine pancreas. II. Dopamine, *Gastroenterology* **72:**719–723.

Bech, K., and Hovendal, C. P., 1982, Effect of dopamine on bethanechol-stimulated gastric antral motility in dogs with gastric fistula, *Scand. J. Gastroenterol.* **17:**945–951.

Behar, J., and Biancani, P., 1976, Effect of oral metoclopramide on gastroesophageal reflux in the post-cibal state, *Gastroenterology* **70:**331–335.

Brock-Utne, J. G., 1980, Domperidone antagonizes the relaxant effect of atropine on the lower esophageal sphincter, *Anesth. Analg. (Cleve.)* **59:**921–924.

Brogden, R. N., Carmine, A. A., Heel, R. C., Speight, T. M., and Avery, G. S., 1982, Domperidone. A review of its pharmacological activity, pharmacokinetics and therapeutic efficacy in the symptomatic treatment of chronic dyspepsia and as an antiemetic, *Drugs* **24:**360–400.

Bron, B., and Massih, L., 1980, Domperidone: A drug with powerful action on the lower esophageal sphincter pressure, *Digestion* **20:**375–378.

Caldara, R., Ferrari, C., Romussi, M., Bierti, L., Gandini, S., and Curtarelli, G., 1978, Effect of dopamine infusion on gastric and pancreatic secretion and on gastrin release in man, *Gut* **19:**724–728.

Cheng, H. C., and Long, J. P., 1974, Dopaminergic nature of apomorphine-induced pecking in pigeons, *Eur. J. Pharmacol.* **26:**313–320.

Chey, W. Y., You, C. H., and Ange, D. A., 1982, Open and double blind clinical trials of domperidone in patients with unexplained nausea, vomiting, abdominal bloating and early satiety, *Gastroenterology* **82:**1033.

Costall, B., and Naylor, R. J., 1981, The hypotheses of different dopamine receptor mechanisms, *Life Sci.* **28:**215–229.

Cox, B., and Ennis, C., 1980, Mechanism of action of dopamine on the guinea pig gastro-oesophageal junction *in vitro, Br. J. Pharmacol.* **71:**177–184.

DeCarle, D. J., and Christensen, J., 1976, A dopamine receptor in esophageal smooth muscle of the opossum, *Gastroenterology* **70:**216–219.

Delcenserie, R., and Laugier, R., 1982, Dopamine effect on electrophysiology and amylase secretion from mouse pancreas, *Digestion* **25:**24.

Delcenserie, R., Devaux, M. A., and Sarles, H., 1982, Action of dopamine and domperidone on the basal meal stimulated secretion of bicarbonate and protein in the dog, *Digestion* **25:**23.

DeLoore, I., Van Ravensteyn, H., and Ameryckx, L., 1979, Domperidone drops in the symptomatic treatment of chronic paediatric vomiting and regurgitation. A comparison with metoclopramide, *Postgrad. Med. J.* **55**(Suppl. 1):40–42.

Donowitz, M., Cusolito, S., Battisti, L., Fogel, R., and Sharp, G. W. G., 1982, Dopamine stimulation of active Na and Cl absorption in rabbit ileum. Interactions with α_2-adrenergic and specific dopamine receptors, *J. Clin. Invest.* **69:**1008–1016.

Dubois, A., Jacobus, J., Grissom, M., Eng, R., and Corral, M., 1981, Prevention of radiation-induced vomiting and altered gastric emptying, *Clin. Res.* **29:**712A.

Ehrlein, H.-J., 1981, Inhibition of reverse peristalsis of the intestine by domperidone, *Scand. J. Gastroenterol.* **16**(Suppl. 67):199–200.

Ennis, C., Janssen, P. A. J., Schneiden, H. J., and Cox, B., 1979, Characterization of receptors on postganglionic cholinergic neurons in the guinea pig isolated ileum, *J. Pharm. Pharmacol.* **31:**217–221.

Eyre-Brook, I. A., Linhardt, G. E., and Johnson, A. G., 1982, The effects of domperidone on antroduodenal motor activity in man: A double-blind study with a new technique. *Br. J. Surg.* **69:**291.

Field, M., and McColl, I., 1973, Ion transport in rabbit ileal mucosa. III. Effects of catecholamines, *Am. J. Physiol.* **225:**852–857.

Fielding, J. F., 1982, Domperidone treatment in the irritable bowel syndrome, *Digestion* **23:**125–127.

Fontaine, J., and Reuse, J., 1978, Pharmacological analysis of the effects of substituted benzamides on the guinea pig ileum. Study of metoclopramide, sulpiride, bromopride, tiapride and sultopride, *Arch. Int. Pharmacodyn. Ther.* **235:**51–61.

Fontaine, J., and Reuse, J., 1979, Pharmacological analysis of the effects of metoclopramide on the transmurally stimulated guinea pig ileum, *Arch. Int. Pharmacodyn. Ther.* **242:**149–158.

Fozard, J. R., and Mobarok Ali, A. T. M., 1978, Blockade of neuronal tryptamine receptors by metoclopramide, *Eur. J. Pharmacol.* **49:**109–112.

Goldberg, L. I., and Kohli, J. D., 1983, Differentiation of dopamine receptors in the periphery, in: *Dopamine Receptors* (C. Kaiser and J. W. Kebabian, eds.), American Chemical Society Publications, Washington ACS Symposium Series 224, pp. 101–113.

Goldberg, L. I., Volkman, P. H., and Kohli, J. D., 1978, A comparison of the vascular dopamine receptor with other dopamine receptors, *Annu. Rev. Pharmacol. Toxicol.* **18:**57–79.

Gorich, R., Weihrauch, T. R., and Kilbinger, H., 1982, The inhibition by dopamine of cholinergic transmission in the isolated guinea pig ileum, *Naunyn Schmiedebergs Arch. Pharmacol.* **318**:308–312.

Hay, A. M., and Man, W. K., 1979, Effect of metoclopramide on guinea pig stomach. Critical dependence on intrinsic stores of acetylcholine, *Gastroenterology* **76**:492–496.

Hoffbrand, B. I. (ed.), 1979, *Domperidone in the Treatment of Upper Gastro-Intestinal Symptoms, Postgraduate Medical Journal*, Volume 55, Supplement 1, Fellowship of Postgraduate Medicine, London, Blackwell Scientific Publications, Oxford.

Holzbauer, M., and Sharman, D. F., 1972, The distribution of catecholamines in vertebrates, in: *Handbook of Experimental Pharmacology*, Volume 33 (H. Blaschko and E. Muscholl, eds.), Springer-Verlag, New York, pp. 110–185.

Horner, H. C., and Szabo, S., 1981, Differential effect of changing central and peripheral catecholamine levels in cysteamine-induced duodenal ulcer in the rat, *Life Sci.* **29**:2437–2443.

Jacobson, E. D., 1982, Physiology of the mesenteric circulation, *Physiologist* **25**:439–443.

Jacoby, H. I., and Brodie, D. A., 1967, Gastrointestinal actions of metoclopramide: An experimental study, *Gastroenterology* **52**:676–684.

Johnson, A. G., 1971, The effect of metoclopramide on gastroduodenal and gallbladder contractions, *Gut* **12**:158–163.

Kahn, T., Elias, E. G., and Mason, G. R., 1978, A single dose of metoclopramide in the control of vomiting from *cis*-dichlorodiammineplatinum (II) in man, *Cancer Treat. Rep.* **62**:1106–1107.

Kauffman, G. L., Jr., 1982, Blood flow and gastric secretion, *Fed. Proc.* **41**:2080–2083.

Kebabian, J. W., and Calne, D. B., 1979, Multiple receptors for dopamine, *Nature* **277**:93–96.

Kilbinger, H., and Weihrauch, T. R., 1982, Drugs increasing gastrointestinal motility, *Pharmacology* **25**:61–72.

Kilbinger, H., Kruel, R., Pfeuffer-Friederich, I., and Wessler, I., 1982, The effects of metoclopramide on acetylcholine release and on smooth muscle response in the isolated guinea pig ileum, *Naunyn Schmiedebergs Arch. Pharmacol.* **319**:231–238.

Lanciault, G., and Jacobson, E. D., 1976, The gastrointestinal circulation, *Gastroenterology* **71**:851–873.

Lanfranchi, G. A., Marzio, L., Cortini, C., and Osset, E. M., 1978a, Motor effect of dopamine on human sigmoid colon. Evidence for specific receptors, *Am. J. Dig. Dis.* **23**:257–263.

Lanfranchi, G. A., Marzio, L., Cortini, C., Trento, L., and Labo, G., 1978b, Effect of dopamine on gastric motility in man: Evidence for specific receptors, in: *Gastrointestinal Motility in Health and Disease* (H. L. Duthie, ed.), MTP Press, Lancaster, pp. 161–172.

Lechin, F., and Van Der Dijs, B., 1979, Effects of dopaminergic blocking agents on distal colon motility, *J. Clin. Pharmacol.* **19**:617–625.

Lux, G., Engel, H., and Rosch, W., 1981, The stimulation of oesophageal motility with bromopride, domperidone, and metoclopramide, in: *Progress with Domperidone, A Gastrokinetic and Anti-emetic Agent, Royal Society of Medicine International Congress and Symposium Series*, No. 36, The Royal Society of Medicine Academic Press, London, pp. 29–36.

Malagelada, J.-R., 1982, Gastric emptying disorders. Clinical significance and treatment, *Drugs* **24**:353–359.

Masso, J. L., and Roberts, D. J., 1980, Comparison of the potencies of clebopride and other substituted benzamide drugs on isolated gastrointestinal tract of the guinea pig and rat, *J. Pharm. Pharmacol.* **32**:727–728.

Milo, R., 1980, Use of the peripheral dopamine antagonist, domperidone, in the management of gastrointestinal symptoms in patients with irritable bowel syndrome, *Curr. Med. Res. Opin.* **6**:577–584.

Mukhopadhyay, A. K., and Weisbrodt, N., 1977, Effect of dopamine on esophageal motor function, *Am. J. Physiol.* **232**:E19–E24.

Niemegeers, C. J. E., and Janssen, P. A. J., 1979, A systematic study of the pharmacological activities of dopamine antagonists, *Life Sci.* **24**:2201–2216.

O'Connor, S. E., and Brown, R. A., 1982, The pharmacology of sulpiride—a dopamine receptor antagonist, *Gen. Pharmacol.* **13**:185–193.

Ormsbee, H. S. III, and Bass, P., 1976, Gastroduodenal motor gradients in the dog after pyloroplasty, *Am. J. Physiol.* **230**:389–397.

Pinder, R. M., Brogden, R. N., Sawyer, P. R., Speight, T. M., and Avery, G. S., 1976, Metoclopramide: A review of its pharmacological properties and clinical use, *Drugs* **12**:81–131.

Pozzessere, C., Materia, E., Corazziari, E., and Anzini, F., 1982, Effects of domperidone on oesophageal motor activity and gastro-oesophageal reflux, *Ital. J. Gastroenterol.* **14**:159–161.

Rattan, S., and Goyal, R. K., 1976, Effect of dopamine on the esophageal smooth muscle *in vivo, Gastroenterology* **70**:377–381.

Reinsberg, J., and Kullmann, R., 1982, The gastric circulation of the rabbit: A model for the *in vivo* characterization of the dopamine vascular receptor, *Naunyn Schmiedebergs Arch. Pharmacol.* **321**:R63.

Richter, J. E., and Castell, D. O., 1982, Gastroesophageal reflux. Pathogenesis, diagnosis, and therapy, *Ann. Intern. Med.* **97**:93–103.

Roberts, D. J., 1982, The pharmacological basis of the therapeutic activity of clebopride and related substituted benzamides, *Curr. Ther. Res.* **31**:(1S):S1–S44.

Sandrock, A. W., 1981, Identification and binding properties of dopamine receptors in the rat gut: Possible role in experimental duodenal ulcerogenesis, *Gastroenterology* **80**:1362.

Satoh, Y., Satoh, H., and Honda, F., 1980, Dopamine receptor blocking activity of sulpiride in the canine exocrine pancreas, *Jpn. J. Pharmacol.* **30**:689–699.

Schrumpf, E., and Linnestad, P., 1982, Effect of cholinergic, adrenergic, and dopaminergic blockade on gastrin secretion in healthy subjects, *Scand. J. Gastroenterol.* **17**:29–31.

Schulze-Delrieu, K., 1979, Metoclopramide, *Gastroenterology* **77**:768–779.

Schulze-Delrieu, K., 1981, Metoclopramide, *N. Engl. J. Med.* **305**:28–33.

Schuurkes, J. A. J., and Van Nueten, J. M., 1981a, Effects of dopamine and its antagonist domperidone cannot be explained by an effect on α_1-adrenergic receptors, *Arch. Int. Pharmacodyn. Ther.* **250**:324–327.

Schuurkes, J. A. J., and Van Nueten, J. M., 1981b, Is dopamine an inhibitory modulator of gastrointestinal motility? *Scand. J. Gastroenterol.* **16**(Suppl. 67):33–36.

Schuurkes, J. A. J., and Van Nueten, J. M., 1982, Dose-dependent stimulation of antroduodenal coordination by domperidone via specific dopamine-receptors, *Arch. Int. Pharmacodyn. Ther.* **256**:311–314.

Snape, W. J., Jr., Battle, W. M., Schwartz, S. S., Braunstein, S. N., Goldstein, H. A., and Alavi, A., 1982, Metoclopramide to treat gastroparesis due to diabetes mellitus: A double-blind, controlled trial, *Ann. Intern. Med.* **96**:444–446.

Sowers, J. R., Stern, N., and Taylor, I. L., 1982, Evidence for dopaminergic modulation of pancreatic polypeptide secretion in man, *Life Sci.* **31**:2971–2975.

Stadaas, J. O., and Aune, S., 1972, The effect of sulpiride on gastric motility, *Scand. J. Gastroenterol.* **7**:717–721.

Szabo, S., 1978, Animal model: Cysteamine-induced acute and chronic duodenal ulcer in the rat, *Am. J. Pathol.* **93**:273–276.

Szabo, S., 1979, Dopamine disorder in duodenal ulceration, *Lancet* **2**:880–882.

Szabo, S., and Neumeyer, J. L., 1983, Dopamine agonists and antagonists in duodenal ulcer disease, in: *Dopamine Receptors* (C. Kaiser and J. W. Kebabian, eds.), ACS Symposium Series 224 American Chemical Society Publications, Washington, pp. 175–176.

Szabo, S., Reynolds, E. S., Lichtenberger, L. M., Haith, L. R., Jr., and Dzau, V. J., 1977, Pathogenesis of duodenal ulcer. Gastric hyperacidity caused by propionitrile and cysteamine in rats, *Res. Commun. Chem. Pathol. Pharmacol.* **16**:311–323.

Szabo, S., Haith, L. R., Jr., and Reynolds, E. S., 1979, Pathogenesis of duodenal ulceration produced by cysteamine or propionitrile. Influence of vagotomy, sympathectomy, histamine depletion, H-2 receptor antagonists and hormones, *Dig. Dis. Sci.* **24**:471–477.

Telford, G. L., Ormsbee, H. S. III, Eisenstat, T. E., and Mason, G. R., 1978, Effect of metoclopramide on delayed gastric emptying and disorders of esophageal motility, *Curr. Surg.* **35**:438–441.

Thompson, B. K., and de Carle, D. J., 1982, The effect of dopamine on human gastric smooth muscle, *Aust. J. Exp. Biol. Med. Sci.* **60**:123–127.

Thorner, M. O., 1975, Dopamine is an important neurotransmitter in the autonomic nervous system, *Lancet* **1**:662–665.

Towse, G. (ed.), 1981, *Progress With Domperidone, A Gastrokinetic and Anti-emetic Agent, Royal Society of Medicine International Congress and Symposium Series*, No. 36, The Royal Society of Medicine/Academic Press, London, Grune & Stratton, New York.

Uvnas-Wallensten, K., Lundberg, J. M., and Efendic, S., 1978, Dopaminergic control of antral gastrin and somatostatin release, *Acta Physiol. Scand.* **103**:343–345.

Valenzuela, J. E., 1976, Dopamine as a possible neurotransmitter in gastric relaxation, *Gastroenterology* **71**:1019–1022.

Valenzuela, J. E., 1981, Effects of domperidone on the symptoms of reflux oesophagitis, in: *Progress With Domperidone, A Gastrokinetic and Anti-emetic Agent, Royal Society of Medicine International Congress and Symposium Series*, No. 36, The Royal Society of Medicine/Academic Press, London, pp. 51–56.

Valenzuela, J. E., Defilippi, C., Diaz, G., Navia, E., and Merino, Y., 1979, Effect of dopamine on human gastric and pancreatic secretion, *Gastroenterology* **76**:323–326.

Van Nueten, J. M., and Janssen, P. A., 1978, Is dopamine an endogenous inhibitor of gastric emptying? in: *Gastrointestinal Motility in Health and Disease*, (H. L. Duthie, ed.), MTP Press, Lancaster, pp. 173–181.

Van Nueten, J. M., Ennis, C., Helsen, L., Laduron, P. M., and Janssen, P. A. J., 1978, Inhibition of dopamine receptors in the stomach: An explanation of the gastrokinetic properties of domperidone, *Life Sciences* **23**:453–458.

Wauquier, A., Niemegeers, C. J. E., and Janssen, P. A. J., 1981, Neuropharmacological comparison between domperidone and metoclopramide, *Jpn. J. Pharmacol.* **31**:305–314.

Weihrauch, T. R., and Ehl, W., 1981, Effect of domperidone on the motility of the antrum, pylorus and duodenum in man, *Scand. J. Gastroenterol.* **16**(Suppl. 67):195–198.

Weihrauch, T. R., Forster, C. F., and Krieglstein, J., 1979, Evaluation of the effect of domperidone on human oesophageal and gastroduodenal motility by intraluminal manometry, *Postgrad. Med. J.* **55**(Suppl. 1):7–10.

Yeh, B. K., McNay, J. L., and Goldberg, L. I., 1969, Attenuation of dopamine renal and mesenteric vasodilation by haloperidol: Evidence for a specific dopamine receptor, *J. Pharmacol. Exp. Ther.* **168**:303–309.

Zar, M. A., Ebong, O. O., and Bateman, D. N., 1982, Effect of metoclopramide in guinea pig ileum longitudinal muscle: Evidence against dopamine-mediation, *Gut* **23**:66–70.

17

The Use of Dopamine Agonists and Antagonists in Neurology

HAROLD L. KLAWANS, CHRISTOPHER G. GOETZ, and CAROLINE M. TANNER

1. Introduction

Both dopamine agonists and antagonists have been used to treat neurological disorders. In some instances, in fact, both classes of drugs have been used in the same disease states (e.g., chorea, dystonia, minimal brain dysfunction). Both agonists and antagonists have also been implicated in the pathogenesis of neurological dysfunction, including one disorder that can be induced by treatment with either class of agent (dyskinesias). A review of all neurological disorders in which dopamine systems may play a role is beyond the scope of this brief chapter, which focuses on two areas of particular interest to our research group: (1) dopamine agonists in the treatment of parkinsonism and (2) dopamine antagonists in the etiology of neuroleptic-induced tardive dyskinesias.

2. Agonists

The first successful use of a dopamine agonist in the treatment of a neurological disorder was the administration of amphetamine in the treatment of parkinsonism (Klawans, 1973). This clinical application antedated both any understanding of the mechanism of action of amphetamine as

HAROLD L. KLAWANS, CHRISTOPHER G. GOETZ, and CAROLINE M. TAN-NER • Department of Neurological Sciences, Rush-Presbyterian St. Lukes Medical Center, Chicago, Illinois 60612.

an indirect dopamine agonist and the demonstration of dopamine deficit in parkinsonism.

Our present understanding of the pharmacology of Parkinson's disease is based on the concept that the primary pathophysiological abnormality in the disorder is a decreased activity of dopamine at striatal dopamine receptors. The major approach to overcoming this deficit has been the use of the precursor, levodopa. The use of direct-acting dopamine agonists is an attractive alternative with several potential advantages:

1. Such agents would not require enzymatic conversion by dopa decarboxylase, which is deficient in the striatum of patients with Parkinson's disease. This relative deficiency of dopa decarboxylase in the striatum could result in a poor therapeutic index for levodopa, with relatively more dopamine being formed and acting outside the striatum. It is also possible that a deficiency in this enzyme may contribute to loss of efficacy. A direct-acting agonist might help to obviate these problems.
2. Since it is possible that all dopamine receptors are not structurally identical, it is easily conceivable that a dopaminergic agonist might be found that has a selective action on those striatal receptors that are primarily involved in the pathological processes underlying parkinsonism. Such an agonist might have a lower incidence of dopaminergic side effects mediated by other dopamine receptors such as psychosis or dyskinesias.
3. It is also possible that a dopamine agonist might be found with a longer half-life than levodopa and that such an agent might be less likely to be associated with the early wearing off of drug effect that is so commonly observed during chronic treatment with levodopa.

Apomorphine is the prototype of such direct-acting dopamine agonists. In the early 1950s, Schwab et al. gave parkinsonian patients subemetic doses of apomorphine subcutaneously (Schwab et al., 1951). This initially produced mild nausea, which was followed by a period of decreased tremor, increased involuntary strength, and reduced rigidity associated with subjective well-being. The short-lived action of the drug (130–180 min) necessitated repeated injections, and the side effects, especially nausea and hypotension, were significant.

More recently, Cotzias et al. reported similar results with subcutaneous apomorphine (Cotzias et al., 1967). They were able to alleviate the cardinal symptoms of parkinsonism in five of six patients. It is of interest that one parkinsonian patient who showed choreoathetoid movements while on levodopa exhibited identical movements after receiving apomorphine. Unfortunately, high oral doses of apomorphine led to prerenal azotemia, so this form of therapy was abandoned.

Most recently the search for a better dopamine agonist has centered on ergot alkaloids, many of which are dopaminergic agonists (Calne, 1978). The ergots are now in three groups:

1. Ergolines, which are substances containing the tetracyclic nucleus of lysergic acid together with any nonpeptide moiety.
2. Naturally occurring ergolines.
3. Ergopeptine, a tetracyclic lysergic acid nucleus combined with a peptide.

2.1. Bromocriptine

Bromocriptine is an ergopeptine that is a direct-acting dopamine agonist.

In the initial studies of parkinsonism, small doses of bromocriptine (up to 20 mg daily) showed somewhat controversial results, but more recent studies with higher intake (up to 150 mg daily) demonstrated definite clinical improvement (Kartzinel *et al.*, 1976a; Lieberman *et al.*, 1976; Parkes *et al.*, 1976). All of the clinical features of parkinsonism improved. The overall extent of the therapeutic response is comparable to that obtained with levodopa, but optimal results are usually achieved by combining submaximal doses of bromocriptine and levodopa. One advantage of bromocriptine over levodopa is reduction in the severity and frequency of "on–off" reactions. There are conflicting reports on whether patients who have become refractory to levodopa gain any benefit from bromocriptine.

Adverse reactions to bromocriptine are similar to those of levodopa, but there is a tendency for dyskinesia to be less prominent. Unfortunately, psychiatric reactions are more common and more severe with bromocriptine, and in some patients hallucinations and delusions have taken several weeks to clear after stopping treatment.

A new problem occasionally encountered with bromocriptine is the induction of erythema, edema, and tenderness of the lower legs, ankles, and feet. This problem can simulate cellulitis or thrombophlebitis. Very rarely, this syndrome is accompanied by livedo reticularis or polyarthralgia. The entire symptomatology disappears within a few days of stopping bromocriptine. Finally, there have been recent reports of pleural thickening and related pulmonary disorders in patients receiving chronic high-dose bromocriptine therapy. Most of these patients were concurrently receiving levodopa. The frequency of these changes appears to be quite low (Calne, 1978).

Overall, bromocriptine does not seem to have a major advantage in site specificity, but combined treatment with bromocriptine and levodopa may have some advantages in overcoming loss of therapeutic efficacy and unevenness of responsiveness. We have recently directed our attention to the latter issue.

Three major types of fluctuations in performance are seen in parkinsonian patients. These are:

1. Episodic freezing episodes, which occur on initiation of large muscle movements such as walking or standing up and can be seen in patients almost any time in the course of the disease.
2. End-of-dose akinesia ("wearing off" phenomenon).
3. Classic "on–off," where there is no clear-cut temporal relationship between dose and onset of akinesia.

Episodic freezing episodes were described prior to the advent of levodopa therapy, but they do appear to be accentuated by this drug. The latter two problems are only seen in patients treated with long-term levodopa therapy and are major limiting problems with this drug. In our study, 23 patients with idiopathic Parkinson's disease with classic "on–off" phenomena were studied prospectively during treatment with bromocriptine. Patients were evaluated for an average of 6 to 12 months and received an average of 56.5 mg of bromocriptine. Nine patients (39%) showed improvement in terms of "on–off." When these cases are evaluated retrospectively, it appeared that the only difference between the responders and nonresponders was a younger mean age (57.1 to 63.2) (Glantz et al., 1981). We also found that bromocriptine was of value over the short term for the treatment of end-of-dose akinesia ("wearing off").

2.2. Lergotrile

Lergotrile is a ergoline that is simpler in structure and easier to synthesize than bromocriptine. Clinically, lergotrile has an antiparkinsonian efficacy comparable to bromocriptine, but dosage must be started at lower levels with a slower build-up because transient hypotension is more common and severe than with bromocriptine (Calne, 1978; Klawans et al., 1978; Lieberman et al., 1975). Cross tolerance between lergotrile and bromocriptine has been demonstrated, so patients can be changed rapidly from one drug to the other without prolonged dose titrations. In one controlled study of lergotrile and bromocriptine, it was found that dyskinesia was less marked with lergotrile. Once again, "on–off" effects often improved during lergotrile therapy. Lergotrile may not result in as much psychosis as bromocriptine. Elevation of plasma transaminase levels

(SGOT and SGPT) occurs quite frequently with lergotrile in the high doses employed for treating parkinsonism (up to 150 mg daily), and these disturbances have been correlated with biopsy evidence of hepatocellular damage. The hepatic changes are reversible on stopping lergotrile therapy, and in some patients the enzyme levels return to normal in spite of continued treatment. Because of the liver involvement, study of this agent has been discontinued.

2.3. Pergolide

Pergolide, like lergotrile, is a synthetic ergoline. Pergolide is a more potent and longer acting prolactin inhibitor than bromocriptine (Kleinberg *et al.*, 1980; Rinne, 1981). By extrapolation, pergolide may also have longer duration, more potent effects at striatal dopamine receptors. Unlike bromocriptine, pergolide has no affinity for serotonin receptors (Kleinberg *et al.*, 1980) and, according to one theory, may thus be less likely to cause psychoses.

The first clinical trials of pergolide were conducted by Lieberman *et al.* (1981). They studied 13 nonambulatory parkinsonian inpatients who had responded poorly to other therapies, including other ergot derivatives. In short (2- to 10-week) trials, nine patients showed statistically significant overall improvement in parkinsonian symptoms when pergolide was added to levodopa. All nine became ambulatory, and duration of levodopa effect (time "on") was prolonged. These patients wore Holter monitors throughout the study; asymptomatic PVCs were recorded in seven patients and were multifocal in only one patient. The five patients with PVCs who continued pergolide for 10 months did not suffer new cardiac symptoms. Three patients also developed psychosis, which resolved with dose reduction.

This promising antiparkinsonian efficacy led to the initation of multiple trials of pergolide in less severely ill parkinsonian patients without known heart disease. Both Calne and Ward (1981) and Parkes *et al.* (1981) compared pergolide, bromocriptine, and lisuride in levodopa-treated parkinsonian patients. In short clinical trials, both groups found pergolide, bromocriptine, and lisuride to be equally effective in treating Parkinson's disease.

Several other groups have conducted open-label trials in parkinsonian patients taking levodopa. Ilson and Fahn (1981) studied seven patients for up to 8 months; Klawans *et al.* (1981) studied 22 patients for 12 months; and Yahr (1981) studied 35 patients for 3 months or more. All investigators reported increased time "on" and improved parkinsonian symptoms during "on" and "off" times. In many patients, levodopa could be decreased

Table I. Data Base on Ten Patients Treated with Bromocriptine and Pergolide[a]

	Bromocriptine	Pergolide
Age at drug introduction	56.1 yr	58.3yr
Levodopa dose equivalence[b]	4.2 g	3.8 g
Hoehn and Yahr stage at drug introduction	3.0	3.3
Duration of drug therapy	25.7 months	23.3 months[c]
Average maintenance dose	45 mg/day	4.05 mg/day
Stage at end of treatment	3.3	3.1[c]

[a] Mean age of onset of Parkinson's disease, 44.8 yr; mean duration of levodopa therapy as of January 1, 1983, 12.5 yr.
[b] Carbidopa/levodopa 25/250 is taken as equivalent to 1 g levodopa.
[c] All patients in this group are currently receiving medication.

and, in a few, stopped. Early side effects were usually transient and included nausea, orthostatic hypotension, nasal stuffiness, increased sweating, and alterations in liver function tests. In our study, levodopa-induced dyskinesias were often less severe. Psychiatric side effects were rare except at very high drug doses and generally resolved with dose reduction. Sustained hepatic enzyme abnormalities or cardiotoxicity were not reported in these later studies.

Whether the PVCs seen in Lieberman's continuously monitored patients were a direct effect of pergolide therapy remains an unanswered question. Our group studied this issue in six parkinsonian patients with known stable heart disease who were treated with pergolide and levodopa. Sixty 24-hr continuous electrocardiographic recordings were obtained for each patient, including pretreatment studies. No significant change in atrial or ventricular rhythmicity, electrocardiograms, cardiac symptoms, or cardiac signs occurred in any patient. Parkinsonian symptoms improved in all patients. All patients have continued pergolide therapy for 12 months or longer without cardiotoxicity and with sustained neurological improvement.

Having established that both bromocriptine and pergolide are efficacious in the treatment of Parkinson's disease, we compared the two medications in the same population. Ten patients (five men and five women) with idiopathic Parkinson's disease were treated first with bromocriptine and subsequently with pergolide; in each case, concurrent treatment with levodopa was continued.

Mean age of onset of Parkinson's disease was 44.8 years. Mean age at the introduction of bromocriptine was 56.1 years, and of pergolide was 58.3 years (Table I). Mean duration of bromocriptine therapy was 25.7 months. All patients showed some improvement in parkinsonism with

Table II. Side Effects Associated with Bromocriptine and Pergolide in Ten Patients

	Bromocriptine		Pergolide	
	N before treatment	N on treatment	N before treatment	N on treatment
Dyskinesia	8	10	10	10
Hallucinations	3	6	5	3
On–off	6	8	10	8

bromocriptine, but the average duration of improvement was less than 9 months. Hoehn and Yahr stage was 3 before bromocriptine and 3.3 immediately prior to terminating the drug. Average daily dose of bromocriptine was 45 mg, with an average levodopa dose (carbidopa/levodopa 25/250 equivalent to 1 g levodopa) of 4.2.

The efficacy of bromocriptine was limited by side effects (Table II). Eight patients with dyskinesia before bromocriptine therapy suffered worsening of this side effect, and the two patients who had no dyskinesia developed this side effect during treatment with bromocriptine. Hallucinations were present in three patients before bromocriptine. They worsened in one, persisted in one, and resolved in one. New hallucinations developed in three other patients, which did not abate. Frequent fluctuations in motor function (both on–off and wearing-off phenomena) were experienced by six patients before bromocriptine was given and were aggravated in four and improved in only one during bromocriptine therapy. Two other patients experienced these side effects for the first time while receiving bromocriptine.

Two patients stopped bromocriptine because hallucinations were disabling, and an additional patient did so because of poor drug efficacy and hallucinations. Five patients stopped bromocriptine because dyskinesias were severe and prolonged and efficacy between dyskinetic episodes was minimal. Two patients stopped bromocriptine because efficacy was poor, although side effects were not disabling.

All ten patients later chose to receive pergolide. Mean Hoehn and Yahr stage prior to pergolide treatment was 3.3. All ten patients have continued to take pergolide (mean duration of pergolide therapy is 23.3 months), and their current mean Hoehn and Yahr stage is 3.1. Although antiparkinsonian efficacy is somewhat less at 2 years than at 6 months, symptomatic improvement persists. The current average maintenance dose of pergolide is 4.05 mg/day, and that of levodopa is 3.8 g/day (in levodopa equivalents as above).

A similar beneficial effect has been noted in drug-induced side effects. Dyskinesia was present in all ten patients before pergolide was started, but this side effect has improved in nine patients and worsened in only one during chronic treatment with pergolide. Hallucinations were present in five patients before pergolide was introduced but are currently present in only three and are improved in one of these. No patient suffered new hallucinations after pergolide was added. All ten patients suffered from wearing-off and/or on–off phenomena before taking pergolide, but only eight suffer from these side effects at present, and all have less difficulty than before.

Thus, although these patients had suffered from and been treated with levodopa for Parkinson's disease for approximately 2 years longer when pergolide therapy was begun than when bromocriptine was started, both their parkinsonian symptoms and their drug-induced side effects were improved on pergolide when compared to bromocriptine. This improvement has been sustained for a mean of nearly 2 years, although the mean daily dose of levodopa is less than that required with bromocriptine. These data suggest that pergolide may prove to be superior to other available ergots in that it is more potent, has longer clinical efficacy, is less likely to cause psychosis, and is less expensive to produce. In continuing clinical experience and in several other studies lasting 6 to 12 months, pergolide does not appear to have serious adverse effects. In particular, early reports of hepatic and cardiac toxicity may well have been overemphasized (Tanner et al., 1982).

In August, 1981, the FDA halted new clinical trials of pergolide in parkinsonism to assess its safety. Their determination of the cardiac or hepatic toxicity of pergolide is still pending despite the accumulation of several years of experience without adverse effects in the small number of patients who could be studied before the FDA deadline.

3. Antagonists

Dopamine antagonists have been used in a variety of neurological disorders, but clear-cut efficacy has only been demonstrated in two movement disorders: Huntington's disease and hemiballismus.

It is generally accepted today that dopaminergic mechanisms play a role in chorea both in Huntington's disease and in other choreatic disorders (Klawans, 1973) and that the efficacy of dopamine antagonists in these disorders result from that specific action.

At the present time, neuroleptics are the most widely employed form of therapy of Huntington's chorea, with haloperidol being the most widely used agent. This is usually used in low doses (2–8 mg/day). Improvement in chorea is mild to moderate and is rarely associated with drug-induced parkinsonism. There is no reason to believe that haloperidol is in fact better than other neuroleptics for this disorder. Individual patients often tolerate phenothiazines such as trifluperazine better than haloperidol with less depression and dysphoria. Because of such problems, reserpine is frequently useful in the control of chorea in Huntington's disease. Reserpine-induced depression can occur but in our experience is infrequent. In the management of patients with Huntington's disease, the physician must keep in mind that both depression and psychosis can be part of the disorder and may respond to appropriate pharmacological treatment.

The role of dopamine in chorea is a bit more complex than this. There are conflicting reports on the effect of bromocriptine on chorea in Huntington's chorea. Some but not all reports using low doses claim sustained improvement, whereas all reports employing higher doses report exacerbation of abnormal movements (Loeb *et al.*, 1979). In order to explain these possibly contradictory results, the concept of a dopaminergic presynaptic autoreceptor has been invoked. This type of receptor is located on the axon terminal of the dopaminergic nigrostriatal neuron. When dopamine is released by this cell, some of it reaches and acts on the autoreceptor to decrease the subsequent release of dopamine. This is a form of negative feedback or self-inhibition. These observations raise the possibility that low doses of bromocriptine act at autoreceptors to secondarily decrease dopamine activity at postsynaptic sites and the high levels also act directly at the postsynaptic sites. It should be noted that in some reports small doses of bromocriptine have no effect or may even worsen chorea (Kartzinel *et al.*, 1976b). It has also been suggested that at low doses bromocriptine may act as a partial dopamine antagonist (Loeb *et al.*, 1979). In this regard, it should also be noted that apomorphine, when given acutely, can also improve chorea (Tolosa and Sparber, 1974). This tends to support the view that the same agonists may (perhaps because of greater affinity) act initially at presynaptic receptors.

The neurological disorder that is of greatest interest in relationship to dopamine antagonists is neuroleptic-induced tardive dyskinesia. Tardive dyskinesia is by definition an iatrogenic disorder caused by the long-term administration of neuroleptics and manifests itself as abnormal involuntary movements that are usually of a choreatic nature.

Since tardive dyskinesia is a complication of long-term neuroleptic therapy, it is only logical that animal models of tardive dyskinesia involve the prolonged administration of neuroleptic drugs (Goetz *et al.*, 1982). Two major types of experimental models exist for tardive dyskinesia, one produced mostly in primates, the other in a variety of rodent species.

Long-term administration of neuroleptic agents to primates elicits actual abnormal movements, whereas in rodents it usually does not.

For the last 10 years we have been studying the rodent model of tardive dyskinesia in both rats and guinea pigs. All of these studies have involved the observation of dopamine-agonist-induced behavior following chronic neuroleptic administration. The theoretical basis behind these studies is the assumption that neuroleptic-induced alterations of dopaminergic function occur in both tardive dyskinesia and these models (Goetz et al., 1982). These models have employed dopamine-agonist-induced stereotyped behaviors as the measure of presumed postsynaptic dopamine receptor site functional sensitivity in the striatum.

In initial behavioral studies, groups of guinea pigs were given daily subcutaneous injections of chlorpromazine (5 mg/kg for 3 weeks in one group, 10 mg/kg for 4 weeks in the other). Beginning 4 days after the last injection of chlorpromazine, amphetamine was given to the two groups of animals (Rubovits et al., 1973). It was found that doses of amphetamine that were too small to produce stereotyped behavior in control animals were effective in producing stereotyped behavior in the chlorpromazine-pretreated animals. The animals were reevaluated weekly for 4 weeks, and it was found that the alteration in threshold for stereotyped behavior persisted. These results were consistent with our hypothesis that the neuroleptic pretreatment in some way altered the sensitivity of the dopaminergic receptors in the striatum to the dopamine released by the amphetamine. An alternative explanation, that the absolute amount of dopamine available to act at the striatum could have been increased as a result of chlorpromazine pretreatment, is unlikely, since the concentration of dopamine in the brain after chronic neuroleptic therapy is not elevated (Guldberg and Yates, 1969; Nyback and Sedvall, 1968).

In a second study, we used the same treatment schedule but used apomorphine, a direct-acting dopamine agonist, as the test drug and found a persistent decrease in the threshold for apomorphine-induced stereotyped behavior (Klawans and Rubovits, 1972) when compared to control animals. Because apomorphine acts directly at dopaminergic receptor sites in the striatum to elicit stereotyped behavior, these results support the hypothesis of a postsynaptic, neuroleptic-induced alteration in sensitivity to dopaminergic agents.

It appears from these initial studies that neuroleptic pretreatment enhanced the sensitivity or lowered the threshold of dopamine receptors to dopamine and hence altered the threshold for the production of amine-induced stereotyped behavior. Likewise, the striatal dopaminergic receptors in patients undergoing neuroleptic therapy may be altered in such a way that, following prolonged therapy, normal amounts of dopamine may trigger an abnormal response.

Since this original description of chlorpromazine-induced behavioral supersensitivity was reported, other investigators have reported similar findings with other neuroleptics in a variety of experimental animals (Tarsy and Baldessarini, 1973; Gianutsos *et al.*, 1974). These studies all indicate that chronic administration of antipsychotic drugs followed by drug withdrawal produces a behavioral state of increased responsiveness to dopamine agonists, consistent with the development of supersensitivity, that lasts for at least several weeks.

In our more recent studies we have used this model to study several epidemiologic issues in tardive dyskinesia. In doing these studies, we have focused on three separate questions regarding neuroleptic-induced dopaminergic hypersensitivity: (1) Is there a relationship between the daily neuroleptic dose and the degree of eventual hypersensitivity produced? (2) Do equipotent antipsychotic doses of different neuroleptics differ in their ability to elicit hypersensitivity? (3) Is duration of treatment a risk factor for the development of hypersensitivity? If the model is an accurate one of tardive dyskinesia in humans, the answers to these questions have theoretical significance but also very practical implications concerning the classes and doses of neuroleptics that are safest in regard to prevention of TD.

Initially, we administered different doses of four neuroleptics (chlorpromazine, prochlorperazine, thioridazine, and trifluoperazine) to groups of guinea pigs or rats for 3 weeks, and the degree of behavioral supersensitivity was evaluated using the dopamine agonist apomorphine. The resulting bar graph dose–response curves are shown in Fig. 1. Chlorpromazine, prochlorperazine, and trifluoperazine showed a definite dose effect, with larger doses causing greater supersensitivity (Klawans *et al.*, 1980). At low doses, no supersensitivity was seen. Thioridazine induced no supersensitivity at the doses studied. These results suggest that exposure dose is a risk factor for the development of dopaminergic striatal supersensitivity for at least some neuroleptics. If applied to TD in humans, the model suggests that keeping the daily neuroleptic dose as low as possible may decrease the incidence of the disorder and, in fact, that very low doses may not be associated with any risk of hypersensitivity. The same data are graphed in Fig. 2 after converting specific milligram doses to chlorpromazine equivalents. This method allows the investigator to compare behavioral effects, in this case, hypersensitivity, caused by different neuroleptics with the milligram doses controlled for comparable antipsychotic potency. The graph demonstrates that at equivalent antipsychotic doses, some drugs appear more likely to induce behavioral hy-

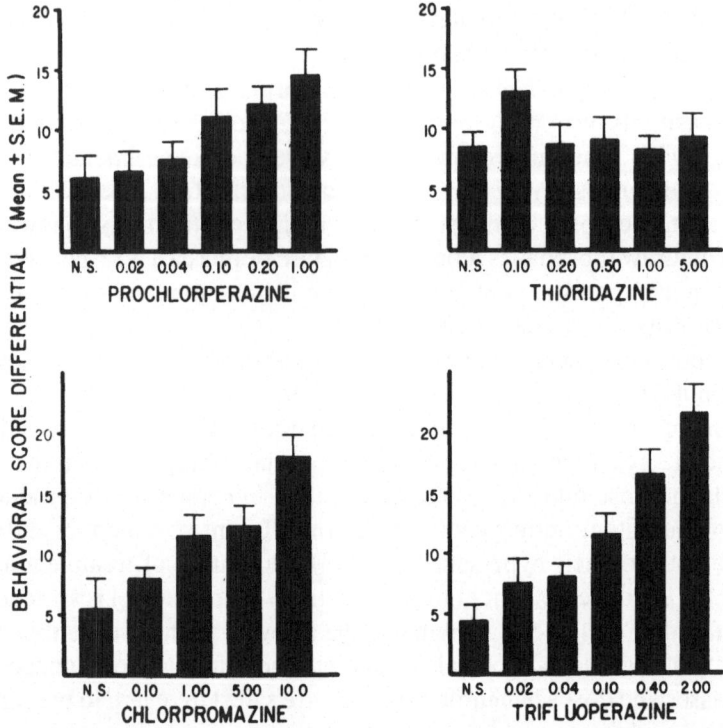

Figure 1. Behavioral hypersensitivity scores to challenge dose of apomorphine after 3 weeks of daily neuroleptic treatment with four different drugs.

persensitivity than others. The direct extrapolation of these data to human incidence of TD has not been confirmed. Such human studies are difficult to perform, since patients commonly receive many different neuroleptic agents over a several-year period.

More recently, we have extended these studies to include the non-phenothiazine neuroleptic haloperidol (Fig. 3). Once again, after 3 weeks of treatment the daily dose of haloperidol administered was directly related to the increase in stereotypic behavioral response (hypersensitivity). It appears from this study that the dose of haloperidol given daily, like that of most phenothiazine neuroleptics, is a risk factor for behavioral supersensitivity in animals and, perhaps by analogy, for TD in man.

This study differed from the earlier studies in that the daily administration of haloperidol was continued for 6 and 9 weeks and the behavioral response to apomorphine was observed three separate times (i.e., after 3, 6, and 9 weeks of continuous neuroleptic treatment) (Fig. 3). This protocol allowed us to look at both daily dose and duration of continuous

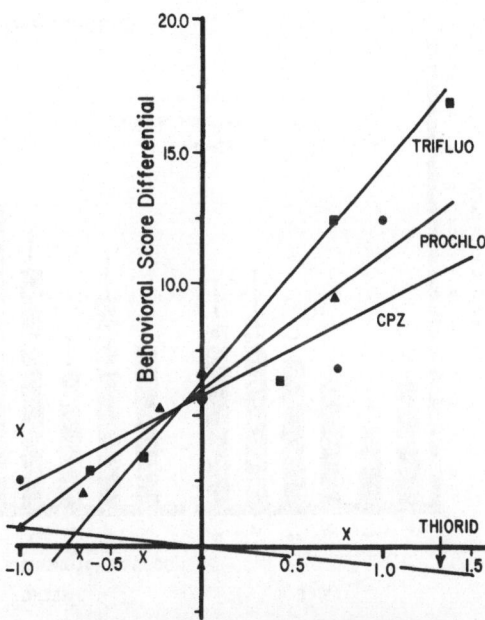

Figure 2. Behavioral hypersensitivity data from Fig. 1 graphed in log dose chlorpromazine equivalents for four neuroleptics.

therapy as risk factors for behavioral supersensitivity. The data demonstrate an increase in behavioral response between 3 and 6 weeks, suggesting that for some period of time duration of therapy is a risk factor. This is not true for the last time period, i.e., between 6 and 9 weeks. We have observed this same time relationship with other neuroleptics—chlorpromazine and trifluoperazine (unpublished observations).

It thus appears that although duration of therapy is a risk factor for hypersensitivity over some time period, this risk factor does not extend as long as the duration of therapy continues but eventually ends. This is most consistent with the human data. That duration is a risk factor for TD is inherent in the definition (i.e., a complication of chronic as opposed to acute exposure). On the other hand, incidence may not be linear with duration of therapy. Many patients, despite extremely long periods of continuous exposure, never develop TD. These observations raise the possibility that the major effect of duration is early in the course of therapy in man and that at some time much later in the course of continuous neuroleptic therapy the duration of therapy is no longer a major risk factor. Unfortunately, it is impossible from our data to suggest the exact time determinants in man.

This model can also be used to study the natural history of neuroleptic-induced hypersensitivity. In these studies, animals were pretreated

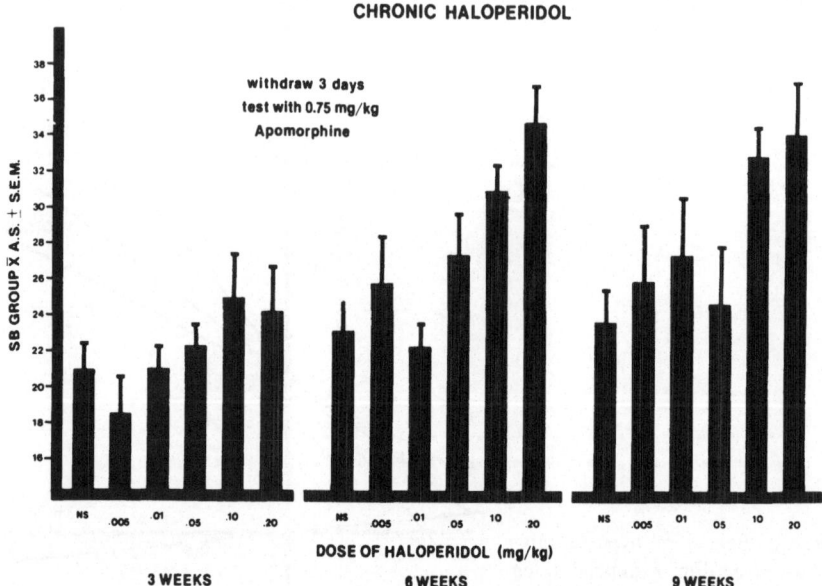

Figure 3. Behavioral hypersensitivity scores to challenge dose of apomorphine after 3, 6, and 9 weeks of daily treatment with haloperidol.

with haloperidol for 3 weeks, and their behavioral responses to apomorphine were observed sequentially for 6 weeks. Figure 4 shows the behavioral response of the haloperidol-treated guinea pigs as compared to controls at various times after discontinuation of the haloperidol treatment (Hitri *et al.*, 1980). The animals exhibited an increased behavioral response to subthreshold doses of the dopamine agonist apomorphine 1 week and 3 weeks after haloperidol therapy, as can be seen from the increased intensity and duration of the stereotyped behavior. However, this increased behavioral responsiveness diminishes 6 weeks after the cessation of haloperidol. These results indicate that the neuroleptic-induced increased behavioral response to a dopamine agonist in animals is reversible with time.

The exact time course of this reversibility is quite long. In animals, 3 weeks of continuous exposure is reversed by a drug-free period of 6 weeks. The analogous time frame in man following years of neuroleptic therapy cannot be predicted. We have, however, seen patients with well-established TD in whom the disorder has proven to be reversible several years after the discontinuation of neuroleptics. For these reasons, we feel that it is best to refer to TD as a persistent disorder, not a necessarily permanent one.

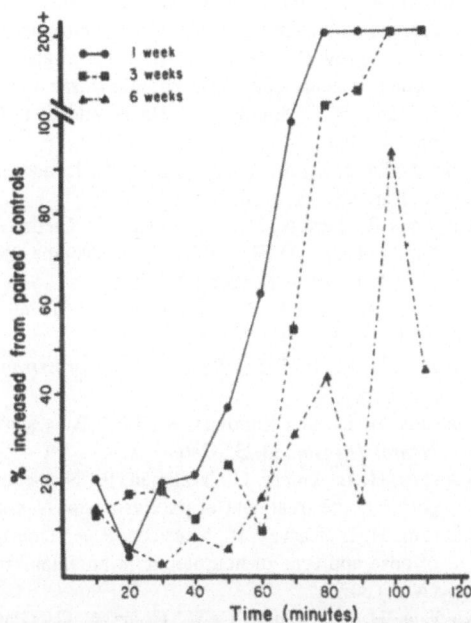

Figure 4. Effect of chronic haloperidol treatment on the behavioral response of guinea pigs to subthreshold doses of apomorphine 1 week, 3 weeks, and 6 weeks after the discontinuation of the treatment. Data are expressed as percent increase over the paired controls.

ACKNOWLEDGMENTS. This work was supported by grants from the United Parkinson Foundation and the Boothroyd Foundation, Chicago, and a bequest from the estate of Clara M. Davis. Dr. Goetz is the recipient of an NINCDS Teacher Investigator Award.

References

Calne, D. B., 1978, Dopaminergic agonists in the treatment of parkinsonism, in: *Clinical Neuropharmacology*, Volume 3 (H. L. Klawans, ed.), Raven Press, New York, pp. 153–166.

Calne, D. B., and Ward, C., 1981, Current concepts on the treatment of Parkinson's disease—the use of dopamine agonists, in: *12th World Congress of Neurology, Kyoto, Japan, September 20–25*, Excerpta Medica, Amsterdam, p. 134.

Cotzias, G. C., Van Woert, M. H., and Schiffer, L. M., 1967, Aromatic amino acids and modification of parkinsonism, *N. Engl. J. Med.* **276**:374–379.

Gianutsos, G., Drawbaugh, R. B., Hynes, M. D., and Lal, H., 1974, Behavioral evidence for dopaminergic supersensitivity after chronic haloperidol, *Life Sci.* **14**:887–898.

Glantz, R., Goetz, C. G., Nausieda, P. A., Weiner, W. J., and Klawans, H. L., 1981, The effect of bromocriptine (BCT) on the on–off phenomenon, *J. Neural Transm.* **52**:41–47.

Goetz, C. G., Weiner, W. J., Nausieda, P. A., and Klawans, H. L., 1982, Tardive dyskinesia: Pharmacology and clinical implications, *Clin. Neuropharmacol.* **5**:3–22.

Guldberg, H. C., and Yates, C. M., 1969, Effects of chlorpromazine on the metabolism of catecholamines in dog brain, *Br. J. Pharmacol.* **36**:535–537.

Hitri, A., Carvey, P., Weiner, W. J., and Klawans, H. L., 1980, Biochemical and behavioral studies of neuroleptic induced behavioral supersensitivity, in: *Tardive Dyskinesia* (W. E. Fann, R. C. Smith, J. M. Davis, and E. F. Domino, eds.), S. P. Press, New York, pp. 145–163.

Ilson, J., Fahn, S., Mayeax, R., Cote, L. J., and Snider, S. R., 1983, pergolide in parkinsonism, *Adv. Neurol.* **37**:85–94.

Kartzinel, R., Perlow, M., Teychenne, P., Gielin, A. C., Gillespie, M. M., Sadowsky, D. A., and Calne, D. B., 1976a, Bromocriptine and levodopa (with or without carbidopa) in parkinsonism, *Lancet* **2**:272–275.

Kartzinel, R., Hunt, R. D., and Calne, D. B., 1976b, Bromocriptine in Huntington's chorea, *Arch. Neurol.* **33**:517–518.

Klawans, H. L., 1973, *The Pharmacology of Extrapyramidal Movement Disorders*, S. Karger, Basel.

Klawans, H. L., and Rubovits, R., 1972, An experimental model of tardive dyskinesia, *J. Neural Transm.* **33**:235–246.

Klawans, H. L., Goetz, C., Volkman, P., Nauseida, P. A., and Weiner, W. J., 1978, Lergotrile in the treatment of parkinsonism, *Neurology (Minneap.)* **28**:699–702.

Klawans, H. L., Carvey, P., Nausieda, P. A., Goetz, C. G., and Weiner, W. J., 1980, Effect of dose and type of neuroleptic in an animal model of tardive dyskinesia, *Neurology (N.Y.)* **30**:95.

Klawans, H. L., Tanner,f C. M., Goetz, C. G., Glatt, S., Nausieda, P. A., and Weiner, W. J., 1981, Pergolide mesylate therapy in Parkinson disease: Report of a three month trial in 20 patients, *Neurology (N.Y.)* **31**(Suppl.):133.

Kleinberg, D. L., Lieberman, A., Todd, J., Greising, J., Neophytides, A., and Keyser-Smith, A., 1980, Pergolide mesylate: A potent day-long inhibitor of prolactin in rhesus monkeys and patients with Parkinson's disease, *J. Clin. Endocrinol. Metab.* **51**:152–154.

Lieberman, A., Miyamoto, T., Battista, A. F., and Goldstein, M., 1975, Studies on the antiparkinsonian efficacy of lergotrile, *Neurology (Minneap.)* **25**:459–462.

Lieberman, A., Kupersmith, M., Estey, E., and Goldstein, M., 1976, Treatment of Parkinson's disease with bromocriptine, *N. Engl. J. Med.* **295**:1400–1404.

Lieberman, A., Goldstein, M., Leibowitz, M., Neophytides, A., Kupersmith, M., Pact, V., and Kleinberg, D., 1981, Treatment of advanced Parkinson disease with pergolide, *Neurology (N.Y.)* **31**:675–682.

Loeb, C., Roccatagaliata, G., Albano, C., and Besio, G., 1979, Bromocriptine and dopaminergic function in Huntington disease. *Neurology (Minneap.)* **29**:730–734.

Nyback, H., and Sedvall, G., 1968, Effect of chlorpromazine on accumulation and disappearance of catecholamines formed from tyrosine C-14 in brain, *J. Pharmacol. Exp. Ther.* **162**:294–301.

Parkes, J. D., Marsden, C. D., Donaldson, I., Galea-Debono, A., Walters, J., Kennedy, G., and Asselman, P., 1976, Bromocriptine treatment in Parkinson's disease, *J. Neurol. Neurosurg. Psychiatry* **39**:184–193.

Parkes, J. D., Schachter, M., Quinn, N., Lang, A., and Horowski, R., 1981, Bromocriptine, lisuride and pergolide in the treatment of Parkinson's disease, in: *Abstracts, 12th World Congress of Neurology, Kyoto, Japan, September 20–25*, Excerpta Medica, Amsterdam, p. 330.

Rinne, U. K., 1981, Dopaminergic agonists in the treatment of Parkinson's disease, in: *Abstracts, 12th World Congress of Neurology, Kyoto, Japan, September 20–25*, Excerpta Medica, Amsterdam, p. 133.

Rubovits, R., Patel, B. C., and Klawans, H. L., 1973, Effect of prolonged chlorpromazine pretreatment on the threshold for amphetamine stereotypy: A model for tardive dyskinesias, *Adv. Neurol.* **1**:671–679.

Schwab, R. S., Amador, L. V., and Lettvin, J. Y., 1951, Apomorphine in Parkinson's disease, *Trans. Am. Neurol. Assoc.* **76**:251–253.

Tanner, C. M., Chhablani, R., Goetz, C. G., and Klawans, H. L., 1982, Pergolide mesylate: Lack of cardiac toxicity in six patients with known heart disease, *Neurology (N.Y.)* **32**:A65.

Tarsy, D., and Baldessarini, R. J., 1973, Pharmacologically induced behavioral supersensitivity to apomorphine, *Nature (New Biol.)* **245**:262.

Tolosa, E. S., and Sparber, S. B., 1974, Apomorphine in Huntington's chorea: Clinical observations and theoretical considerations, *Life Sci.* **15**:1371–1380.

Yahr, M. D., 1981, Treatment of Parkinson's disease, in: *Abstracts, 12th World Congress of Neurology, Kyoto, Japan, September 20–25*, Excerpta Medica, Amsterdam, pp. 134–135.

Index

373